Food Science

Experiments and Applications

Second Edition

Food Science

Experiments and Applications

Second Edition

Mohini Sethi PhD

Former Reader
Department of Food and Nutrition
Institute of Home Economics
University of Delhi

Eram S. Rao PhD

Reader
Department of Food Technology
Bhaskaracharya College of Applied Sciences
University of Delhi

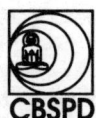

CBSPD

CBS Publishers & Distributors Pvt Ltd

New Delhi • Bengaluru • Chennai • Kochi • Kolkata • Lucknow • Mumbai
Hyderabad • Jharkhand • Nagpur • Patna • Pune • Uttarakhand

Food Science
Experiments and Applications

ISBN: 978-81-239-1693-4

Second Edition: 2011
Reprint: 2013, 2019, 2021, 2024

First Edition: 2001
Reprint: 2005

Published by **Satish Kumar Jain** and produced by **Varun Jain** for

CBS Publishers & Distributors Pvt Ltd
4819/XI Prahlad Street, 24 Ansari Road, Daryaganj, New Delhi 110 002, India.

Ph: 011-23289259, 23266861

Website: www.cbspd.com
e-mail: delhi@cbspd.com

Corporate Office: 204 FIE, Industrial Area, Patparganj, Delhi 110 092
Ph: 011-4934 4934   Fax: 011-4934 4935 e-mail: publishing@cbspd.com;publicity@cbspd.com

Branches

- **Bengaluru:** Seema House 2975, 17th Cross, K.R. Road, Banasankari 2nd Stage, Bengaluru 560 070, Karnataka, India
  Ph: +91-80-26771678/79   Fax: +91-80-26771680   e-mail: bangalore@cbspd.com
- **Chennai:** 7, Subbaraya Street, Shenoy Nagar, Chennai 600 030, Tamil Nadu, India
  Ph: +91-44-26680620, 26681266   Fax: +91-44-42032115   e-mail: chennai@cbspd.com
- **Kochi:** 42/1325, 1326, Power House Road, Opp KSEB, Ernakulam 682 018, Kochi, Kerala, India
  Ph: +91-484-4059061-67   Fax: +91-484-4059065   e-mail: kochi@cbspd.com
- **Kolkata:** 147, Hind Ceramics Compound, 1st Floor, Nilgunj Road, Belghoria, Kolkata 700 056, West Bengal, India
  Ph: +91-33-25633055/56   e-mail: kolkata@cbspd.com
- **Lucknow:** Basement, Khushnuma Complex, 7-Meerabai Marg (Behind Jawahar Bhawan), Lucknow 226 001, UP, India
  Ph: +0552-4000032   e-mail: tiwari.lucknowi@cbspd.com
- **Mumbai:** PWD Shed. Gala no. 25/26. Ramchandra Bhatt Marg, Next to JJ Hospital Gate no. 2, Opp. Union Bank of India, Noorbaug, Mumbai 400 009, Maharashtra, India
  Ph: 022-66661880/89   e-mail: mumbai@cbspd.com

Representatives

• Hyderabad	0-9885175004	• Jharkhand	0-9811541605	• Nagpur	0-8692091830
• Patna	0-9334159340	• Pune	0-9664372571	• Uttarakhand	0-9716462459

Printed at: Sanjay Printers, Sahibabad, Delhi, India

Foreword

Experiential learning is considered to be the best, yet practical laboratory work which is conducted in small groups tends to be varied and falls short of expectations.

As a teacher I feel that good practical guidebooks that provide sufficient theoretical base are urgently needed to upgrade practical experiential teaching–learning.

This guidebook of food science developed and prepared after years of work by two teachers with commitment is a welcome entry. I congratulate Dr. Mohini Sethi who has an impressive track record of writing and a commitment to elevate undergraduate practical teaching.

Dr. Eram Shahid Rao with her bright insight into food science is also a dedicated teacher with concern for good training. I have no doubt that students will benefit from this book which is comprehensive in content and well presented with colourful plates that are appealing. This book will go a long way in upgrading the laboratory teaching of food science. I recommend that teachers and students make the best use of it.

Dr. Satinder Bajaj, PhD
Ex-Director
Head, Department of Home Science
Lady Irwin College
University of Delhi

Acknowledgements

Our special thanks go to Iksha Chabbra and Sukhneet Suri for their valuable suggestions and inputs for this edition.

The authors wish to express their gratitude to all users of the first edition who communicated their suggestions along with their appreciation of the efforts involved in bringing the second edition to them.

Preface to Second Edition

Food Science: Experiments and Applications provides the scientific basis for the changes that are observed in different foods as they occur in nature, on cooking, processing and under controlled laboratory conditions.

The second edition has attempted to incorporate changes which became necessary to keep in line with the changes in syllabi of practical courses now being taught in colleges of home science and institutes of food technology and catering of which food science forms an essential base.

This publication now includes a new unit on *Food Preservation* along with inputs that have resulted from research and feedback of teachers from various colleges and universities. In addition, some new experiments as well as practice exercises have been included to encourage creativity in the learning and teaching experience. This effort should assist teachers and students to guide their food science laboratory work as well as, understand the theory on which the practical work is based.

The text is divided into six units, each containing 2–5 chapters, which discuss the structure, composition and properties of foods and the theory that relates to the experiments that follow. Each experiment is followed by practice exercises geared to enhance application of the subject to daily food preparation, processing and purchasing activity, as well as encourage creative thinking among the students.

The book offers the first practical experience in food science, and deals with the basic reactions and changes that take place in foods when combined, cooked, treated and stored as required. It provides an understanding of the physics, chemistry and microbiology of foods and the ways of enhancing their acceptability while at the same time providing a variety in meals. It thus enables one to gain control over the characteristics of foods which can then be produced at will. When anything goes amiss in storage, cooking in terms of texture or other sensory qualities, the reason can be identified and corrective action taken without wasting the food and or other ingredients.

It is hoped that this effort will make the basics of food science sound, and provide a practical, interesting and motivating experience for students and teachers as well as other users. We look forward to further interaction with the users of this edition.

Mohini Sethi
mohinisethi@hotmail.com

Eram S. Rao
eramrao@hotmail.com

Preface to First Edition

Foods by their very nature change colour, flavour and texture as they mature, affecting acceptability. Those that are generally not eaten in their raw form, are subjected to cooking or processing bringing about changes in their physical and chemical properties. While all processing methods aim at enhancing palatability and aesthetic quality of foods, they may not always increase their nutritional value.

Food Science: Experiments and Applications is an attempt to provide a scientific basis for the changes that are observed in different foods as they occur in nature, and to see what changes take place when these foods are handled, cooked or processed for consumption at home or under controlled laboratory conditions.

The text is divided into five units, three relating to carbohydrates, proteins and fats and two to food evaluation and adulteration. Each unit contains 2–5 chapters, which discuss the structure, composition and properties of foods and the theory that relates to experiments designed at the end of each chapter. Each experiment is followed by practice exercises to enhance knowledge of the science of food, and its applications in everyday food preparation. A number of ideas have been presented for encouraging creative thinking among students.

For teachers of food science, it is hoped that the publication will be a helpful guide for planning practicals because the theory applicable to practical work has been discussed in each chapter.

The text offers the first practical experience in food science, and deals with the basic reactions and changes that take place in foods when combined, cooked, treated and stored for use as required. An understanding of the physics, chemistry and microbiology of foods and the ways of enhancing acceptability through variety in preparation makes one gain control over the characteristics which can be produced at will. When anything goes wrong in storage, cooking, or in texture and other sensory qualities, we know why, and can perhaps rectify the defect without wasting the food or other ingredients.

It is hoped that this publication will help to make food science a practical, interesting and motivating experience.

Mohini Sethi
Eram S. Rao

Introduction

The science of food is the study of food components, and how they react or behave when their natural environment is changed, as in the process of harvesting, cutting, peeling, cooking, exposure to air, sun, heat, acids, alkalis and so on. In food processing operations too, food handling alone affects the sensory and keeping qualities of the final products along with their general acceptability. For each food the processing methods evolved are based on their composition in terms of carbohydrates, proteins, fats, organic and inorganic components.

Pre- and post-harvest activities bring about many changes depending on the nature of the foods and the handling processes required. These changes may occur in the macro components such as starches, sugars, proteins, water content or micro components like enzymes, minerals, vitamins, antioxidants and so on, affecting their colour, taste, flavour and textural properties.

In some foods like corn, the sugars decrease and starch content gradually increases post-harvest, whereas in unripe fruits the opposite changes take place. The degree of change depends on the preuse storage temperatures and environmental conditions as in the case of potatoes which tend to become sweeter if stored at temperatures above 10°C. Foods stored for dehydration, therefore, require changes from starch to sugars to be minimized, to prevent browning reactions from taking place during processing.

The changes in pectins are greater after harvesting, being characterized by decrease in insoluble pectic substances and increase in the water-soluble pectin leading to gradual softening of fruits and vegetables and a reduction in turgor.

The organic acids present in fruits generally decrease on storage and during ripening. In citrus fruits and vegetables the amount of acid and sugar present have significant effects on the sensory quality of the fruits and the amount and quality of the juices extracted from them.

In meats caution has to be exercised because the palatability depends on factors like rigor mortis and ageing, as well as the methods used in butcheries to maintain sanitary quality. The age of the bird or animal and storage temperatures are all vital to quality on cooking or processing, as these influence the methods to be selected for tenderizing the final products.

New food processing technologies now aim at not only increasing the shelf-life through innovative food preservation techniques but also retaining maximum organoleptic and nutritional qualities. This has led to the emergence of minimally processed foods such as purees, pasteurized products, cleaned, cut, prepared and packaged meats, vegetables and fruits all for the consumer's convenience. Minimal processing coupled with cryogenic freezing helps to inactivate enzymatic degradation and retain the natural colour and flavour of foods.

Today, research in the field of food science has progressed from basic physical, chemical and biological reactions that take place in foods during cooking and processing, to the fields of biotechnology, food engineering, packaging and its effect on the product received by the consumer. In fact, biodegradability is at present a pressing field of research in efforts to protect the exhausted natural environment.

Performing Food Science Experiments

Studying food science through experiments helps to integrate theory with laboratory work. The exercises strive to create an understanding of the influence of food ingredients, the amounts in which they need to be used for a required product and how methods of preparation and processing can be altered for desired results.

The compositional and behavioural characteristics of different types of foods can be identified and measured through sensory or objective tests in the laboratory. The process involves preparation of a product according to a standard recipe, called the basic sample which is known to have high acceptability. Certain variations are then planned in the ingredient, brand, quantity added, method of addition, temperature, time of cooking, addition of other substances, pH and so on, to determine the effect of each variation on the end result.

Each sample prepared needs to be clearly labelled as soon as it is ready so that observations recorded with respect to acceptability standards laid down for the product are accurate. A comparison is then made with the basic and each sample is test scored. In this manner it is possible to arrive at a product which is suitable in composition and behaviour for different end uses,

When an experiment is conducted by a number of students, more samples can be prepared to demonstrate the effects of any variables studied than when an individual sample is prepared for each variable. Group results also counterbalance any uncontrolled features that may have been introduced by some individuals in performing the experiment. In some experiments an assembly line arrangement for each step helps to reduce errors offering better control because the same individual performs the same step for all the samples.

Experiments make students inquisitive about the nature and behaviour of foods and their components, and create in them a longing to search for new ways and means of making food interesting and enjoyable. The intellectual curiosity and power of discrimination developed also protects against unscrupulous or indifferent food marketers.

The susceptibility of foods to constant change provide new challenges to the food scientist who then tries to control variable closely to assure quality of the final products for users.

The equipment basic to a food science laboratory has been classified under 6 basic categories such as preparation equipment, testing equipment, storage and display equipment, glassware, reagents and stationery. The details of basic equipment necessary is as follows.

PREPARATION EQUIPMENT

- Heating mantle
- Cooking pans
- Utensils
- Ladles and spatulas
- Oven
- Food processor
- Strainer
- Juice extractor
- Blender
- Whisks
- Chopping board
- Cutting and peeling tools
- Tripod stand
- Burners
- Holders
- Clamps
- Measuring cups and spoons

TESTING EQUIPMENT

- Weighing scales
- Lactometer
- Microscope
- Stopwatch
- Dryer
- Thermometer
- Refractometer
- Hygrometer
- Humidifier
- pH meter
- Filter paper
- pH strips
- Standard measures

STORAGE AND DISPLAY EQUIPMENT

- Refrigerator
- Freezer
- Tables
- Stools
- Cutlery
- Crockery
- Table mats or covers

GLASSWARE

- Volumetric cylinder
- Flasks
- Pyrex beakers
- Test tubes
- Petri dishes
- Funnels
- Glass rods
- Pipettes
- Dropper
- Tumblers
- Slides and coverslips

REAGENTS

- Sodium chloride (NaCl)
- Potassium metabisulphite ($K_2S_2O_5$)
- Hydrochloric acid (HCl)
- Benzoic acid or sodium benzoate
- Acetic acid
- Citric acid
- Tartaric acid
- Sodium hydroxide (NaOH)
- Sulphuric acid (H_2SO_4)
- Baking soda
- Alcohol
- Benzene

STATIONERY

- Filing cabinet
- File covers
- Writing pad
- Marking pens
- Glass pencil
- Chalk
- Board
- Food science book
- Record file
- Brown paper
- Foil
- Food wrap

The above list of equipment is only a basic guide and needs to be updated according to space available, course requirements, newer technologies developed, the level of accuracy desired and the number of students performing the experiments at one time.

It may be noted that volumetric and weight measures given in the experiments may vary slightly when laboratory conditions change. These may be with respect to external temperature, atmospheric pressure, quality of food and other ingredients, water quality, humidity and so on.

Contents

LIST OF TABLES, FIGURES AND PLATES

CARBOHYDRATES

Carbohydrates are composed of macrocompounds such as sugars, starches, pectins, gums and celluloses. Each group of compounds exhibits characteristic properties depending on the ratio in which they are present in a food. Every food therefore, has different physical and chemical properties, that change during cooking and processing when heat is applied or the pH is altered and so on. Carbohydrates can thus be classified as indicated in Fig. 1.0.

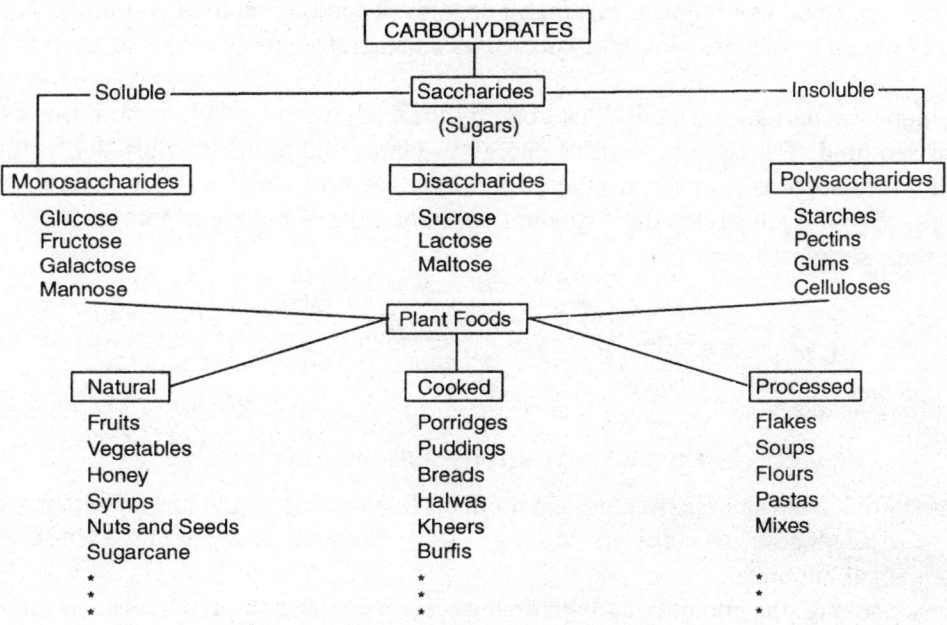

Fig. 1.0. Classification of carbohydrates.

The classification in figure 1.0 is by no means complete as there are a large variety of carbohydrates occurring naturally in foods, both in free and combined forms, each serving functions that provide structural as well as palatability and aesthetic characteristics to foods. A knowledge of the behaviour of these components during cooking and processing is essential to understand how variety can be introduced into foods and meals. These components have been dealt with in chapters 1-4.

Sugars

Sugars in their simplest forms are present as single hexose units called monosaccharides, which have the ability to combine with other single units to form double sugars or disaccharides. When more than two units combine together complex units are formed termed as polysaccharides, which under certain conditions of temperature and pH can be reverted to simple units. The mono- and disaccharides possess a sweet taste varying in degrees depending on their solubility. As the structural size of the units increases solubility decreases and therefore these are progressively less sweet in taste.

The monosaccharides are easily absorbed by the body where they are stored or used up for energy as required. The storage form of energy in plants and animals is usually in the form of polysaccharides such as starch and glycogen, which are reversible on hydrolysis to circulating single units. Fig. 1.1 illustrates the structural configuration of hexose sugars and their ability to revert to their simplest forms.

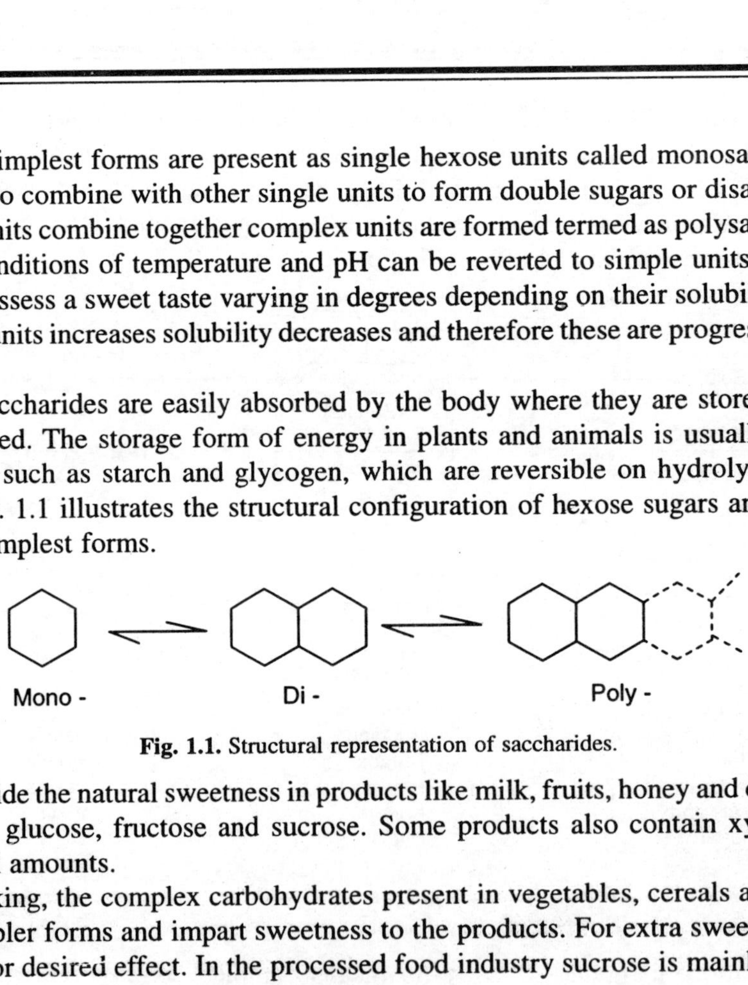

Mono -   Di -   Poly -

Fig. 1.1. Structural representation of saccharides.

Sugars provide the natural sweetness in products like milk, fruits, honey and other foods which contain lactose, glucose, fructose and sucrose. Some products also contain xylitol, xylose and sorbitol in small amounts.

During cooking, the complex carbohydrates present in vegetables, cereals and pulses get hydrolysed to simpler forms and impart sweetness to the products. For extra sweet desserts sucrose may be added for desired effect. In the processed food industry sucrose is mainly used for manufacture of fruit syrups, candies, confections and preserves.

CANDIES

Candies are of two main types, crystalline forms like fudges, fondants, *burfees* and the like, and noncrystalline forms such as caramels, brittles, chewy and gummy products. Candies are also made

2

from mixtures of a foam and gel as in marshmallows, a syrup and gel as in *karachi halwa,* or through a combination of crystals and foams as in frostings often used as coating for nutty candies.

Crystalline candies

These are basically prepared from saturated sugar syrups in which some crystals are suspended. Methods may involve varying the conditions so that a partial recrystallisation takes place and the crystals get surrounded by the syrup. On cooling it sets to give specific textural qualities.

Noncrystalline Candies

Noncrystalline products are prepared using syrups of varying consistencies, usually described as 1, 2 or 3 thread consistencies.

Tests for syrup readiness

Tests for syrup readiness are important in sugar cookery because on cooling a syrup, it may set to varying degrees and the product may not always be as desired. Therefore, one needs to know when to stop boiling a sugar solution to get the right results after it cools. A number of quick household tests as well as objective accurate tests have been devised which are followed for repeated successful results.

Thread test

A drop of the syrup is cooled and taken between the thumb and index finger, which are then pulled apart. The syrup gets pulled in one, two or three threads according to the thickness of the syrup and its readiness for different kinds of confections as required. Fig. 1.2 shows this simple method for determining the end point in boiling sugar solutions used for the preparation of different sweets and desserts.

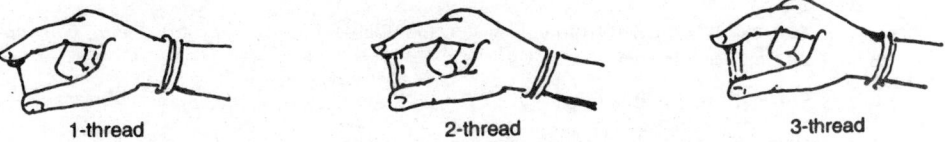

1-thread   2-thread   3-thread

Fig. 1.2. Household test for sugar concentration.

Cold water test

In this a drop of hot syrup is dropped into cold water, and then picked up between thumb and index finger. If the drop cannot be picked up and spreads in the water, the syrup can be used only for the

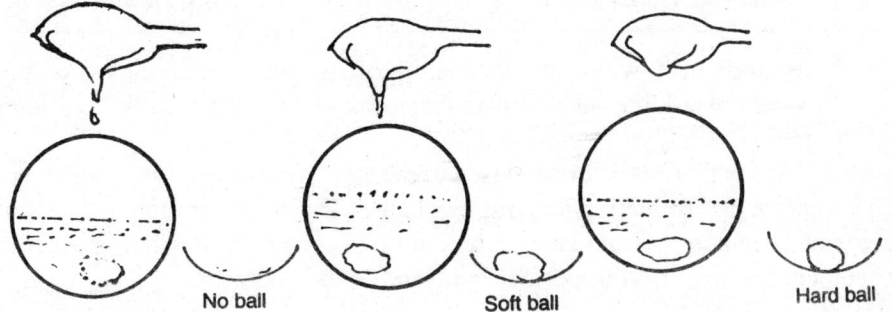

No ball   Soft ball   Hard ball

Fig. 1.3. Stages of cold water test for boiling sugar solutions.

preparation of syrupy products like squashes, *rasagullas, halwas* and so on. If it can be picked and manipulated to a soft ball which changes form with slight pressure it is suitable for making fondant, fudge, *burfees, halwas* and the like. Further heating will give a firm ball with this test, indicating that the syrup is ready for hard candies like caramels. For toffees a soft crack stage or hard ball is desirable. Figure 1.3 indicates the various stages of cold water testing.

Plate Test

This is an alternative test for determining the setting point of a sugar product such as jam. The method involves spooning a very small amount of boiling jam on to a chilled plate and allowing it to cool. On cooling if the sample forms a skin that is firm enough to wrinkle when pushed with the fingertip, the jam is ready to set. If it remains fluid, continue boiling the jam, and retest till done.

These tests are however approximate and do not ensure the same product consistency at all times except with experience. However, the temperature recorded for the different stages of the above tests act as a guide for better accuracy. Table 1.1 gives the temperature guidelines for syrup readiness along with their applications in candy making.

Table 1.1 Temperature guidelines for syrup readiness

Temperature°C	Response of syrup to cold water and thread tests	Application in food preparation
105	Readiness for bottling jam	Preparation of jams, jellies
110	Drop dissolves in cold water Start of thread formation	Making *Rasagulla*
113	Drop dissolves not identifiable Short thread	*Halwa* preparation
118	Identifiable film in cold water, no ball formation elastic single thread	*Gulabjamun* syrup
120	Soft ball when lifted from cold water, mouldable, 2-thread consistency	*Ladoo, Pinni, Chenna murki*
122	Soft ball, stretchable thread	Candy
132	Hard ball, multiple elastic threads set on pulling or stretching	Caramel
145	Hardball, set immediately, brittle threads, break with soft crackle	Candies, *Chikki*, Butterscotch
160	Hardball, golden yellow, many threads which crackle	*Chikki*, Caramels, Brittles
170-180	Burnt molten mass	Not usable

From the above guidelines, which are for heating of sucrose, alterations in colour and texture of candies can be made by adding interfering substances like acid, fat, milk at different stages to provide desired results in candy or *mithai* making.

In the industry, sugar thermometers are used to measure the temperatures which thus act as the guidelines for accurate determination of syrup readiness. The concentration is then verified by the use of refractometers which indicate sugar strength of the syrup for desired product use. For jam making the temperature test is an important indicator of its readiness.

Temperature test

As the term indicates this test involves measuring the temperature of a boiling liquid to determine the end point of the cooking process, after which the heating is discontinued. Thermometers of different calibrations are used as required. Those used for sugar syrups and mixtures are called sugar thermometers. For making jam a temperature of 105°C is registered on the thermometer when ready. The temperature test gives consistent quality products each time.

Noncrystalline candies are usually hard and glassy, break with a crackling sound and do not melt in the mouth as easily as crystalline candies. Those prepared with very thick syrups are brittles and lollipops which have a low moisture content.

The sugar used most commonly for the confectionery industry is sucrose or crystal sugar commonly known as table sugar. The size of the crystals can be varied by changing the conditions under which crystallization takes place. On hydrolysis sucrose breaks down to give one molecule each of glucose and fructose.

Properties of Sugars

Sugars exhibit a number of useful properties which help in providing variety in meals and processing of candies and confections.

Solubility

Sugars are soluble in water but to different extents, sucrose being more soluble than glucose and less than fructose. The solubility however, increases with rise in temperature.

Hygroscopicity

Sugars possess water binding capacity which is useful in retaining quality of foods as also preventing attack by fungi and moulds.

Crystallization

Sugars crystallize out from supersaturated solutions on cooling and this is an important phenomenon in sugar cookery. The degree of agitation affects the stage of crystallization and size of crystals formed. The size in turn depends on their rate of growth around a nuclei. If only one or two nuclei are formed the size of the crystals are large. The rate of nuclei formation and crystallization are modified by the nature of the crystallizing substrate, its concentration, presence of interfering substances, degree of agitation and temperatures employed in the process. These can also affect the sensory attributes of the products formed to various extents.

Melting

Sugars contain a certain amount of water of crystallization. On heating, this is released and the sugar syrups become watery at first followed by evaporation of all the moisture. The sugar then melts at temperatures varying between 150-160°C and is known as molten sugar. This form if left undisturbed super cools into a clear, shiny, brittle solid.

Caramelization

If molten sugar is heated above the melting temperature, it breaks down into a complex mixture in which 5-hydroxylmethyl furfural and furfural are prominent, giving rise to a strong odour and a dark brown colour. If heated further a black-brown colour results emitting an irritating burnt sugar aroma, the mass having a bitter taste.

In food preparation and processing, the undesirable features are minimized to obtain the desired colour and flavours of caramel in products. Caramelization is an important non-enzymatic reaction.

Inversion

When sucrose is heated in the presence of acid or the enzyme *invertase,* equal amounts of *dextrose* and *levulose* are formed. This mixture is known as invert sugar. The process by which invert sugar is prepared either in the laboratory or in nature by enzyme or acid hydrolysis is called *inversion.* Invert sugar is usually considered superior to sucrose in food processing operations because of its sweetness and the special textural properties it imparts to baked products because of its moisture retention qualities.

Hydrolysis

Enzymes bring about hydrolysis of sugars for example, invertase acts on sucrose and converts it to glucose and fructose, maltase converts maltose to glucose (dextrose) and lactase acts on lactose to convert it to glucose and galactose. Enzymes also bring about the hydrolysis of oligo saccharides and polysaccharides. They however get inactivated when food is cooked at high temperatures.

Weak acids like lemon juice, vinegar, fruit juices, cream of tartar and others also bring about inversion of sucrose. Like acids alkalis too decompose sugars. Weak alkali present in hard water makes sugars yellow or brown in colour.

Reducing potential

Sugars have the property of removing oxygen from other substances thus acting as reducing agents. They easily give up H ions which bind with free oxygen and make it unavailable.

Uses of Sugars

There are innumerable uses of sugars in nature, food preparation and in processing.

   (*i*) They add sweetness, flavour, colour and texture to foods.

  (*ii*) Being hygroscopic in nature, sugars possess water retention properties and thus prevent foods from drying out.

 (*iii*) They also help in preservation by binding the moisture thus inhibiting the action of micro-organisms.

 (*iv*) Sugars provide the medium for action of yeast in fermented products.

  (*v*) Unrefined sugars are a source of minerals like calcium, potassium and iron in the diet.

Thus, with an understanding of the behaviour of sugars on heating and the effects that can be produced by the addition of other substances in a mixture containing sugar, the properties of sugars can be used very creatively in food preparation and processing.

Experiments 1-5 have been designed to provide some first hand knowledge and practical experience of the properties of sugars and create interest in developing ideas for their application in food preparation.

EXPERIMENT 1

Aim

To study the effect of sugar on the boiling point of water.

Equipment

Measuring cup, beakers, burner, thermometer, clamp, glass rods, holder, gauze, stop watch.

Materials

Sucrose, distilled and tap water.

Principle

Sugar dissolves in water and raises the boiling point of water. Every molecule of sucrose (mol. wt. 342 g) dissolved in a litre of water increases the boiling point of water by 0.52°C, provided the atmospheric pressure and humidity remain the same. As the concentration rises so also the boiling temperature, and the increase becomes more pronounced as the sugar concentration increases beyond 70%.

Procedure

A. (*i*) Prepare 8 beakers each containing 100 ml sugar solution with the following concentrations—0, 10, 20, 40, 60, 80, 85, 90% of sucrose respectively, using distilled water.

  (*ii*) Taking one sample at a time heat to bubbling boil, switch off the burner, and record the temperature immediately.

 (*iii*) Note the time taken to bring each sample to boiling point.

B. (*i*) Repeat (*i-iii*) using tap water.

Observations

Enter the results according to the format in Table 1.2.

Table 1.2 Effect of addition of sugar on boiling point of water

Sucrose (g)	D. water (ml)	Tap water (ml)	Concentration (%)	Boiling temperature DW (°C) TW	Time taken DW (min) TW
0	100	100	0		
10	90	90	10		
*	*	*	*		
*	*	*	*		

From the observations recorded, calculate the increase in the boiling point at each concentration. Graphically depict your results and see if they prove the principle of this experiment. Use the X and Y-axis for concentration and boiling temperatures respectively. Draw your inferences and state the applications of this experiment in food preparation. Record any difficulty if encountered in bringing higher concentrations of sugars solutions to their boiling points.

Precautions

1. Use medium heat throughout the experiment.
2. Switch off the flame before taking temperature readings.
3. Dip thermometer in hot water before taking syrup temperature to prevent its breakage.
4. The solutions should be brought to bubbling boil before taking the temperatures.
5. The amount of solution prepared should be enough to allow the bulb of the thermometer to be immersed.
6. The volume of water should be kept constant for all samples.

Practice Exercises

1. Perform the experiment learnt with salt instead of sugar and see if the increase in boiling temperatures is the same as for sucrose. If they are different try to explain the reasons.
2. Prepare sugar solutions using at least 2 concentrations of sucrose as learnt. Observe and record any colour changes which take place till boiling temperature is reached. Suggest any dishes in which the solutions made can be used effectively.

EXPERIMENT 2

Aim

To study the effect of temperature on solubility of sugar and determine the concentrations at which the solutions become saturated.

Equipment

Weighing scale, measuring cup, beakers, sugar thermometer, clamp, glass rods, holder, burner, gauze, stop watch.

Materials

Sugar and water.

Principle

Sugars are soluble in water but at any one temperature there is a point at which no more than a certain amount of sugar can dissolve. At this point the sugar solution is said to be saturated. However, the amount of sugar that can dissolve in water increases with increase in temperature, and when cooled the sugar recrystallizes from the super saturated solution. The percentage of saturation of a sugar solution also varies with the temperature. According to Charley, (1982) a 67% sucrose solution is saturated at 20°C as against 87% at 115°C. The increase in solubility of sugar with rise in temperature is mainly due to the OH groups on sugar molecules, and the number of such groups in the structures of various sugars determines their solubility.

Procedure

A. (*i*) Weigh out 100 g of sugar in 5 separate lots.
  (*ii*) Measure out 100 ml water in 5 different beakers. Note the temperature and keep aside till required.
  (*iii*) Take one beaker, place it over a burner and suspend a thermometer with the help of a stand so that its bulb dips into the water. Heat the water over a steady flame to 25°C.
  (*iv*) Switch off the flame and gradually dissolve sugar in the water a little at a time till the last spoon does not dissolve completely. Take care to monitor the temperature and light the burner if temperature begins to fall below 25°C.
  (*v*) Stop adding sugar and note the time taken for saturation. Weigh the amount left unused from the first lot.
  (*vi*) Calculate the amount dissolved and the % concentration of the sugar solution using simple arithmetic.

B. (*i*) Use the second beaker and heat the water to 30°C and repeat A (*iii-vi*)
  (*ii*) Record the concentration at which saturation takes place.

C. (*i*) Repeat experiment A (*iii-vi*) but heat the water to 40°C.

D. (*i*) Repeat A (*iii-vi*) but heat the water to 50°C.

E. (*i*) Repeat A (*iii-vi*) but bring the water temperature to 100°C.
      Note the colour of the sugar solutions at the various concentrations.

Observations

The observations may be recorded as per the sample format given in Table 1.3.

Table 1.3. Solubility of sugar.

Temperature °C	Sucrose (g)	Time taken (min.)	Concentration (%)	Applications in cooking
25				
30				
40				
50				
100				

From the observations recorded inferences regarding the use of sugar solutions at each temperature in cooking and food processing may be drawn. The results obtained may be graphically illustrated with sugar weight on the X-axis and temperature on the Y-axis. Similarly, a graph may be plotted for concentration against time taken for saturation.

Precautions

1. Beakers used for heating sugar solutions should be made of heat resistant pyrex glass.
2. Temperatures should be recorded carefully for accuracy.
3. Measurement of weights and volumes should be standardized to avoid variations in the results.
4. Switch off the burner while attempting to read the temperature of a nearly saturated solution, to prevent spurting of hot liquid.
5. Hot sugar solutions should not be handled with bare hands.
6. Use medium heat for the experiment.

Practice Exercises

1. Use different types of sugars and perform the experiment to examine the differences with respect to the concentrations required to reach supersaturation. Then cool each sample and observe if recrystallization takes place. Note the nature of the crystals formed with each sugar.
2. List the foods you have eaten which are prepared using sugar syrups.

EXPERIMENT 3

Aim

To determine the effect of heat on sugar solutions and observe their behaviour corresponding to the *thread and cold water tests.*

Equipment

Weighing scale, measuring cup, beakers, burner, gauze, petridishes, sugar thermometer, clamp, glass rod, holder and stop watch.

Materials

Distilled and tap water, sucrose.

Principle

When sugar is dissolved in water the volume of the resulting solution increases approximately by the weight of sugar added. This is because the sugar contains water of crystallization which becomes free when the sugar dissolves. On heating, it gradually changes colour from pale to yellowish and then brown depending on the amount of moisture evaporated, and the concentration of the sugar in solution. When the solution loses enough water to change its viscosity it is termed as a syrup. A point comes when all the water evaporates leaving a very viscous liquid called molten sugar, which has a characteristic brown colour and a discernible odour.

Procedure

A. (*i*) Measure out 100 ml of tap and distilled water in 2 separate beakers.

  (*ii*) Dissolve 30 grams sugar in each beaker and note the clarity and colour of the two solutions.

  (*iii*) Place the beaker with distilled water solution on medium heat over a gauze and suspend a sugar thermometer from a stand, as learnt.

  (*iv*) Heat the solution and observe the changes that take place at 111°C, 113°C, 118°C, 122°C, 132°C, 140°C making note of the time taken for each change.

  (*v*) At each temperature perform the thread test as learnt, and put a drop of the sugar solution into cold water placed in petridishes marked suitably, using a glass rod.

  (*vi*) Examine the sugar drops in each petridish and observe for colour, viscosity and consistency and describe the texture of the ball formed.

B. (*i*) Repeat A (*iii-vi*) using the tap water solution.

Observations

Record your observations according to the format indicated in Table 1.4 and draw inferences with respect to the applications to which each stage of the solution can be put in food preparation.

Table 1.4 Effect of heat on sugar solutions

Sugar °C solution	Clarity	Colour	Viscosity/ threads/ball	Behaviour in water	Time (min/sec)	Applications
110						
113						
116						
122						
132						
140						

Variations can be planned taking into account various kinds of sugars in different concentrations for comparison and study of suitability for creating desirable characteristics in food products.

Precautions

1. The thermometer should be suspended to the right height before heating is started.
2. Heat one solution at a time because as the temperature rises it will become difficult to make accurate observations on more than one sample.
3. The temperature reading should be taken at the level of the upper miniscus when the solution becomes too viscous.
4. Use a stop watch to note the time at each stage of change.
5. Do not put your face on top of the beaker to note the temperature, because as the sugar gets more and more concentrated even a drop on the skin can cause a serious burn.
6. Use beakers of a size that are stable on the flame.

Practice Exercises

1. Make a list of the sweets which are prepared using syrups of different concentrations and colours commensurate with those which you have identified in this experiment.
2. Compare the syrups of *rasgulla* and *gulabjamun* and comment on their differences in the light of the experiment learnt.
3. Prepare any sweet or a dessert using a syrup. Describe the thread consistency of the syrup used.

EXPERIMENT 4

Aim

To demonstrate the process of sugar recrystallization through the preparation of fondant, fudge *shakarpara* and *chenna murki*.

Equipment

Weighing scale, measuring cups and spoons, cooking utensils, kadai (wok), strainer, wooden spoon, stainless steel knife, cooking range, perforated ladle, plates, dishcloths, butterpaper.

Materials

Maida, fat, sugar, oil, milk, butter and water, cottage cheese, cream of tartar, kewra essence (optional).

Principle

Sugars are soluble to different extents depending on the temperature of the water or liquid in which they are dissolved. However, when the solution is heated it becomes capable of dissolving a greater amount of sugar than at room temperature. This capacity increases with rise in temperature, but when the solution is cooled the sugar recrystallizes. This phenomenon is utilized to different extents in the preparation of sweets, candies and desserts to provide varying textures, colours and other sensory qualities. The acceptability of a product depends largely on the size of the crystals and the amount of interfering substances added in a particular preparation.

Procedure

In this experiment 3 recipes have been chosen to demonstrate the type of crystallization that takes place in food preparation. The first one is made purely from sugar and water, while the other two show crystallization when interfering substances are added.

A. Fondant

(*i*) Measure out 200 g sucrose and add to it 100 ml water in a pan or enamel bowl.

(*ii*) Cover and heat the pan for 4-5 minutes on medium heat without stirring the contents.

(*iii*) Keep boiling the sugar till it reaches a temperature of 114°C.

(*iv*) Remove from fire, cool to 60°C, and then beat the mixture continuously with a wooden spoon till it all comes together around the spoon and crystallization is complete.

(*v*) The mass can now be kneaded and pressed or rolled on a greased flat surface, cooled and cut into any shape.

(*vi*) Make observations with respect to clarity, colour, mouthfeel, texture and size of crystal under the microscope.

(*vii*) Keep some pieces wrapped in grease proof paper for 12-24 hours, and repeat the observations, to find out if any differences occur in the quality of the product.

B. Fudge

(*i*) Stir 200 g sugar, 15 g butter and 20 g chocolate into 120 ml milk in a pan.

(*ii*) Heat the pan to bring contents to 112°C and remove from fire.

(*iii*) Cool the mixture to 60°C and proceed as for fondant.

C. Shakarpara

(*i*) Rub 10 g fat lightly into 50 g *maida* (refined wheat flour) till it is evenly grainy in texture.

(*ii*) Add a small quantity of water to make a dough, without kneading excessively. Let it rest.

(*iii*) Make syrup of 2-thread consistency using 100 g sugar and 50 ml water. Keep aside.

(*iv*) Roll the dough, cut into squares, and fry them in hot oil over medium heat till golden brown.

(*v*) Drain the oil and put the fried pieces in syrup for 5-10 minutes.

(*vi*) Remove the pieces from the syrup and place in a sieve to drain and air-dry.

(*vii*) Observe the size of the crystals formed on the surface of the pieces using a microscope and note the colour and other characteristics of the preparation.

(*viii*) Keep aside for a few hours and observe again. Note the difference in the crystals.

D. Chenna Murki

(*i*) Cut 100 g *paneer* (cottage cheese) into 1 cm cubes.

(*ii*) Heat 2T water and 50 g sugar to one-thread consistency.

(*iii*) Add $\frac{1}{8}$t cream of tartar to the syrup and remove from fire.

(*iv*) Add the *paneer* cubes and leave for 5 minutes.

(*v*) Replace on heat and stir constantly till the sugar starts to recrystallize on the cubes.

(*vi*) Remove from fire add essence and continue stirring till all the cubes are coated with crystals and separate out.

(*vii*) Keep aside for a few hours and observe any changes in the crystals.

Observations

Record all the observations made for the recipes as per the format in Table 1.5, and compare the type of crystals formed in each preparation.

Table 1.5 Crystal formation in different foods

Preparation	°C	Time	Colour	Appearance	Texture	Taste	Mouthfeel
A. Fondant							
B. Fudge							
C. Shakarpara							
D. Chenna Murki							

Draw inferences and conclusions regarding the application of the property of sugar recrystallisation in food preparation and processing. Explain the reasons for the different textures, tastes and mouthfeel of products and the role that acid plays in the preparation of D. Variations in the experiment may be made by changing the method of addition of the ingredients, the quantities added, temperatures and deletion, addition or substitution of certain ingredients.

Precautions

1. Cooking pan should be of the same type and size with a smooth inner surface.
2. Cover the pan during the initial phase of cooking as this will allow the steam to wash down the crystals from the sides of the pan, and prevent immature recrystallization.
3. Syrups should not be over heated otherwise they will give rise to large crystals which destroy the smoothness of the product and its mouthfeel.
4. Do not scrape the sides of the pan, stir or roll the thermometer while the syrup is being cooled as this may cause crystals that may seed the entire mass.
5. Candies must always be allowed to mature before being consumed.

Practice Exercises

1. List 4 items prepared or manufactured where fondant plays a special role. What functions does it perform as far as shelf life of the product is concerned.
2. Prepare *ladoos* by any recipe, using a syrup in one and crystal sugar in the other. Compare the colour, texture, taste, mouthfeel and general acceptability of the two sweets. Give reasons for the differences and state which qualities you identified that you liked or did not like.

EXPERIMENT 5

Aim

To study the process of inversion, melting and caramelization in sucrose and their usefulness in food products.

Equipment

Cooking pans, wooden spoon or stirrer, burner, stop watch, thermometer, non-stick board, pH paper.

Materials

Sucrose, water, cream of tartar, alkali and fat or oil.

Principle

Inversion

This is the process by which sugar gets hydrolyzed to an equimolar mixture of glucose and fructose, called *invert* sugar. The hydrolysis may be brought about by addition of acid or presence of enzymes during cooking. The invert sugar acts as an interfering substance to crystal formation in the syrup, which therefore remains in liquid form. Natural products of inversion are honey and corn syrup. Textures can be altered in candies by varying the amount of acid or enzyme added, and thus controlling the degree of crystallization in the product. A high proportion of interfering substances may prevent crystallization totally as in non-crystalline candies.

Melting

Sugar crystals melt when placed in a heavy pan and heated gradually on low fire. Melting starts when all the water of crystallization has been evaporated, at about 160°C. To prevent scorching at the bottom shaking the pan occasionally to turn the sugar over is necessary. This can also be prevented by adding a table spoon of water to the sugar before heating. When removed from heat and left undisturbed the molten mass supercools into a clear, glass-like solid which breaks with a crackling sound.

Caramelisation

If the melted sugar is heated beyond 160°C begins to change to a deep brown colour giving off a pleasant caramel odour, that turns to a strong smell of burnt sugar, if the heating is continued beyond 170°C. These changes are due to the breakdown of sugar molecules to a complex mixture in which 5-hydroxymethyl furfural and furfural predominate. If baking soda is added to caramelized sugar, the heat and acids present give rise to carbon dioxide which escapes resulting in a porous texture on cooling, often seen in brittles and candies.

Procedure

A. Inversion

(*i*) Make fondant as learnt in experiment 4 and keep aside.

(*ii*) Prepare another sample of the fondant but add a pinch of cream of tarter dissolved in a little water, to the boiling syrup.

(*iii*) Compare the results of (*i*) and (*ii*) and record the differences observed in the texture and other characteristics of the fondant.

B. Melting

(*i*) Place 20 g sucrose in a pan and sprinkle 15 ml water on it.

(*ii*) Put the pan on medium heat and as the bubbles of water become visible, lift pan and shake its contents. Return to heat, and when bubbling stops the sugar will begin to melt.

(*iii*) Immediately pour out the hot mass on to a pre-greased wooden or non-stick chopping board. In a few minutes the mass will set.

(*iv*) Just before it totally sets lines may be cut lightly on the surface, horizontally and vertically, and the mass allowed to set.

(*v*) When set, pass the knife under the mass to release it from the board.

(*vi*) Press with finger at the markings to break into pieces of glossy brittle or *chikki*. This is a non-crystalline candy.

Variations may be made by altering the type of sugar used, or adding substances like nuts or dried fruits and observing the end product for sensory properties. Inferences can be drawn and the knowledge gained applied to food preparation in creative ways.

C. Caramelization

(*i*) Repeat as above till the molten sugar is formed.

(*ii*) Continue heating a few minutes longer till a characteristic odour of caramel is sensed. The viscous mass may then be directly set or cold water may be added to it drop by drop and stirred to prepare a caramel syrup.

The heating may be stopped when the desired colour and odour have been obtained. The resultant syrup can be used as an ingredient in food preparation or as a topping to desserts.

Observations

The observations made with respect to time, temperature, colour, clarity, crackle, may be recorded in a suitable format as learnt in earlier experiments.

Precautions

1. When heating sugar protect hands and face well, to avoid the chance of burns from splashing syrup.
2. Flame must be lowered as the syrup thickens.
3. Pour hot sugar out on lightly greased surface before it sets.
4. Keep all equipment ready at hand before starting the experiment.
5. Ensure that the cold water is added dropwise at first when preparing caramel syrup, and the mixture is constantly stirred during addition till the syrup consistency is reached.

Practice Exercises

1. Prepare molten sugar by adding a pinch of soda to the syrup when bubbling. Note the changes in the final product as compared to that in the experiment.

2. Prepare a caramel custard. Comment on the texture and use of the caramelized sugar used in the preparation.

3. Prepare caramel syrup and explain why recrystallization does not occur in it. Mention 3 food products in which the syrup can be used in food preparation and processing.

SUGARS

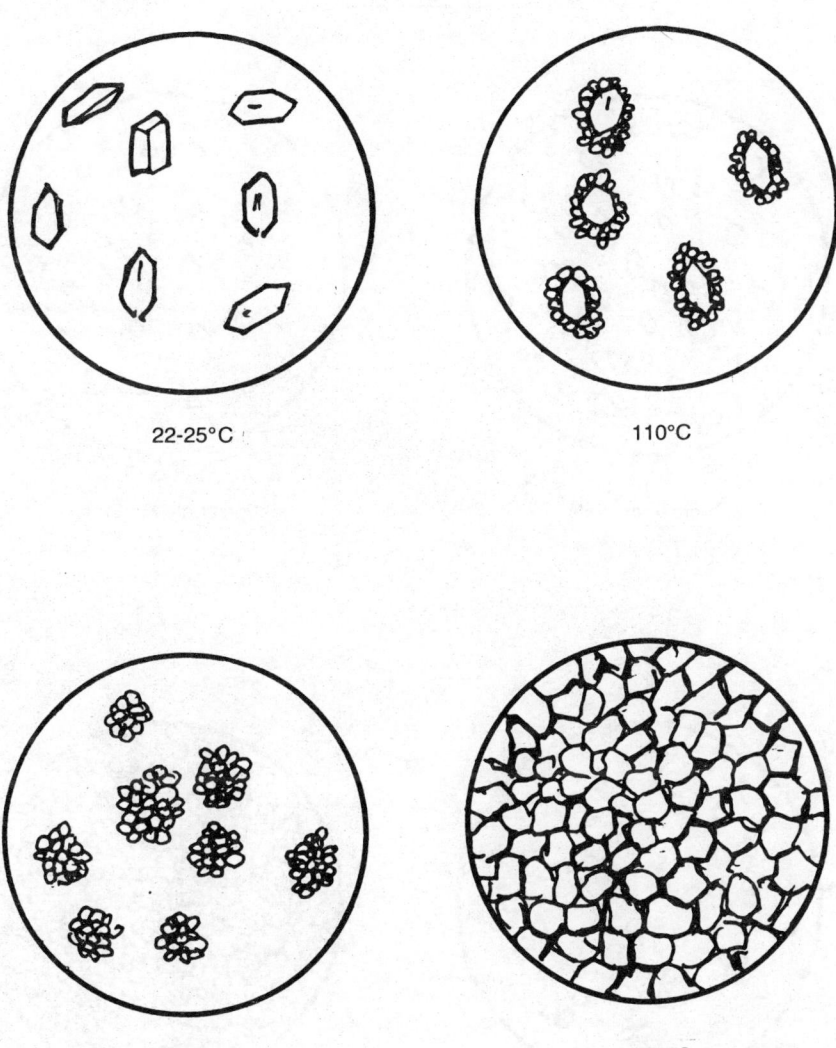

22-25°C

110°C

120°C

180°C

Plate I: Microscopic structure of sugar solutions at different temperatures corresponding to the cold water test.

FUDGE

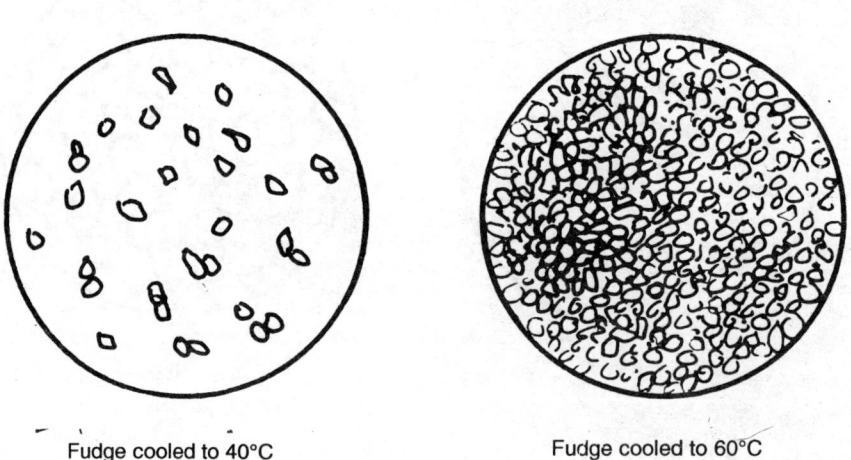

Sucrose crystals   Fudge cooled to 30°C

Fudge cooled to 40°C   Fudge cooled to 60°C

Plate II: Microscopic view of sugar recrystallization in preparation of fudge.

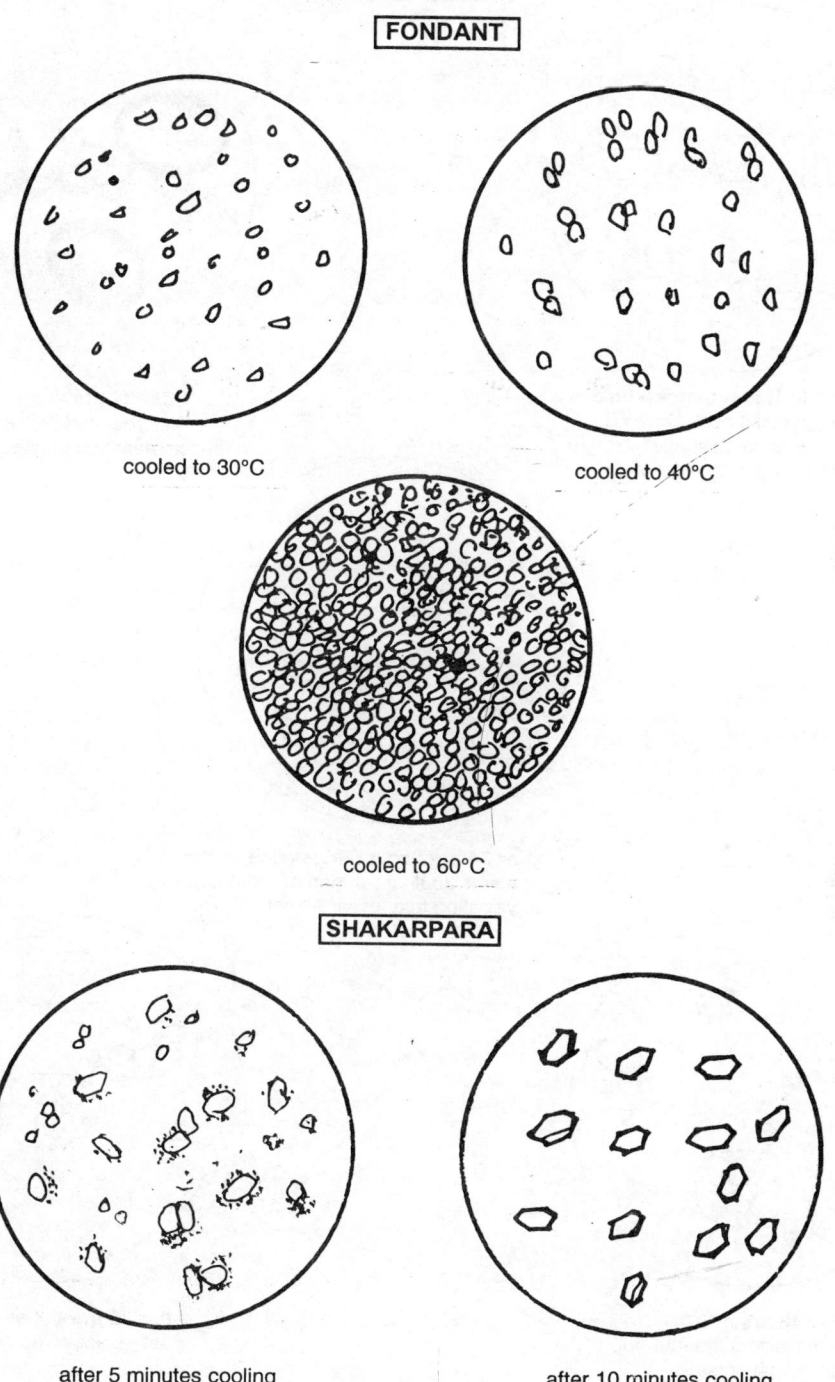

Plate III: Microscopic view of recrystallization in fondant and *shakarpara*.

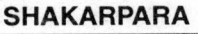

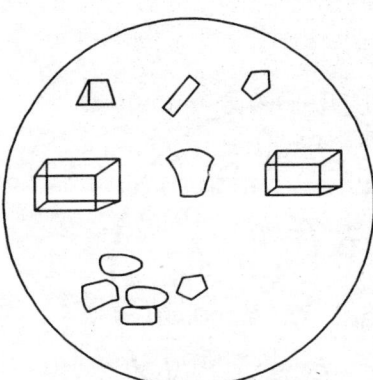

Cooled to Room temperature
Large (crystals) non clustered
clear hexagonal in shape
recrystallizing in the pan of sugar.

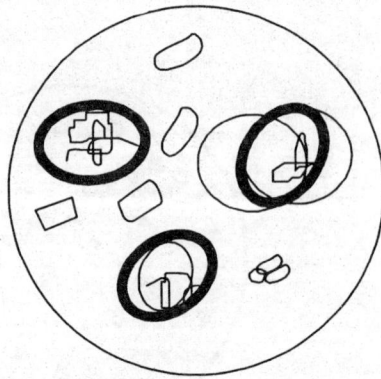

After 24 hrs at room temp.
Size reduced with aggregation of
crystals and subsequent growth.

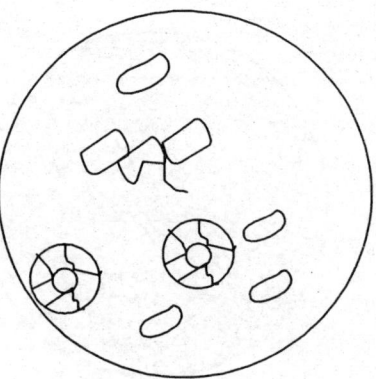

After 24 hrs under refrigeration
Size small but larger than at room temp.
aggregation to a lesser extent.

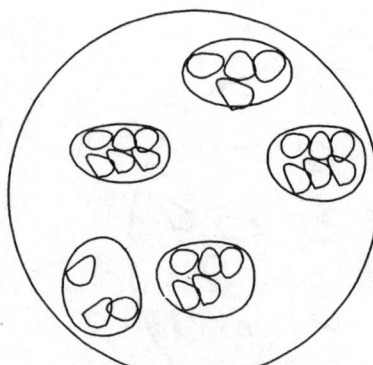

After 48 hrs at 60°C
Form clusters that are not
well defined in size.

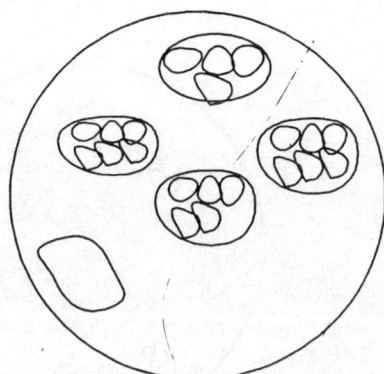

After 48 hrs under refrigeration
clusters observed are smaller.

Plate IV: Microscopic view of *shakarpara* crystals

CHENNA MURKI

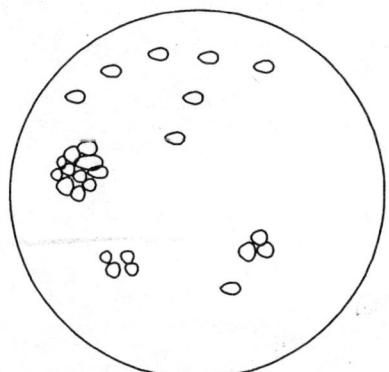

Cooled to Room temperature
Polygonal crystals with some clusters.

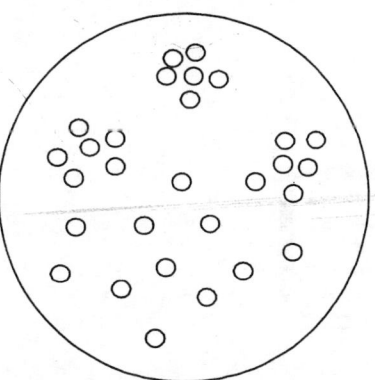

Under Refrigeration at 7-10°C.
Aggregation of crystals observed.
Crystals size larger than that of room temp.

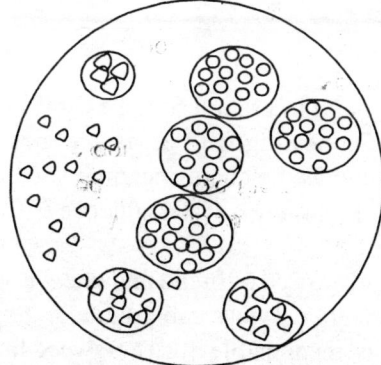

After 48 hrs at 60°C
Crystal size very small. Shape could not be identified
as too much aggregation occurred. Crystal growth
was observed.

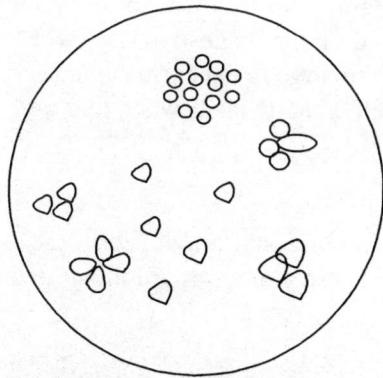

After 24 hrs under refrigeration.
Circular and polygonal crystals formed clusters
that were less dense, but slightly bigger
than those at room temperature.

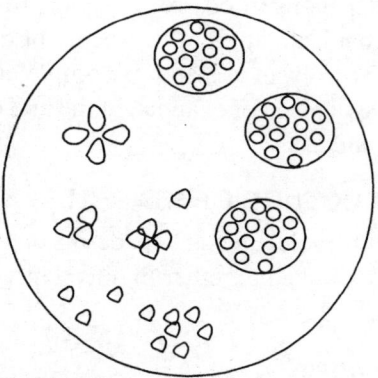

After 24 hrs.
Small circular crystals with aggregation.
Shape not well defined.

Plate V: Microscopic view of *Chenna Murki* crystals

2

Starches

Starch is a polymer of glucose units, found in granules, and exhibiting characteristic shapes, sizes and arrangements in different foods. On heating with acids starches hydrolyze to dextrins which are shorter polymers of glucose units and as the chains become smaller the solubility of the starch increases. On completion of the starch breakdown 100% glucose is formed. Such reactions are not reversible.

It is for this reason that when we eat a piece of bread and chew it well it tastes sweeter, because the starch in bread gets mixed with salivary amylase and gradually gets hydrolyzed to more soluble forms and finally to glucose which is responsible for the sweet taste. Again, when you lick a postage stamp to paste it, a sweet taste remains in the mouth. This is due to the soluble dextrin used on the back of stamps, which gets hydrolyzed to glucose with time and the taste buds respond.

Chewing food well is good for health, because the starches are broken down not only by mechanical action of the teeth but the burden of digestion is reduced on the disgestive tract when the hydrolysis of starch is completed in the mouth. Further, there is no urge to eat extra sugar. Try eating a piece of chappati at the end of your meal and see for yourself what happens when it is well chewed.

STRUCTURE OF STARCH

Starch molecules are made up of two types of structures called amylose and amylopectin molecules linked together in different ways in a particular food starch. These structures are illustrated in Fig. 2.1.

Amylose

As seen from Fig. 2.1 amylose is a very flexible molecule usually made up of glucose units which are linear in their arrangements. It can therefore very quickly change into different shapes because of the many OH groups available for easy bonding, and form a 3-dimensional gel structure in starchy food products. The amylose content of a starch affects its properties of gelatinization pasting and retrogradation. A waxy starch for example, contains only about 2-3% amylose.

Amylopectin

Amylopectin structures are usually branched and therefore impart different characteristics to food starches than do amylose predominant starches. Amylopectin represents 70-80% of the total starch content of a food, although many starches are composed totally of amylopectin molecules. The crystalline nature of raw starch granules is attributed to allignment of the linear segments into crystalline miscelles, but many different theories for this exist.

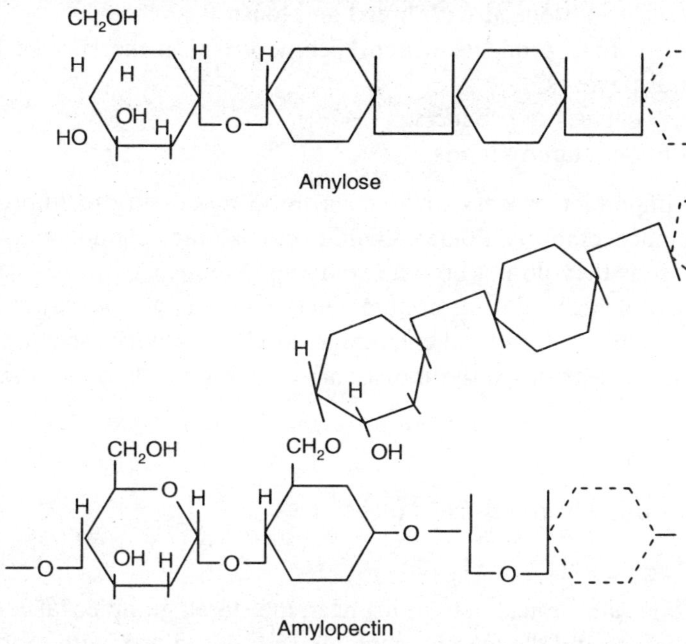

Fig. 2.1. Amylose and amylopectin linkages.

Starches like potato and tapioca which have a high percentage of amylopectin molecules impart high viscosity and low gelling properties as compared to amylose predominant starches. The former also have a slight tendency towards retrogradation. With iodine, amylopectin gives a red purple colour whereas amylose gives a characteristic blue.

EFFECT OF COOKING ON STARCH

Starchy foods may be cooked by dry or moist heat methods depending on the taste, colour and textural properties desired. The foods with a high proportion of starch in their structure are cereals, legumes, vegetables followed by fruits and nuts.

Effect of Dry Heat

Some examples of dry heat cooking are making of toast, roasting or cereals and nuts prior to preparation or direct consumption. Application of dry heat initiates the process of starch break-down through a process called dextrinization.

Dextrinization

Dextrinization is the process by which the large starch structure enmeshed together is broken down into smaller polysaccharides till dextrins are formed. This process has the following effects:

(*i*) Dextrins reduce the thickening power of the starches in the foods

(*ii*) Bring about surface browning and add colour to foods like toasted, roasted and baked products.

(*iii*) Change the flavour as experienced with bread and toast.

(*iv*) Change the texture of final products which become crisp on the surface but retain their juiciness and natural flavours.

(*v*) Imparts a delicate sweetness to products.

(*vi*) Improves digestibility of starchy foods.

Dextrinization is an important process involved in food processing to improve the sensory qualities of foods and their acceptability. Potatoes held in cold storage cannot be used immediately for fried or baked products as they do not brown evenly and are also sweet to taste due to starch breakdown and formation of dextrins during storage. On the other hand, sweet potatoes are held in a warm place to increase their sweetness and encourage amylase activity especially in high moisture varieties. The amount of dextrins in the moist variety is higher than in those which are dry when cooked.

Browning

Due to dextrimization browning of foods takes place.

Effect of Moist Heat

When starch or starchy foods are subjected to moist heat, the starch granules take up the water and swell. The granular wall bursts and the starchy contents spill out to mix with more water to form a sol which is milky in appearance.

Gelation

Every starch has a temperature range within which it thickens, becomes more viscous and forms a gel, which is a 2-phase system that resists flow. The process by which this takes place is called gelation. According to Hermansson (1986), gel is the intermediate state between a solution and a precipitate.

Gelatinization

On further heating, the sol becomes translucent and forms a network of amylose, amylopectins and water held together by intermolecular bonds. All the free water gets enmeshed in a matrix, indicated by a coating on the back of a spoon. The hot mixture when poured into a mould and allowed to cool, sets into a firm structure which when unmoulded, retains the shape of the ontainer. This process is called gelatinization.

Syneresis

When a moulded starch is kept for a time in the refrigerator or cut and stored, some of the water starts to ooze out of the structure, which is disturbed. This process is referred to as syneresis which was first observed in 1861 by T. Graham, who described the process as an exudation of small amounts of liquid on standing because of a slight contraction of the gel. With certain gels however, syneresis is observable with increase in substrate concentration whereas with others a dilution is necessary as in the case of gelatin and agar-agar gels. Although no net volume change occurs in the gel, syneresis cannot be described as a reversible process.

Retrogradation

When, some cooked gels showing syneresis exhibit further realignment of the amylopectin fractions to further alter the structure, the process is termed as retrogradation. This phenomenon is observed on cooling, but only in some cooked starches such as wheat and corn where recrystallization of the gelatinized starches occurs, as in the cooling of bread or corn preparations. Waxy starches do not exhibit retrogradation.

Malting

The effect of applying of both dry and moist heat are seen in a process called malting. This is a process in which grains are dampened to allow them to germinate. They are then dried, dehusked and milled. Malting breaks down the starch to sugar, as well as increases the content of riboflavin, niacin and iron. A gruel made from malted flour is less thick because of the presence of amylase, and more flour can be used in preparing the food than ordinary flour. Malting increases the energy density of food, a factor important for feeding young children.

Use of Starches in Food Preparation

Starches may be used for various reasons as ingredients in cooking, because they act as agents for thickening, binding, coating, gelling and so on.

Thickening

Starches used for thickening gravies, soups, puddings etc. need to have clarity, viscosity and pasting properties depending on the quality of the finished product required. Commonly used are corn, refined wheat and rice flours and arrowroot. Corn has twice the thickening power than wheat flour, but if the flours are roasted or browned this power decreases due to dextrinization. Liquids thickened with potato or other waxy starches are more elastic.

Binding

Any of the above mentioned starches or foods containing them may be mixed with other ingredients that need to be closely bound together. For example, in the preparation of vegetable cutlets, a wide variety of vegetables which do not mix together are made to do so by adding refined flour, breadcrumbs or potato to the mixture. The starch helps to bind the ingredients together and prevent the cutlets from splitting during frying.

Coating

Starches are often used in the from of batters to coat foods before frying. This gives the product crispness, and seals-in the flavours by forming a barrier to evaporation of food contents, and provides a smooth golden appearance to the product by filling any crevices or irregularities on the surface.

Gelling

Starches form the main ingredients in preparation of porridges and puddings which require good gelling, moulding and cutting qualities. Some examples are rice and bread puddings, *halwas* and so on.

Browning

When subjected to dry heat starchy foods brown as in the preparation of toast or *chapati*, due to dextrinization. The colour may be due to sugar-protein reactions in food containing these components as well.

Thus, starches and starchy foods play an important role in providing not only energy in our diet but variety in food as well, behaving differently each time the ingredients, cooking time and temperature and the type and concentration of the starch are changed. However, it is important to understand that all the changes that take place during cooking are not necessarily desirable. Knowledge of such changes and why they take place, can help in preventing them, and avoiding unnecessary wastage of ingredients, time and other resources.

Modified starches

Today, starches are extensively modified for use in the food industry with the idea of producing certain desired qualities in finished products. Such starches are called modified starches, the modifications being brought about by physical changes, molecular degradation and addition of chemicals. All these methods alter the molecular properties of the natural starches, enabling them to be used for a wide range of applications (Dias et al., 1997). There are basically four ways in which starches are modified.

Thin boiling

In this method, modification is based on hydrolysis of the natural starch by boiling with acid which results in debranching the amylopectin molecules. This forms a thin sol when hot, which sets to a strong gel on cooling. This modification is used in the manufacture of gum drops or *karachi halwa*.

Pregelatinization

This involves precooking and vacuum drying. Such starches thus acquire the property of dissolving and swelling easily in cold water and are used in preparation of instant foods such as soups and other premixes providing convenience to the user.

Cold water-swelling (CWS)

In this method the starch is instant in use but remains as an intact granule, offering stability, clarity, texture and convenience, Such starch may be gelling or non-gelling and are used in preparation of cold process salad dressings. They provide the thick creamy mouthfeel in fat-free dressings.

Oxidation

The starch solutions are subjected to reaction with sodium hypochlorite. Such products exhibit properties similar to thin boiling starches but form softer gels. Oxidized starches however, have limited use in food processing.

Cross-linking

This is a process which involves the production of starches under alkaline conditions, usually in combination with acetic or succinic anhydride. The starches produced in this manner are known for their thickening and stabilizing properties, and the products prepared undergo minimal retro-gradation.

The purpose of cross-linking is to enable the starch to withstand conditions of low pH, high shear or high temperaturer. The starch becomes more resistant to rupture. It is largely used in acid sauces. Stabilized starches are used in preparation of frozen foods as they prevent gelling or syneresis in foods stored at low temperatures.

Starches are also being modified for non-food uses such as in pharmaceutical delivery systems, as flavour and odour enchancers and filtering agents for removal of off-flavours in fruit juices.

It is with this in view that food science has developed, to promote an understanding of the physical, chemical and biological changes that can occur right from harvesting processing and till the products reach the consumer for cooking, service and final consumption.

Experiments 6-9 have been designed to provide familiarity with the properties and behaviour of starches as used in food preparation, and to provide a feel of the importance of Food Science, through its applications in daily life.

EXPERIMENT 6

Aim

To study the microscopic structure of food starches.

Equipment

Electron weighing balance, microscope, slides, cover slips, droper, burners, food thermometers, clamp, measuring spoons, standing cups, test tubes and stand, petridishes, filter paper, cooking pans, wooden spoons, and toothpicks.

Materials

Wheat, rice arrowroot, potato, bengal gram.

Reagents

Iodine solution, alcohol, glycerine, distilled water.

Principle

Starch occurs in small particles known as granules. The size and shape of each kind of starch is characteristic for each food type, hence microscopic examination of a starch isolated from any food, can usually help to determine the food source of the starch, or the presence of any adulterants in the food especially when it is bought in powdered form as flours.

Starches are usually insoluble in water at room temperature, but when subjected to moist heat they swell up and get held together by hydrogen bonds between the branches of the amylopectins in the structure of the starch. This process leads to changes in the texture and setting qualities of the different starch products, when prepared under controlled conditions of temperature, time of cooking, amount of heat and quantities of materials used.

Procedure

This experiment is divided into 3 parts as follows:

A. *Preparation of slides*

(*i*) Take lg each of corn, wheat, pulse, rice and arrowroot flours in different test tubes.

(*ii*) Add 5ml of distilled water, shake vigorously and let stand for a few seconds.

(*iii*) When the sediment settles slightly, take a drop of the turbid sol on a slide, spread it out thinly with the help of another slide, cover with slip and view under the microscope.

For preparing slides from roots and tubers like potato, sweet potato etc. grate the starchy portion and proceed as described for other starches.

B. (*i*) Repeat slide preparation as in A (*i*) but before placing the cover slip add a drop each of alcohol and diluted glycerine (diluted 50:50 with water). Spread as instructed cover and observe under the microscope at low as well as high power.

(*ii*) Repeat (*i*) but add a drop of iodine solution. Observe the blue to purple starches under the microscope.

C. *Effect of cooking on starch structure*

(*i*) Stir 15g of each starch in 240ml water and bring to boil on medium heat stirring constantly till the mixture coats the back of the spoon.

(*ii*) Cool, prepare a slide and observe under the microscope.

(*iii*) Record the changes observed and compare the effect of cooking on the microscope structure of the starches.

Observations

Record your observations with respect to structure, size, shape, arrangement and nucleation of the various starches observed in experiments (A), (B) and (C) according to the format presented in Table 2.1.

Table 2.1 Microscopic Identification of raw starches

Starch	Description			
	Size	*Shape*	*Arrangement*	*Nucleation*
Corn				
Wheat				
Rice				
Potato				
Pulse				

Microsopic examination can help to identify adulterant powders in flours.

Repeat these observations in every class when you prepare any starch food and learn to recognize the structures and the changes that occur in them after cooking. Prepare suitable illustrations for each starch according to the format indicated in Table 2.2.

Table 2.2 Structural comparison of raw and cooked starches

Starch	*Microscopic* raw	*Structure* cooked	*Applications in food* preparation
Corn			
Wheat			
*			
*			

Precautions

1. The microscope lens, slides and cover slips should be thoroughly cleaned before use.
2. Just a drop of the starch extract should be used for the slide preparation.
3. All cooked starches should be cooled to room temperature before the slide is prepared.

Practice Exercises

1. Take a mixture of corn and wheat flours, prepare a slide as learnt and observe under the microscope. See if you can identify the two starches distinctly. List the food that can be prepared in the home using such mixtures of starchy foods.

2. Prepare slides from raw and cooked whole and dehusked pulses, legumes, roots and tubers and observe under the microscope. Record your observations and interpret your results with respect to the practical applications of the starches in pure or mixed forms in everyday food preparation and processing.

EXPERIMENT 7

Aim

To study the gelatinization properties of food starches.

Equipment

Refrigerator, weighing scale, pans, wooden spoons burners, thermometer and clamp, measuring cup and spoons, petridishes, toothpicks.

Materials

Corn, wheat (refined flour), rice, arrowroot starches.

Principle

Starches have the characteristic property of thickening food mixtures in the presence of moist heat, the effects varying with the structure of the starches present. Those starches which contain more amylose tend to have better gelation properties compared to starches in which amylopectins predominate. Amylose is not truly soluble in water but forms hydrated micelles in which the long chains get twisted to form a coil-like structure. It is this structure that is responsible for the gelling characteristics of cooked and cooled starches. The amylopectins in starches of roots and tubers are more brush like because of their branched structure, and usually provide high viscosity, lending to thickening properties in foods, but do not contribute to effective gel formation.

Procedure

A. Prepare a starch sol using 15 g starch and 240 ml water in the following manner :

(i) Take the starch in a container using a small quantity of the measured water to make a smooth paste.

(ii) Add the remaining water gradually with stirring to prevent lump formation. Note the clarity of the sot.

(iii) Cook the mixture over direct medium flame with constant stirring till the mixture begins to thicken. Note the time taken and the temperature at which thickness is first felt. This is the temperature at which gelatinization starts.

(iv) Continue cooking for another few minutes till the mixture becomes suddenly thick enough to coat the back of a spoon.

(v) Remove from heat and note the time taken and temperature at which gelatinization was completed. Note the clarity of the paste at each stage.

(vi) Pour the hot mixture into two petridishes, placing one at room temperature (RT) and one in the refrigerator (FT) to set.

(vii) When set, calculate the percentage sag of the gel to determine its firmness. For the calculation proceed as follows:

(a) Pierce a toothpick vertically in the centre of the petridish, then pull it out and measure the moist level using a mm scale. This reading is R1.

(b) Loosen the sides of the gel in the petridish with a moist knife and invert the gel on the centre of a plate. Again take the reading as in (a). This is R2.

(c) Calculate the % sag using the formula $\% \text{ sag} = \dfrac{R_1 - R_2}{R_1} \times 100$.

B. Repeat A (i-vii) using *maida* (wheat starch).
C. Repeat A (i-vii) using Rice flour.
D. Repeat A (i-vii) using arrow root starch.

Observations

Record your observations with respect to solubility of the starch in cold water, changes in colour, transparency and solubility on heating, the time and temperature range for gelatinization to occur in each starch, stability of the gel, its viscosity when poured into petridishes to set and its cutting quality when lunmoulded. The observation may be recorded according to the format indicated in Tables 2.3 and 2.4.

Table 2.3 Changes on heating of starches

Starch	Solubility			Viscosity	Colour	Transparency
	Cold	H_2O	Hot			
A Corn						
B Wheat						
C Rice						
D Arrowroot						
*						

Table 2.4 Gelatinization properties of starches

Starch	Gelatinization		% Sag		Cut		Application in
	Time	°C	R. T.	F.T.	R.T.	F.T.	Cooking
A. Corn							
B. Wheat							
C. Rice							
D. Arrowroot							
*							

Draw your inferences and discuss the suitability of each starch in food preparation.

Precautions

1. Prepare starch sols always in cold water and then heat.
2. Even heating with constant stirring in essential to prevent lump formation.
3. The bulb of the thermometer should be immersed in the sol and not touch either the sides or bottom of the beaker or pan.

4. The time for cooling should be the same for all samples.
5. The measurement of readings for the % sag, should be taken from the centre of the gel in the petridish or when unmoulded.

Practice Exercises

1. Prepare a porridge from broken wheat (*dalia*) or semolina (*suji*) using any standard recipe, and comment on the sensory and gelation properties of the products when hot and cold.
2. Using the method learnt prepare the porridge with rice flour and sago. Compare your observations using the various kinds of starches and indicate your acceptability for the products in order of preference. Give reasons why one porridge is liked more than the other and how your knowledge of starches can help to improve the acceptability.

EXPERIMENT 8

Aim

To study the various factors affecting the gelatinization properties and setting quality of food starches.

Equipment

Same as in experiment 7.

Materials

Corn, wheat, rice and arrowroot flours.

Principle

A number of factors affect the gelatinization properties of the different starches such as their structure, amount used in cooking, temperature, presence of other substances such as sugar, salt, acid, fat and the type of heat applied. All these and other factors therefore produce varying results in food preparation, and by understanding these one can alter the factors to achieve desired results in a product. For example, if starch is required only as a thickening agent in food, one can choose a starch that has more amylopectins in its structure. Since they do not form as good gels as amylose based starches.

Procedure

This experiment is intended to provide a feel of what the science of food can do for us and how we can correct an unacceptable product by varying anyone or more of the factors that are under our control. The experiment covers a number of variations, and the results observed applied to every-day experiences with food.

A. *Effect of starch concentration*

(*i*) Take different starches and prepare 100 ml sols at 5%, 10%, 15% and 20% concentrations in cold water, in separate beakers.

(*ii*) Heat each sample one by one to 90°C and remove from burner.

(*iii*) Pour the hot starch of each concentration into 2 petridishes, leave one at room temperature and the other in the fridge till set.

(*iv*) Calculate the % sag as learnt in experiment 7.

(*v*) Prepare a slide at each concentration and examine under the microscope. Compare structure of raw and cooked starches. Comment on the differences.

(*vi*) Label all the samples accurately and keep aside for evaluation.

B. *Effect of temperature*

(*i*) Make 5% solutions of each starch and cook to 60, 70, 80, 90 and 100°C.

(*ii*) Proceed as in A (*iii-vi*).

C. *Effect of added substances*

   (*a*) *Sugar*

      (*i*) Heat a 5% starch sol to 90°C and then add 10,30 and 60 g sugar in separate samples.

      (*ii*) Cook till sugar dissolves and remove from heat.

      (*iii*) Proceed as in A (*iii-vi*).

   (*b*) *Effect of Salt*

      Proceed as for (*a*) except replace sugar with 1/2, 1 and 2T salt in each sample.

   (*c*) *Effect of Acid*

      Proceed as for (*b*) but replace salt by 1/2, 1 and 2T acid either in the form of lemon juice or vinegar.

   (*d*) *Effect of Fat*

      Repeat as in (*c*) replacing acid with 1/2, 1 and 2T fat or oil.

   Note the effect of all the added substances on gelatinization properties of starches comparing them to a standard in which no additional substances were added.

Observations

Tabulate the observations obtained through experiments A-F, using the format presented in Table 2.5.

Table 2.5 Effect of starch concentration on gelatinization

Starch	Concentration %				Colour	Time	%sag	Cut	Application
	5	10	15	20		mins			
Corn									
Wheat									
Rice									
A. root									

Precautions

Same as for experiments 6 and 7.

Practice Exercises

1. Cook any two dishes using wheat, potato or sago starches in both sweet and salt preparation. Keep the time, temperature and cooking conditions the same. Record your observations for gelation and gelatinization properties of the products.
2. What differences do you observe when given boiled or fried rice. Explain why you prefer one to the other.
3. Make a list of dishes that you eat at home in which a starch or a food containing it has been used to provide thickening, coating or gelling properties.

EXPERIMENT 9

Aim

To determine the gluten content and water absorption of different flours.

Equipment

Porcelain or stainless steel flat bottom dish, weighing balance, spatula, burette, muslin cloth, butter paper, oven, beaker.

Materials

Whole wheat, water, other cereal flours.

Principle

Gluten is predominantly a wheat protein composed primarily of gliadin and glutenin. At a neutral pH, it is insoluble in water whereas, in an acidic or alkaline medium, it becomes soluble. Other protein fractions present in wheat are soluble in water even at a neutral pH. Thus, gluten can be obtained by washing away starch and bran from the kneaded dough. Hydrated gluten (as in kneaded dough) contains 65-70% water therefore on kneading it becomes sticky to touch. It provides structure to the product when heated due to coagulation and helps in holding gas or air in the product as seen during baking cake or preparing a chappati. Based upon the gluten content, flours can be categorized as soft, medium or strong. Compared to *all-purpose flour* (9-10% protein) which is considered to be a medium flour, *bread flour* (atta) has 12.0 to 13.5% protein. *Cake flour* on the other hand is considered to be a weak flour as it has only 7.0-8.5% protein.

The approximate strength of the flour can be assessed by mere physical examination too. If on squeezing the flour in our hand it crumbles away, it is a strong flour whereas, a weak flour tends to stick to the hands due to its low protein and high starch content.

Procedure

1. Weigh accurately 25 gm of flour sample.
2. Put in a china dish.
3. Add water through a burette and knead the dough using a spatula.
4. Measure the volume of water used to make a soft dough, accurately.
5. Keep the ball of kneaded dough immersed in water in a beaker for 1/2 hour.
6. Take out the dough using a spatula, wrap in a small muslin cloth and wash under running chlorine free tap-water, till the starch gets completely removed and water coming out is clean.
7. Add a drop of iodine to confirm complete removal of starch.
8. Weigh the gluten after removing muslin cloth.
9. Place on butter paper and dry it in an oven (130 ± 1°C) for 2 hrs.
10. Keep in the dessicator to cool and weigh.
11. Calculate the gluten content using the standard formula:

$$(i) \quad \text{Gluten content}(\%) = \frac{\text{Dry weight of gluten}}{\text{wt. of flour}} \times 100$$

(*ii*) Water absorption power of flour is determined by estimating the quantity of water used in dough preparation during the experiment. For example:

25 gm of flour required x ml of water to make a soft dough.

∴ 100 gm of flour required $= \dfrac{x \times 100}{25}$ ml water.

% water absorption $= \dfrac{\text{water used}}{\text{wt. of flour}} \times 100$

Observations

Record your observations as indicated in the Table 2.6.

Table 2.6 Gluten content and water absorption capacity of different flours

Sample	Gluten content	% water absorption
1. Wheat flour		
2. Refined wheat flour		
3. Rye/rice flour		
4. Cake flour		
5. Maize flour		

Precautions

1. Weigh the flour, gluten and measure the water accurately.
2. Make sure that all the starch gets washed away before keeping the gluten in the oven.
3. Use a spatula and not your fingers to knead or hold dough.

Practice Exercises

1. Repeat the above experiment using different cereal flours such as refined wheat flour, rice flour, maize flour etc. Record your observations as learnt.
2. Experiment with pulse fours and compare their gluten content with cereat flours.
3. List food products that are gluten free.

A
Raw

B
Cooked

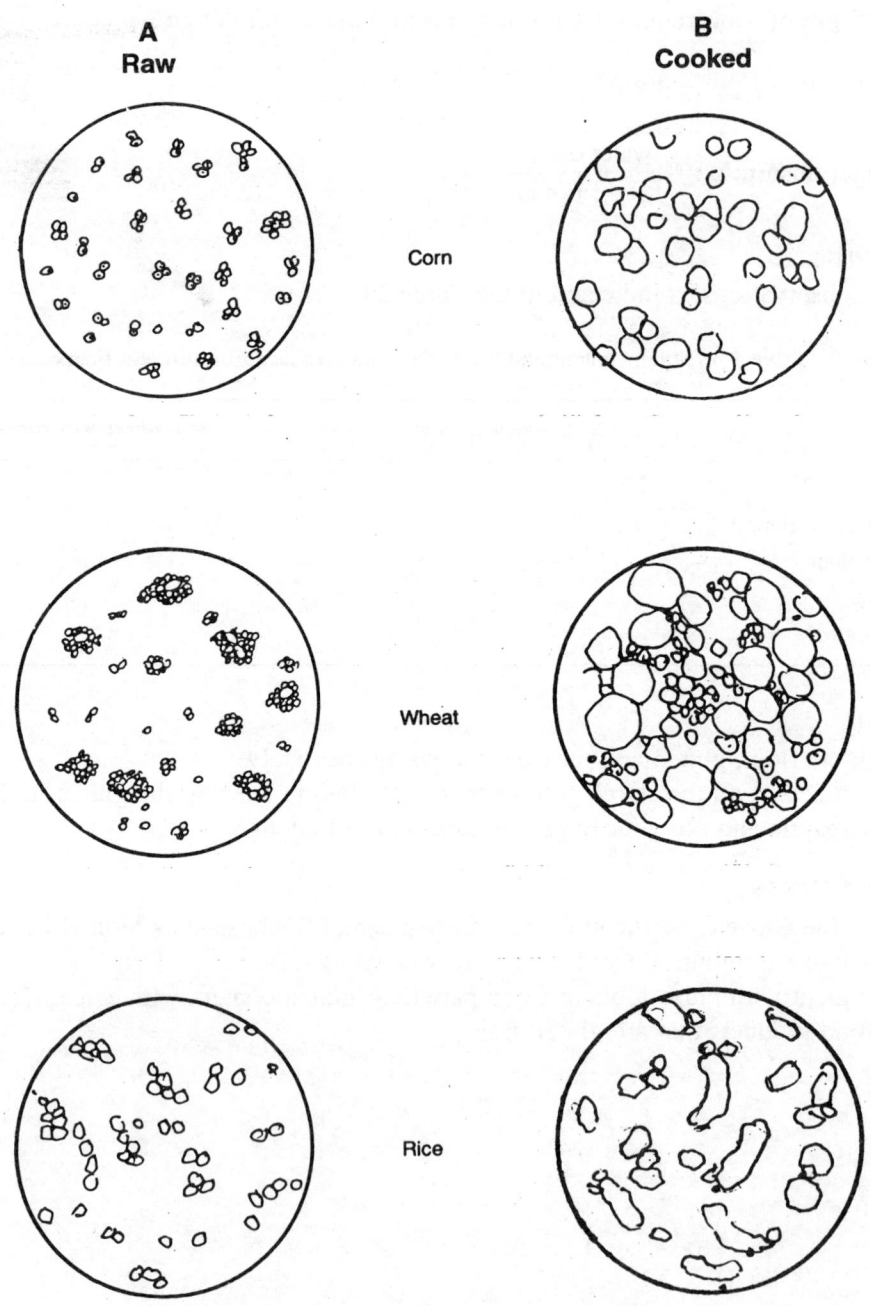

Corn

Wheat

Rice

Plate VI A: Microscopic structure of raw and cooked starches.

A
Raw

B
Cooked

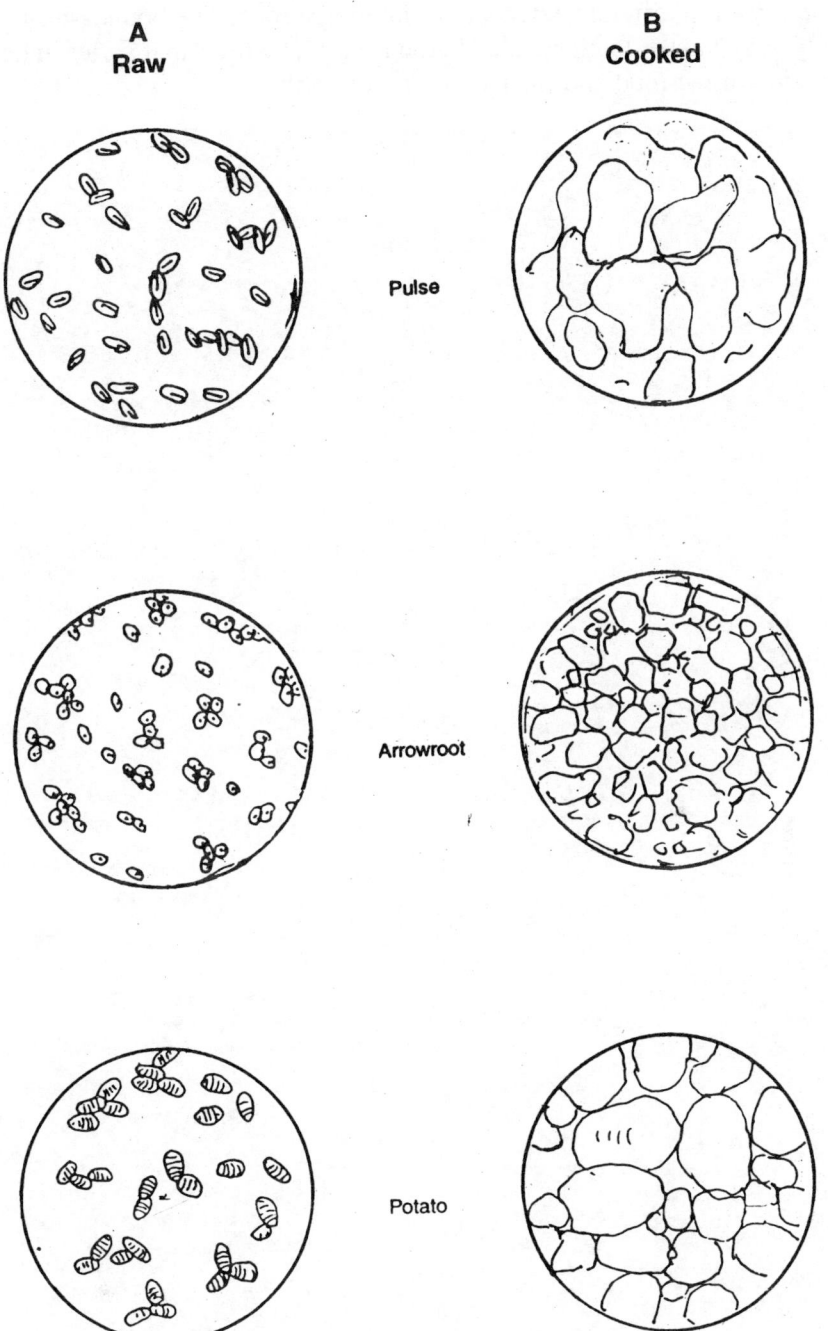

Pulse

Arrowroot

Potato

Plate VI B: Microscopic structure of raw and cooked starches.

It will he noticed from plates VI A and B that, in the case of all cereals, pulses and tubers tested, the shape of the starch granules is well defined and characteristic of the food material used while on cooking they swell to different extents amd soften the food. The boundaries therefore get less defined as cells carrying the starch burst and produce a sticky mass that varies in texture according to the composition of the food and the nature of the starch.

3

Pectins and Gums

Pectic substances represent a group of compounds which are carbohydrate derivatives found in the middle lamella of all plant tissues. They are (polysaccharides of galacturonic acid or of its methyl ester, being) polymers of D-galacturonic acid united by the α-1, 4-glycosidic linkage. These substances include pectic and pectinic acids or pectin and protopectin which act as intercellular cementing material in the form of calcium and magnesium pectinates or pectates in plants. Pectinic acids have methyl ester groups attached to carboxyl groups in the galacturonic polymer. If half or more of the COOH groups are esterified, the substances are designated as pectins. The pectin linkage is illustrated in Fig. 3.1.

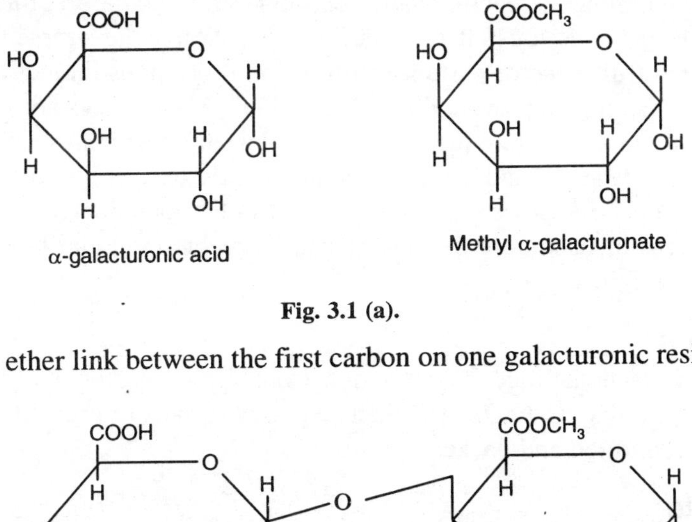

α-galacturonic acid

Methyl α-galacturonate

Fig. 3.1 (a).

The 1-4 link is an α ether link between the first carbon on one galacturonic residue and the fourth carbon on another.

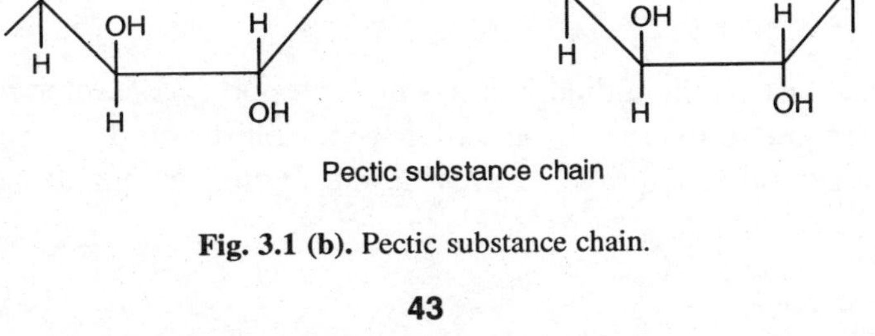

Pectic substance chain

Fig. 3.1 (b). Pectic substance chain.

43

Pectic acid

This is found in abundance and contains COOH group in its structure which is not esterified, and can therefore react with metallic ions to form salts which then get deposited as pectates.

Protopectin

Protopectins are the insoluble pectic substances found in immature plants and unripe fruits and vegetables. However, when immature plant foods are heated the insoluble protopectin gets converted to pectin which easily disperses in the water. It is for this reason that just ripe or green immature fruits are boiled in water and the extracts containing the pectin are used for preparation of jellies. As ripening takes place the pectin gets gradually demethylated and unable to form gels. Fruits and vegetables also contain an enzyme *pectin methyl esterase* which hydrolysis the pectin reducing its ability to gel. Overripe fruits therefore have little or no gelling power.

Pectins

Pectins are water soluble and when heated in certain ratios with sugar and acid form gels. This property is used in the manufacture of fruit jellies, jams, gels, candies and the like. Low methoxyl pectins however, can form gels in the presence of divalent ions such as calcium, and therefore milk can be made into mouldable puddings without the addition of sugar and acid. The gelling in milk is either colloidally dispersed casein or calcium caseinate.

Pectins from different food sources exhibit different characteristics due to their varying molecular size, structure and degree of esterification. Jellies prepared from citrus fruits are more friable and less elastic than those from apple.

At constant pH and temperature there is an optimum time for pectin extraction. When heating is continued beyond that time the pectin quality gets degraded. Therefore, for best results, pectin quality needs to be tested at various intervals during extraction using simple tests.

If freshly prepared fruit juice or paste is left to stand it becomes thinner due to the action of *methyl esterase* on the pectin. To prevent this processed juices and pastes are suitably subjected to heat as in pasteurization to inactivate the enzyme. Apples and the spongy white albedo of citrus fruits are high pectic substances and therefore commercially used in the manufacture of pectin. Other foods which are good sources of pectin are used in the manufacture of pectin. Other food which are good sources of pectin are berries, guava, *karonda, amla* and many other indigenous plant foods of Indian origin.

Commercial Pectin

Commercial pectin is manufactured by extraction from apple pulp or orange skin pith as a by product of the juice industry. The extract is then heated with salts to precipitate the pectin which is then washed, filtered, dried and packed.

Fruit Pectin Gels

Theory

A gel behaves like an elastic solid although it has high proportion of water enmeshed in it. While pectin is essential for gel formation, by it self it is unable to bind the water to form a three dimensional structure. Acid is required to provide the hydrogen ions to neutralize the charges enough so that the dispersed pectin molecules do not repel each other. Further, sugar is necessary in a concentration that lowers the water activity initiating the formation of cross links between pectin molecules. The proportion of hydrogen ions, sugar and pectin determine whether the gel will set on cooling.

Hydrogen ion concentration

The hydrogen ion concentration represents a measure of the acid in a solution. Most fruit pectins form gels within a pH range of 2.8-3.4, the higher pH values being non-conducive to gel formation. If at all gels do form, they take much longer. When the pH is less than 2.8 the high hydrogen ion concentration raises the temperature at which a gel sets. Thus, if the gel begins to set even before the hot mixture is poured out into containers for setting, the structure is disturbed and the final product is a weak jelly.

There is no optimum hydrogen ion concentration for all jellies, as this depends on the quality of pectin in the fruit extract, especially its methoxyl content and the salts present. Usually tartaric acid is favoured to citric acid in promoting gel formation because of its higher ability to ionize. Grapes therefore make good jelly on account of their tartaric acid content.

Sugar concentration

The boiling point of a jelly mixture may be used as an index of the amount of sugar concentration in the jelly. The sugar concentration in jellies may vary from 40-70% but is usually 60-65%, indicating the doneness of the product. Most pectin gels are ready when the sugar concentration is enough to raise the boiling point of the mixture to 103°C – 105°C. The exact concentration of a mixture can be measured using a digital refractometer.

Inversion of some of the sugar as well as the presence of pectin prevents the recrystallisation of sugar in the jelly as it cools and sets. Sugar crystals may form in jellies made with commercial pectin which requires a short cooking time and therefore inversion is not complete.

Pectin concentration

The concentration of pectin in a jelly is dependent on the amount of water evaporated during cooking. Weak pectin sols require less sugar as against high concentration of pectin in the extract. However, jelly formation depends not only on the quantity but also quality of the pectin present.

Tests for pectin

There are two simple tests for measuring pectin concentration which can be used at household level, in the laboratory and in food processing.

Jelmeter test

Pectin concentration is tested by using a simple instrument called a jelmeter, which records the rate of flow of the sol. The time taken for the sol to flow through the capillary tube is recorded. The greater the time taken the higher is the pectin concentration.

Alcohol test

A 5ml sample of the extract is taken in a test tube and cooled to room temperature. The tube is then held in a tilted position and 10ml of alcohol is poured down the side of the tube till the alcohol makes contact with the extract. The test tube is then allowed to stand undisturbed for a minute or two. After that, the tube is closed with the thumb and again tilted slowly till the contents touch the thumb. In this process if one large clot moves in the test tube the pectin content is high, if two small clots are visible the pectin is of medium strength, if a number of tiny clots are seen then the pectin is weak and requires addition of extra pectin before a good jelly can be made.

Quality of Pectin

The greater the methylation in the pectin structure the greater is the sugar requirement for setting fruit jellies and vice versa. The presence of divalent ions such as calcium, are however necessary to form cross linkages between pectin molecules through the COOH groups. When more than 50% of the COON groups are not methylated, the divalent ions may help to form the network resulting in a gel without addition of sugar.

Testing Jelly Readiness

It is difficult to judge when enough water from a jelly mixture has evaporated to form a gel on cooling. A few tests can therefore be useful to judge the readiness of a hot fruit-pectin-acid mixture before it can be poured out to set.

Boiling point test

Usually a mixture that reaches a temperature of 3-5°C higher than the boiling point of the sugar solution alone is the right temperature for setting jellies. For example, if 200g of sugar is added to the fruit extract being boiled, then make a solution of 200g of sugar in water and note its boiling point. Heat the fruit extract 3-5°C higher than the determined boiling point of the sugar solution. Remove from heat and pour into the required container and air cool to set the jelly. The usual temperatures for readiness range from 102-107°C.

Plate test

Pour a spoonful of the boiling jelly mixture on a plate and allow it to cool. If it sets on cooling and no water separation is seen, the mixture is ready for bottling.

Sheet test

This can be conducted as a household test as well and requires no sugar thermometer. When the fruit mixture starts to break into large heavy bubbles during boiling, a wooden spoon may be used to take a little of the hot mixture, and raise the spoon above the cooking vessel. Now tilt the spoon so that the mixture drops back into the pan, till the last drop remains like a sheet hanging from the edge of the spoon. Repeated tests may be necessary at intervals, to reach the sheet point on air cooling of the last drop. At this juncture the hot syrup is poured into sterilized containers and left to set undisturbed. The various stages of the sheet are depicted in Fig. 3.2.

If a jelly mixture does not respond to the sheet test it may be due to a lack of hydrogen ions, which can be corrected by adding a little lemon juice. Another reason for the failure of the test can be addition of excess sugar in the mixture, or overheating in which case some of the pectin may have been hydrolysed to soluble forms. In such case one teaspoon of liquid pectin per cup of original extract may be added and the mixture boiled for 1/2 to 1 minute to set the gel.

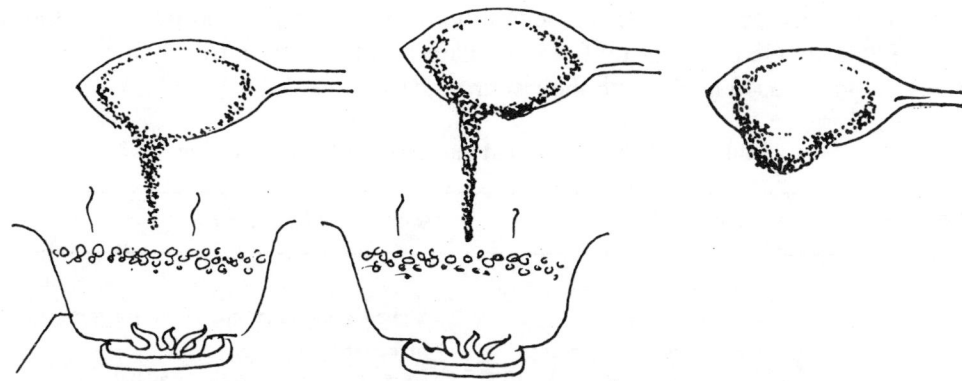

Fig. 3.2. Stages of the sheet test.

Refractometer test

A drop of jelly may be placed on the refractometer disc and doneness tested by reading off the sugar percentage in the mixture.

Gel Quality

The qualities of a good fruit gel are :

  (*i*) Attractive colour
  (*ii*) Transparency
  (*iii*) Sets well and quivers gently on being disturbed
  (*iv*) Produces a clean firm cut
  (*v*) Soft texture with good spreadability

It may be noted that to obtain the above qualities not more than 2-3 cups of fruit extract should be cooked at a time as the setting quality as well as its sensory attributes will be grossly affected.

Gums

Gums are secretions of plants found on leaves, roots and barks and are also called exudates or derivatives. These are usually obtained from quince seed, karaya, acacia, tragacanth, irish moss, guar, sodium alginate, ammonium alginate and propylenealginate. All gums are subject to deterioration and require preservatives. Gums act as liquid emulsions and are used to thicken products and make them creamy. Vegetable gums are plant polysaccharides and composed of complex polymers of various sugars and their derivative uronic acids. All gums are hydrophillic, some yielding clear viscous sols while others are valued for their gelling properties. Gums swell in water but tend to get moldy and therefore when manufactured, require the addition of preservatives. When extracted from seaweeds and mosses the secretions are slimy in character and known as *mucilages*.

Uses of Gums

Although gums were used in their natural forms for thickening in foods, their easy perishability made the products prone to spoilage. They are now widely used for the manufacture of processed food products in which preservatives are added to prolong shelf life and improve other qualities. Gums are used as stabilizers in many food emulsions and as non-nutritive thickeners. Table 3.1 summarizes the gums used along with their sources and usage.

Table 3.1 Uses of gums and mucilages in food processing

Gum/Mucilage	Source	Usage in food processing
Gums		
Arabic	*Acacia* tree bark	Thickener and creaming agent for gum confectionery
Ghatti	Stems of *Anogeissus* plants	Thickener for creams
Guar	Seeds of *Cyanopsis*	Stabilizer for Icecream and desserts
Karaya	*Sterculia* plant	Creaming agent for salad creams
Locust bean	Fruit of carob tree-*Ceratonia*	Thickener for puddings, salad creams and frozen desserts
Tragacanth	Shrub bark - *Astragalus*	Stabilizer for salad creams and dips.
Mucilages		
Agar-agar	Red seaweed	Gelling agent for soups, jellies, icecreams and meat pastes
Alginates	Brown seaweed	Same as agar-agar
Carrageen	Moss from seaweed extract - *Chondrus*	Emulsifier for beverages

Adapted from O.F.G. Kilgour, *Complete Catering Science*. (1986). p. 110

Table 3.1 is by no means complete as newer sources come to light with progressive research on plant and weeds. However, they will continue to be used in the food industry as stabilizers, thickeners, emulsifiers, creaming agents and so on.

Gums are permitted up to 0.5% level by weight of finished product according to Indian food standards, especially for foods with high moisture and fat content. They give body to cheese, free flowing properties to evaporated milk and juice, prevent crystallization in jellies and stabilize suspended matter in beverages.

EXPERIMENT 10

Aim
To test the pectin strength of different fruits and vegetable extracts.

Equipment
Cooking pans, steel knife, test tubes, dropper, muslin cloth.

Materials
Alcohol, citric acid, guava, cooking apple, tomato, pumpkin, karonda and amla.

Principle
The formation of a gel is dependent on the pectin content of a fruit or vegetable. The strength of the final product however, varies with concentration of pectin, sugar, pH, temperature and the salts present in the fruit extract. The physical characteristics of pectins as well as their insolubility in alcohol and acetone form the basis of testing the pectin strength of extracts and consequently their power of gelation.

Procedure
A. (*i*) Wash fruit remove any blemishes or dark spots and cut into thin slices using a stainless steel knife.
  (*ii*) For 1 kg fruit add 1/5 teaspoon citric acid and $2\frac{1}{2}$ cups water to just cover the fruit.
  (*iii*) Heat the pan to boiling and then cook at simmering temperature (97°C) for 30-40 minutes or until the fruit becomes tender.
  (*iv*) Remove from fire and cool slightly, then strain the contents through a muslin cloth without using pressure to expel the extract so that it is clear.
  (*v*) Test for pectin strength using the alcohol test described on page 45.

B. (*i*) Repeat A (i-v) for apple and other fruits and vegetables.
  (*ii*) Compare the pectin strength of each fruit and vegetable extract.
  (*iii*) Measure the extract obtained from the same quantity of each fruit and use for experiments 10 and 11.
  (*iv*) Strain the pulp of each fruit separately and place in refrigerator for use in experiment 12.

Observations
Tabulate your observations with respect to each food extract commenting on colour, clarity, and pectin strength. Also note the time taken to prepare each extract and draw inferences as to suitability for jam or jelly making.

Precautions
  1. Foods should be sliced very thinly for maximum pectin extraction.
  2. Stainless steel knife should be used.
  3. Only enough water to cover the fruit should be added.
  4. The fruit should be cooked at simmering and not boiling temperature.

5. The extract should be allowed to drip through the muslin without pressing it out.

Practice Exercises

1. Prepare extracts from a wide variety of fruits and vegetables and test their pectin strengths.
2. Classify the foods as low, medium and high pectin fruits and vegetables.
3. Puree the pulp of the fruits separately and add a spoon of butter and sugar and cook till a mass of fruit mixture comes around the ladle while heating. Transfer the hot mixture on to a light greased chopping board, flatten with a palette knife and let it cool to set. Cut into candy sized pieces wrap in grease proof paper and serve as candy. Observe the differences in colour, texture and taste of the different fruit cheeses prepared, when fresh and after 24 and 48 hours.

EXPERIMENT 11

Aim

To prepare a fruit jelly.

Equipment

Same as in experiment 10.

Materials

Fruit extracts prepared in experiment 10, sugar.

Principle

Fruits like guava are high in pectin and also contain an appreciable amount of ascorbic acid. Depending on the stage of ripeness of the fruit and the resultant pH of the extract, jelly can be set with the addition of sugar followed by cooking of mixture. The setting quality is directly related to the pectin strength of the extract. The greater the pectin strength the lesser is the sugar required to form a good jelly.

Procedure

Jelly is made in two stages, one is the preparation of the fruit extract and two, cooking of the jelly. Taking the fruit extracts prepared in experiment 9 proceed as follows:

(*i*) Take 200 ml of each fruit extract and add 65% sugar to it.
(*ii*) Bring it to a vigorous boil without stirring.
(*iii*) Continue boiling till. the bubbles become large and viscous.
(*iv*) Test for readiness using the boiling point and sheet tests periodically.
(*v*) When the mixture is ready, pour it hot into sterilized jars and leave undisturbed to set.
(*vi*) Seal airtight when set.

Preservatives are only added if the product is to be stored for long periods at room temperatures as in the case of manufactured products.

Observations

Make observations with respect to temperature at readiness, time taken, colour, clarity, volume or weight, cut and spreading quality of the set products from each fruit extract. Grade the quality of the products according to the following acceptability criteria.

Excellent 5; Good 4; Fair 3; Satisfactory 2; Unsatisfactory 1. Comment on the products and indicate why some were unsatisfactory. Also state how products which are not good can be utilized in food preparation and processing to prevent their wastage.

Precautions

1. The jelly should be cooked at bubbling boil without stirring.
2. Sugar thermometer should dip into the boiling mixture without touching the bottom or side of the pan.

3. Pour the jelly mixture out while it is still hot.
4. Small lots should be prepared at a time.

Practices Exercises

1. Buy a manufactured jelly and comment on its texture, spreadability and other sensory qualities. Read the label and note the extra ingredients added by the manufacturer. Comment on the reasons for their addition.
2. Prepare jelly using *karonda* and compare it with the jellies prepared in this experiment.

EXPERIMENT 12

Aim

To determine the effect of varying the proportions of acid, sugar, temperature, pectin and cooking time on formation of guava jelly.

Equipment

As in experiment 10, pH paper, watch and Brix refractometer or jelmeter.

Materials

Guava extract, citric acid, sugar and water.

Principle

A pectin sol is stabilized by hydration and a negative charge on the pectin particles. Increase in acidity or alkalinity bring about destabilization of the molecule, stability being best in the neutral pH range of 6.8-7.0. In jelly making sugar acts as a dehydrating agent and therefore the lower the pH of the extract the lesser is the sugar required for precipitation of the pectin. Salts may aid or hinder precipitation depending on whether they increase or decrease the pectin stability. The amount of pectin required for good gel formation is between 0.7-1.8%. Commercial jelly is usually stiffer containing as much as 1.25% pectin as against 0.75-1.0% in home made products.

Procedure

  (*i*) Prepare the fruit extract as learnt using 5 kg guava.

  (*ii*) Test for pectin strength, and keep aside for use.

  (*iii*) Return the fruit pulp to the pan, and prepare a second extract.

  (*iv*) Test pectin strength and set aside for use.

  (*v*) Perform experiments with the variations according to instructions in A-D below using the first extract.

A. *Effect of varying the amount of sugar*

  (*i*) Boil 100 ml of extract in a suitable pan without adding any sugar and heat to 103° C. Record the time taken and pour the same into 2 petridishes and keep aside to set, one at room temperature and one in a fridge.

  (*ii*) To 100 ml extract add 60 g sugar and boil the mixture without stirring to 103°C, keeping the mixture at bubbling boil. Proceed as in (*i*)

  (*iii*) Proceed as in (*ii*) but add 120 g sugar in 100 ml extract.

  (*iv*) Proceed as in (*ii*) but add 180 g sugar in 100 ml extract.

B. *Effect of varying the cooking time*

  (*i*) To one cup extract add 3/4 cup sugar and heat rapidly for 15 minutes. Pour the hot mixture into a petri-dish and keep aside.

  (*ii*) Repeat (*i*) but heat for 25 minutes.

  (*iii*) Repeat (*ii*) but heat for 30 minutes.

  (*iv*) Pour out each sample as in A (*i*) and keep to set.

C. *Effect of varying the temperature of cooking*

(*i*) Take quantities as in B and heat to 107°C

(*ii*) Repeat as in (*i*) and heat to 105°C

(*iii*) Repeat as in (*i*) and heat to 103°C

(*iv*) Pour out each each sample as in A (*i*) and keep to set.

D. *Effect of varying the pectin content*

(*i*) Take amounts as in (B) using the first fruit extract and heat to 103°C

(*ii*) Repeat using the second extract

(*iii*) Pour and allow to set as in A (*i*).

(*iv*) Compare results of (*i*) and (*ii*) as learnt.

Label all the samples of jelly poured out in duplicate in different petridishes. Let one sample set at room temperature and one in the fridge for one hour. Then compare the results of the various samples.

Observations

Record your observations with respect to appearance, colour, clarity, gloss, set, cut, spreadability taste texture and grade of jelly formed as learnt. Draw inferences with respect to the best method for making guava jelly.

Precautions

As for experiment 10 and 11.

Practice Exercises

1. Prepare jelly using a fruit and a vegetable. Record your observations, and compare the quality of the two samples.
2. Name the fruits and vegetables that are rich in pectin and will form good jellies.

EXPERIMENT 13

Aim
To prepare toffee from fruit pulp or puree.

Equipment
Cooking pan, burner, ladle, chopping board.

Materials
Fruit pulp, milk sugar, glucose, hydrogenated fat.

Principle
When sugar is heated with fruit puree it first turns brown or the original colour of the fruit may in some cases get enhanced. With the addition of interfering substances like milk or glucose and fat, the sugar does not recrystallize and results in a pliable mass which can be shaped or moulded as desired. Due to the effect of heat on melted sugar the toffee acquires a little plasticity, and a rich brown colour. Commercially prepared candy or *mithai* usually have flavour and colour added to resemble that of the original fruit.

Procedure
The fruit pulp left over from experiment 9 may be used for this experiment and different fruit toffees prepared as follows:

A. *Guava toffee*
   (*i*) Mix together 1 kg fruit pulp, 600g sugar, 100g fat, 100g glucose and cook till it reaches the soft ball stage. Test periodically.
  (*ii*) Prepare a thick paste using 150g milk powder and water, and mix with the other ingredients in the pan.
 (*iii*) Cook till thick and mixture comes around the ladle.
 (*iv*) Transfer to lightly greased chopping board roll out into a rectangle or square and let it cool.
   (*v*) Cut into squares and wrap each in grease proof paper.
  (*vi*) Divide into 3 parts, opening 1 part immediately for evaluation, one after 24 hours and the 3rd after 48 hours.

B. *Apple toffee*
Repeat procedure as in A (*i-vi*).

C. *Tomato toffee*
Repeat as in A (*i-vi*).

D. *Pumpkin toffee*
Repeat as in A (*i-vi*).
Label all samples clearly for evaluation.

Observations

Evaluate the samples from A-D for colour, texture, taste, plasticity and sheen, Tabulate your observations and comment on the quality of the toffee after 24 and 48 hours.

Precautions

1. Strain the fruit solids to get a smooth pulp.
2. The fruit mixture should be cooked on medium heat to prevent spurting of the hot mixture.
3. The toffee mixture should be molded when hot, and marked into sqares when cooled at room temperature.
4. Toffee should be stored at room temperature.

Practice Exercises

1. Prepare a banana and ginger toffee and compare the results. Comment on the quantities of the ingredients required and the sensory qualities of the products.
2. Make a carrot preserve using any basic recipe. Show how its shelf life can be prolonged over 6 months.
3. Prepare guava cheese using 200g guava pulp, 200g sugar, 15g butter, 1/4 teaspoon citric acid, 30g skimmed milk powder and a pinch of salt. Use the method for toffee learnt. Comment on the differences between a toffee and fruit cheese.

4

Celluloses

Cellulose along with pectins and gums, forms the structure of plant foods, and is the material that makes up the fibrous part of fruits and vegetables, the husks and bran of cereals which are to a large extent indigestible. The amount of cellulose in each plant varies with different foods according to their variety, age and growing conditions. For examples, spinach has less cellulose than carrots, young vegetables in season less than the older end-of-season crops. Similarly, those grown under good soil and climatic conditions are tender, juicier and have less cellulose than varieties grown under drought conditions.

Structure

Cellulose is a β-D-glucose polymer responsible for the toughness or pliability of cell walls. It is deposited as fibres connecting cell walls, and within intersticial spaces-as a noncrystalline matrix composed of hemicelluloses and pectic substances. The thicker skin of fruits and vegetables and examples of protective tissue which contains a higher proportion of celluloses and hemicelluloses than the fruit itself. The fruits and vegetables contain celluloses only as supporting substance in vascular tissue for the easy flow of food and water through the plant.

Hemicelluloses

Some are polymers of the 5-carbon sugar xylose together with the some glucuronic acid derived from glucose and known as "xylans". Others are polymers of pentose, arabinose and galacturonic acid derived from galactose (arabans). Hemicellulose is less polymerized than cellulose and breaks down in the presence of alkali. Figure 4.1 indicates the structural dimensions of various plant foods.

Lignin

In addition to celluloses, molecules of substances known as *lignin* are present to give support to plants. Lignin is an aromatic substance derived from benzene, and is responsible for the woodiness of plants. It is deposited between the crystals of cellulose in the secondary cell wall after the plants stop growing. Lignin is indigestible material as it cannot be hydrolysed by acids, alkal is or digestive enzymes and therefore only adds bulk or roughage to the diet.

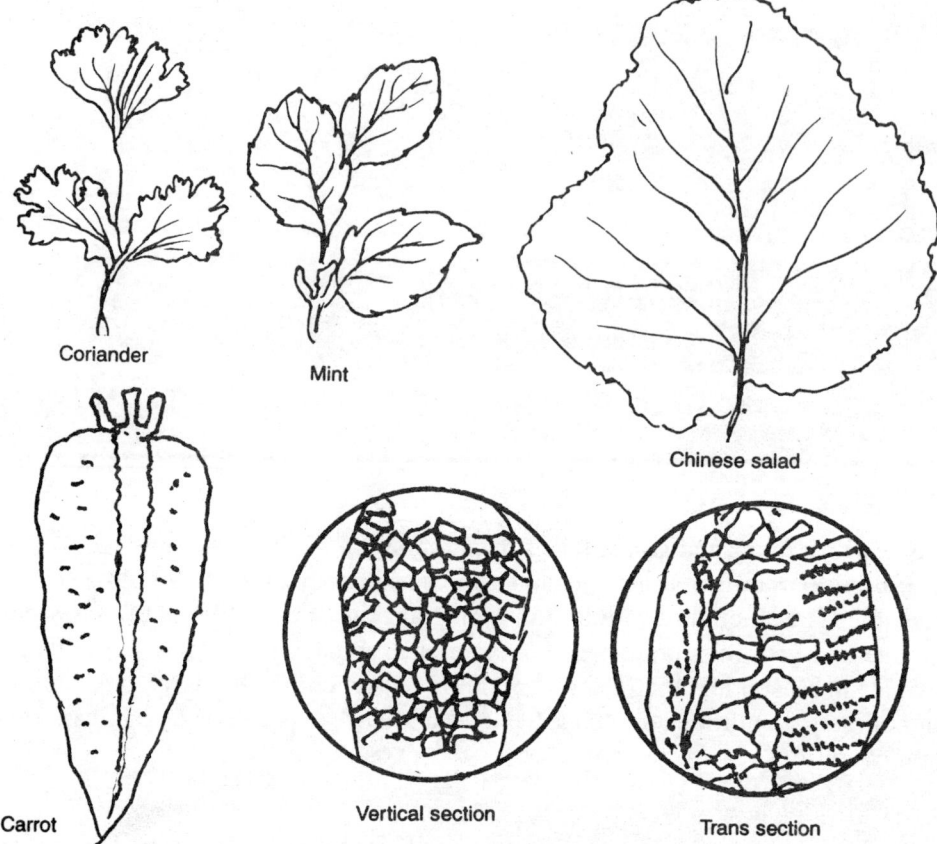

Fig. 4.1. Cellulosic structure of plant foods.

Edible parts of plant food do not contain heavily lignified tissue, and it can only be found as deposits in pears and other gritty fruits. The cell vacuoles contain water with dissolved sugars, acids, salts and other low molecular weight constituents.

The structures show the arrangements of the cellulosic fibres in different foods indicating the extent and areas of protection and support offered in each case.

Modification of Cellulose

Chemically, cellulose has been modified to produce sodium carboxy-methyl-cellulose (CMC) which is used extensively in the food industry.

Properties of Celluloses

Celluloses exhibit characteristic properties of imparting rigidity to plants, but get affected easily when subjected to heat, acids, alkalis and enzymes.

Firmness

Addition of sugar or calcium chloride strengthens the cellulose, making the food more firm. On the other hand treatment with alkali softens it, as seen when vegetables are cooked in hard water which is alkaline in reaction. Acids also contribute to firming of cellulose in plant foods.

Digestibility

Those fibres which breakdown easily on hydrolysis to simple, carbohydrates get easily digested as

Against woody parts of plants, because they become more soluble and enzymes can act on them.

Effect of heat

The properties of celluloses can be effectively utilized to provide a wide variety in vegetarian cooking. Heat softens the cellulose making foods easily digestible. Plant foods are best cooked using moist heat methods, as they get easily charred when subjected to dry heat.

High moisture foods like green leafy vegetables shrink when heat is applied because the cellulose and other cementing materials breakdown to release the bound water and the structure collapses. Heat however, also releases the pigments, electrolytes and flavour compounds affecting the colour, taste and flavour of the foods. At the same time any starch present gets gelatinized to give body to the vegetable, while a part of it may get hydrolyzed to simpler more soluble saccharides imparting a sweet taste.

Effect of pH

Tough vegetables can be cooked in slightly alkaline water to tenderize them quickly, reducing the cooking time. On the other hand very tender vegetables can be subjected to an acid cooking medium to enable the shape and form of the vegetables to be retained.

Any discussion of celluloses focuses on the properties of edible plant foods which are dealt with under fruits and vegetables.

Fruits and Vegetables

Fruits and vegetables are recognised for their aesthetic and nutritive contributions to the diet in addition to the variety of aromas and tastes they provide throughout the globe.

India has a long history of eating fruits raw rather than cooked, except when they are preserved in the form of jams and jellies, candied fruit or *murraba,* or dehydrated. In contrast the vegetables provide a large variety in colour form when added to cooked, largely cereal based vegetarian diets. It is only a very recent trend that frozen fruits and vegetables are now becoming available to the consumer, but the demand and the supply is still limited to very few items.

Structure

All plant foods consist of a cell wall mainly composed of cellulose deposited as fibres interspersed with a noncrystalline matrix of hemicelluloses and pectins that support the contents of the plant cells and give rigidity or turgor to vegetables and fruits. There is a parenchymatous secondary wall which is thinner than the outer cellulosic wall, and are porous and permeable to water. The walls of some of the plant cells contain a group of substances called *lignin* which gives the woody character and aroma to the plant. Edible parts of fruits and vegetables do not usually contain *lignin* and therefore can easily 'be softened by cooking and subsequently digested by the body. The grittiness in some fruits such as pears is due to lignin deposits present in appreciable amounts. Pectic substances serve as cementing material between cells. (see pectins p. 44).

Composition

Water

Fruits and vegetables contain 70–90% water which is the vehicle for carrying soluble sugars, salts, organic acids, pigments and vitamins. The water also acts as the continuous phase for dispersion of insoluble substances that may be present in the fruits.

Carbohydrates

Besides water, carbohydrates are present in appreciable quantities in soluble and insoluble forms, as sugars, starches, pectins, hemicelluloses and celluloses, As the fruits ripen the starch gets hydrolysed to sugars and therefore tastes sweeter than unripe fruits. This is specially noticeable in bananas, guavas, apples etc. Which contain higher quantities of starch by weight of fruits, as compared to juicy citrus varieties.

Carbohydrates in the form of celluloses, pectins and the like, contribute to the texture of fruits and vegetables, besides providing the fibre necessary for good health. The textural changes are due to the enzymes present in plant foods. (see pectic enzymes. p. 44).

Proteins

Fruits and vegetables contain very small amounts of proteins, providing only about 1g or less in every serving. However, textured proteins are manufactured from plant sources such as oil seed residues, wheat, soya bean and so on.

Textured vegetable protein

Soyabean protein is widely used in the manufacture of products, being converted into fibrous forms with a biological value of 70%, which is equivalent to that of red meat. Textured proteins are manufactured by being spun or extruded and therefore a number of different textures can be made available for the supplementation of vegetarian diets. Some inedible materials are also used as source material for processing textured vegetable proteins such as grass, molds, leaves and weeds.

Single cell proteins

These are manufactured by feeding *Fusarium,* a yeast mould, on hydrocarbon oil waste or carbohydrate waste material. The mould growth is then harvested and processed to produced a fibrous product containing 45% protein.

Leaf proteins

Leaf proteins are manufactured after extraction from grass, water weeds and leaves of trees, and provide 3-5% protein, a useful source of textured vegetable protein.

Fat

Fruits and vegetables are low in fat with few exceptions such as avocados and olives, which are not commonly consumed in India.

Minerals and vitamins

Fruits are not good sources of calcium, phosphorus and iron, although the dark green leafy vegetables do contribute these minerals to the diet.

Citrus fruits, berries, guava and most salad vegetables are good sources of Ascorbic acid (vitamin C), though they are low in B-vitamins. Yellow fruits and vegetables however contain appreciable amounts of carotenes, the precursors of vitamin A. For example, peaches apricots, mangoes, pumpkin and carrots.

Organic acids

In addition to the above nutrients, fruits and vegetables contain a number of organic acids as such or in combination. Some examples in fruits are citric acid in citrus fruits and tomatoes, malic acid in apples and peaches, malic and tartaric in grapes, malic and oxalic in rhubarb, citric and malic in pineapple and citric and benzoic acids in certain berries. In vegetables at least 10 organic acids have been clearly identified. These are formic, succinic, citric, malic, aconitic, benzoic, tartaric, fumaric and oxalic.

The pH of fruits varies widely from 2.0-2.2 in lemons to 2.7 in berries, and 3.0-3.4 in plums, apples, grapefruit etc. In other fruits like pears, oranges the pH may lie between 3.5-3.9. The average for bananas is 4.6 depending on the variety. Figs and watermelons may record up to 6.0.

The pH of vegetables however is much higher, ranging between 5.0-5.6. the highest concentration of acid in vegetables like tomatoes may vary between 4.0-4.6. Vegetables like potatoes, peas and corn however, have pH of over 6.0.

Pigments

Fruits and vegetables are an attraction mainly because of the different colours they provide in the diet. These are due to different kinds and amounts of pigments present in them, which give characteristic colours, shades and hues to each fruit and vegetable. Basically there are three types of pigments present of pigments in plant foods namely chlorophyll, carotenoids, and flavonoid pigments.

Chlorophyll

This is the pigment responsible for the green colour in plant foods, and is found dissolved in fat within the plastids of cells, where the chlorophylls are bound to protein molecules in the form of organised complexes. Chlorophylls also play an important role in the production of carbohydrates from carbon dioxide and water through the process of photosynthesis. Chlorophyll may be present together with other pigments in the same plant and therefore when green fruits and vegetables mature the chlorophyll gets masked by other pigments to give the product its characteristic colour and hue.

Chlorophylls are present mostly in unripe or immature fruits and vegetables. On ripening, processing or cooking the protein gets denatured and the pigment becomes highly unstable changing to olive green or even brown. For this reason the colour of a fruit or vegetable has come to be associated with its stage of ripeness. A green tomato will never be associated with ripeness. Similarly a green guava is associated with crisp texture and not an overly sweet taste, and when a pale yellow fruit is selected it is expected to be sweet, soft in texture and possesses other sensory qualities associated with a ripe fruit.

Chlorophyll is insoluble in water at room temperature but undergoes changes when subjected to heat. acids, alkali or other added substances. The changes that occur are indicated in

Plate VII A and B, and form the basis on which cooking conditions are controlled in order to achieve the desired characteristics in the cooked product.

Carotenoids

Carotenoids are found along with chlorophyll in the plastids of plant cells and impart the yellow to orange colour present in food such as peaches, apricots, muskmelons, pumpkin and so on. The changes in the colours of yellow orange fruits are not so pronounced as in the case of chlorophyll.

Carotenoid pigments are of two types, the carotenes and the xanthophylls. Carotenes are hydrocarbons which contain 40 carbon atoms per molecule, whereas the xanthophylls contain one or more oxygen atoms in addition. Carotenes appear in alpha and beta forms and as *licopene,* the pigment in tomato. The xanthophylls most commonly distributed are *lutein* in green leaves, *cryptoxanthin* in yellow corn, *zeaxanthin* being more widely distributed. *Cryptoxanthin* yields vitamin A; while *lutein* and *zeaxanthin* have no vitamin A value.

Flavonoids

These pigments are water soluble and found in the cell sap of plants. They can be grouped into three distinct categories:

(*i*) *Anthocyanins:* They impart the blue to purple colour to fruits and vegetables as in brinjals, bluish red cabbage, plums and grapes. The colours of foods may vary from red, purple to blue depending on the position of the carbon to which they are attached in the structure. If there is an increase in the number of hydroxyl groups the colour shifts from red to blue, indicating the changes that may take place with a change in the pH of the cooking medium of a fruit or vegetable containing fiavonoid pigments.

(*ii*) *Anthoxanthins:* These are responsible for the creamy yellow colour of cauliflower, white onions, turnips etc. Anthoxanthins are more widely distributed than anthocyanins, and include (flavones, flavanols and flavanones, indicating slight differences in structural arrangements of the molecules. Most anthoxanthins occur as glycosides such as *naringin* which is the bitter substance in grapefruit peel. The flavonol *Quercetin* is also commonly present.

(*iii*) *Tannins:* This group constitutes a number of related colourless phenolic compounds which play an important role in colour and flavour of fruits and vegetables. They react with metallic ions to produce colours ranging from red to black, the shades depending on the tannin present and other added substances.

Some tannins are water soluble and therefore responsible for the colour changes that take place in fruit juices and in tea and coffee decoctions, Tannins also provide astringency and body to the beverages and therefore when tea or coffee are overbrewed they cause a puckery sensation in the mouth enjoyed by same people in the case of wines and beer.

Both anthocyanins and anthoxanthins occur in the same plants, causing colour differences which are seen in fruits and vegetables, depending on the dominance of a particular pigment. In the presence of anthoxanthins the blue colour becomes more intensified and vice versa. This phenomenon is referred to as co-pigmentation.

Effect of Heat on Pigments

On cooking of vegetables noticeable changes take place in the pigments, affecting their sensory qualities. These changes are quite pronounced in the case of chlorophyll containing vegetables.

(*i*) When a green vegetable is cooked at first the green colour becomes brighter. This is attributed to the expulsion of intercellular air from the plant tissue making it more translucent.

(*ii*) As cooking continues the organic acids are released into the cooking water and the intense green colour gets masked by the carotenoid pigments present in green plant tissue resulting in a muddy olive green colour.

(*iii*) There is a consequent change in the structure of the pigment, the magnesium being easily displaced when heated in the presence of organic acids. Hydrogen replaces the magnesium in the chlorophyll molecule resulting in the formation of a compound known as *pheophytin* 'a' which is a green-grey compound, or *pheophytin* `h' which gives an olive green colour to the vegetables.

The effect of heat on the other pigments is negligible.

Effect of Acid and Alkali on Pigments

Chlorophyll: Vegetables which contain low amounts of organic acids such as spinach and peas, retain their green colour to a greater extent than low pH vegetables like green beans. It is therefore important to use cooking methods that will minimize the effect of acids present. The effect of acid on chlorophyll during cooking make vegetables aesthetically unacceptable if heated for long periods by methods that involve condensation. If the green vegetable is cooked in water containing alkali like sodium bicarbonate, it displaces the phytyl and methly groups of the chlorophyll to form *chlorophyllin,* which imparts a bright green intense colour. In addition the texture becomes soft and mushy due to breakdown of hemicelluloses in cell walls. Fortunately fruits are usually eaten uncooked in India and therefore their bright pigments are an asset to meals.

Carotenoids: When unsaturated carotenoids are heated in the presence of acid they isomerize changing the linear configuration of the molecule, and the colour of foods from the bright orange-red to paler yellow-orange. The higher the temperature and time of cooking the greater is the loss of intensity of the colour.

Anthocyanins: The anthocyanins are responsible for the blue to purple colour in fruits and vegetables such as plums, grapes, *jamun*, red cabbage, beetroot and brinjals. The pigments are soluble in water and therefore easily extracted for colouring foods naturally, during cooking and processing.

These pigments as in red cabbage and beetroot show dramatic changes when cooked with acid, alkali or metallic salts. On heating the bright red colour formed is due to the formation of flanyllium cations. While on cooking with alkali these turn blue due to quinone cations. Both reactions are reversible as the pigments are highly sensitive to pH changes. The presence of alkali has the same effect on other pigments as with chlorophyll. It intensifies the colours and destroys texture of all plant foods.

Anthoxanthins: These are responsible for imparting the creamy yellow colour to veg⋯ les like cauliflower, mushrooms, white onions, radish and the like. On cooking the vegetables become whiter in acid medium and creamier at alkaline pH, as when soda is added during cooking.

Both anthocyanins and xanthins may occur in the same plants and are responsible for the colour changes that take place in fruit juices if anthoxanthins are present. The blue colour of fruit gets intensified or reduced depending on the dominance of a particular pigment in the foods.

Tannins: The term is used for a number of colourless phenolic compounds which play an important role in colour of foods. They basically impart brown colours. Tannins are water soluble and responsible for the brown colour of tea and coffee.

Together anthocyanins, xanthins and tannins form the group of pigmenting compounds called *flavanoids* which also impart astringency and body to beverages including wines and beer.

Browning in Fruits and Vegetables

Browning in foods during cooking or processing is a common phenomenon, and may result from enzymatic or non-enzymatic reactions that take place given conducive conditions of temperature, oxygen humidity and the presence of other substances.

Enzymatic browning

This is commonly observed when vegetables and fruits containing poly-phenolic compounds are cut and exposed to air. The oxidizing enzymes present in the fruits of vegetables act on the phenols to produce quinones, which are responsible for the brown colour. Some common examples are cut and exnosed brinial, potato, banana and apple.

Non-enzymatic browning

This is the browning in foods which occurs due to a reaction between a free amino acid group from protein and a carbonyl group from the carbohydrate component of the food when it is subjected to cooking. This reaction is well documented as the *Maillard's Reaction* named after its discoverer. An example of such browning is seen in the colour of sweetened condensed milk which is rich in protein and contains sugar. In the process of such browning reactions, unsaturated polymers are formed called *melanoidins*.

Browning is also seen to occur when reaction between the carbonyl and alcohol groups takes place. This is called hydrolytic browning and is commonly noticed in fruit juices when they are kept unused for some time.

When foods are cooked at very high temperatures, they get denatured resulting in different levels of browning varying with the time and extent of exposure to the different temperatures. This is effectively used to produce foods of different textures and flavours, as seen through methods such as toasting, roasting, grilling and scorching the latter being generally unacceptable.

Based on the qualities required in a finished product degrees of browning can be controlled by mixing various foods together and then heating at required temperature and time.

Preventing Browning

There are many ways of preventing undersirable browning in foods. Enzymatic browning can be prevented by changing the optimum conditions for the activity of the various enzymes present in the food. This can be achieved through:

- Coating cut surface of fruits and vegetables with an antioxidant like ascorbic acid found naturally in lemon juice and many other citrus fruits.
- Applying meta-bi-sulphites which gradually release sulphur dioxide that acts as a reducing agent and cuts off contact of oxygen with the cut surface.
- Removing moisture from food through drying or dehydration.

- Lowering storage temperature to freezing, if texture is not of consequence when the product used after thawing.

- Dipping in water, sugar solution or brine to cut off oxygen supply by preventing direct contact with air.

- Coating with oil to avoid oxidative reactions.

Controlling browning therefore, basically involves control over temperature, pH, humidity, moisture content and oxygen supply with the object of inhibiting enzyme activity.

Experiments 14-17 are designed to understand these changes in raw vegetables and fruits as well as those occuring during cooking.

EXPERIMENT 14

Aim

To study the effect of browning in fruits and vegetables.

Equipment

Stainless steel knife, plates, bowls, iron knife.

Materials

Apple, banana, potato, brinjal, lemon salt, sugar, water, potassium meta-bi-sulphite (KMS), baking

Principle

Certain fruits and vegetable turn brown when their cut surface is exposed to air for a while. A number of oxidizing enzymes are involved in the process of oxidation and reduction in plant cells. A number of compounds like tannins, anthocyanins, catecholamines, phenols and their derivatives which are present in different concentrations and in different parts of plants have the ability to catalyze the oxidation of phenols in the presence of oxygen and thereby cause browning. This enzymetic browning is an undesirable change that occurs often and should be avoided or prevented, the methods for which have been discussed on p. 64 . The factors which are necessary for browning to take place are presence of oxygen, phenolic compounds enzymes and an optimum pH for enzyme activity.

Procedure

A. (*i*) Select just ripe apples without blemishes.
　(*ii*) Cut the fruit into slices and using the following variations, expose them to the air for about one hour each.
　(*a*) Cut few slices with a steel knife and expose to air in one plate.
　(*b*) Cut the slices with an iron knife.
　(*c*) Cut and dip in water to cover the slices completely.
　(*d*) Apply lemon juice to the cut surface.
　(*e*) Dip in salt solution.
　(*f*) Apply baking soda to cut surface.
　(*g*) Dip in sugar solution.
　(*h*) Blanche in boiling water.
　(*i*) Dip in KMS solution.
B. Repeat experiment A using banana.
C. Repeat experiment A using potato.
D. Repeat experiment A using brinjal.
　Label plates and bowls carefully so as to evaluate the samples accurately.

Observations

After one hour observe any changes in the colour of the slices give the various treatments. Record your observations and give reasons for the differences in colour and pattern of browning is observed. State how you would apply the knowledge gained to preparation of vegetables and fruit.

Precautions

1. Fruit or vegetables should be freshly peeled and or cut for the experiments.
2. All equipment and ingredients should be kept ready before starting the experiment.
3. Only stainless steel knife should be used unless otherwise stated.

Practice Exercises

1. Prepare a fruit salad using apple, banana, and apricot.
   Divide the above preparation into three separate bowls.
   In one do not add anything, in the second mix french dressing and in the third add salt, pepper and lemon juice. Evaluate the three samples in the light of experiment performed.
2. Prepare a plate of cut boiled potato and expose to air for one hour. Record your observations with respect to its sensory qualities. Explain your results.
3. Name three dishes in which cut vegetables are cooked after treating them in any one of the ways mentioned under (*a*)-(i) of the experiment for the purpose of preventing browning.

EXPERIMENT 15

Aim

To study the effect of heat on vegetables and fruits.

Equipment

Cooking pans, steel knife, weighing balance, bowls, measuring cylinders, cooking stove, thermometer.

Materials

Spinach, cauliflower, carrot, red cabbage or beetroot, apple.

Principle

When fruits and vegetables are subjected to heat as in cooking, they loose their selective permeability and osmosis is inhibited due to the denaturation of the cell membranes. Water and other solutes therefore enter and leave the cells by the process of diffusion, which is slow and uncontrolled. Also the cells of heated tissue loose their turgidity and become limp, resulting in the loss of crispness. Cooked fruit is therefore tender, translucent, sinks to the bottom of the pan as intercellular gas gets replaced by water. While the insoluble pectic substances change to water dispersible forms, the adhesion between the cells gets reduced although the lignin remains unaltered.

Procedure

A. Effect of dry heat

(*i*) Wash 100g each of spinach, cauliflower and carrot thoroughly. Peel or trim and cut appropriately into separate pans.

(*ii*) Place the pan on source of heat and cook for 3, 5, 7, 10 and 15 minutes, stirring periodically without covering the pan. Remove a sample from the pan after each time period into a bowl for evaluation.

(*iii*) Repeat A (*ii*) but keep the pan covered. Keep samples aside in separate bowls.

B. Effect of moist heat

(*i*) Repeat A(*i-iii*) but add enough water to cover the vegetables. Note the temperature of the liquid at the different time periods. Keep samples aside as instructed.

(*ii*) Drain the liquid from the pan into a measuring cylinder for each sample. Note the volume and colour.

C. (*i*) Perform experiments A and B with beetroot and apple, removing samples as learnt.

(*ii*) Cook the beetroot and apple whole without peeling, and proceed as in A(*ii*) and (*iii*). Peel cut and keep aside.

Observations

Lay out all the samples neatly labelled, and observe the differences in the cooked products. Tabulate Your results as indicated in Table 4.1.

Table 4.1 Effect of temperature on the cooking of vegetables and fruits

Fruit/Veg.	Veg (Wt.) Raw Cooked	Time Min.	Colour	Flavour	Texture	Taste	Applications
A. Spinach							
(i)							
(ii)							
B. Carrot							
(i)							
(ii)							
C. Cauliflower							
(i)							
(ii)							

Compare the results and draw your inferences with respect to the best method of cooking vegetables and fruits.

Precautions

1. The source of heat should be kept constant throughout the experiment, varying only the time of heating.
2. Temperature should be recorded accurately at each time period, ensuring that the bulb of the thermometer dips in the liquid without touching the base or side of the pan.

Practice Exercises

1. Cook the vegetables without covering for 3 minutes as learnt and then cover and cook till tender. Observe the time taken to cook each type of vegetable and fruit. Record your results and comment on the acceptability of the products.
2. Vary the amount of water and cook vegetables and fruit for a fixed time only. Record your observations, and comment on the applicability of each method in everyday cooking.

EXPERIMENT 16

Aim

To observe the effect of changes in pH during cooking of vegetables and fruits.

Equipment

As in experiment 14, plus pH paper.

Materials

Salt, vinegar, citric acid, sodium bicarbonate, milk curd, and vegetables.

Principle

The pH of the cooking medium affects the colour, taste, texture and general acceptability of the prepared dish. Raising the pH of the cooking water of vegetables retains the green colour but destroys vitamins of the B group and C. It also affects the turgidity of the vegetables and fruits. Low pH values on the other hand retain firmness in vegetables. Chosen cooking methods therefore, need to be adjusted to provide the desired characteristics in cooked or processed products.

Procedure

Choose vegetables containing different pigments such as spinach, carrots, beetroot and cauliflower. "fake 100g of each vegetable, wash, peel and cut into uniform pieces. Keep aside till required.

A. Spinach

(i) Take 25 g of prepared spinach in each of 6 pans.

(ii) Add 100 ml of one of the following ingredients to each pan, and note their pH.

    (a) Distilled water
    (b) Tap water
    (c) Tap water containing 1/2 t citric acid
    (d) Tap water containing a pinch of cooking soda
    (e) Milk
    (f) Beaten curd

(iii) Place pan with (a) on the burner, and cook the spinach till tender. Note the time taken.

(iv) Repeat the cooking with each of the pans containing (b)-(f) for the same time as recorded in (iii).

(v) Drain any liquid remaining and measure it for volume and pH, keeping the liquid and vegetable separately in bowls for evaluation.

B. Carrot

(i) Repeat as in A (i-v) replacing spinach with carrot.

C. Beetroot

(i) Repeat as in A (i-v) using beetroot.

D. Cauliflower

(i) Repeat as in A (i-v) using cauliflower.

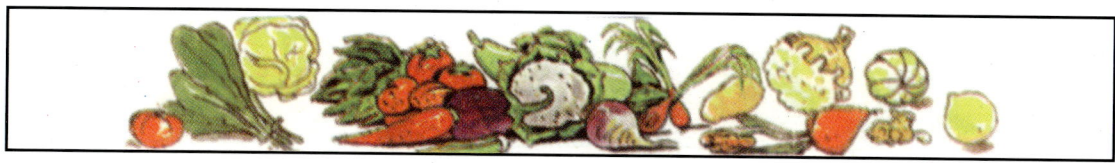

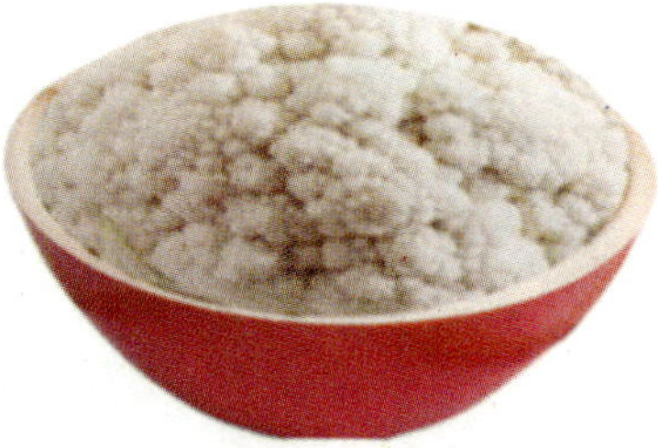

(a) Cauliflower Uncooked

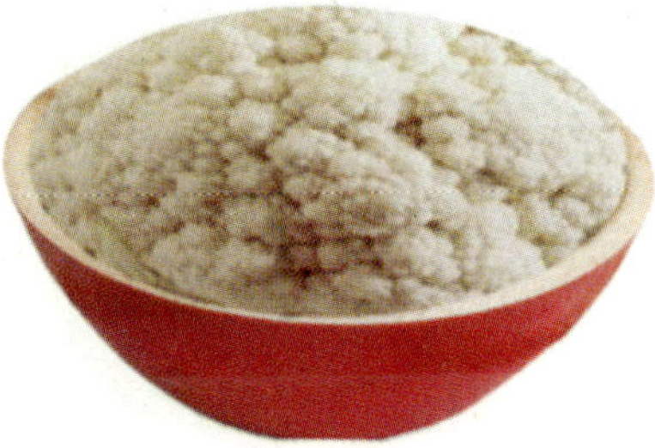

(b) In Acid pH

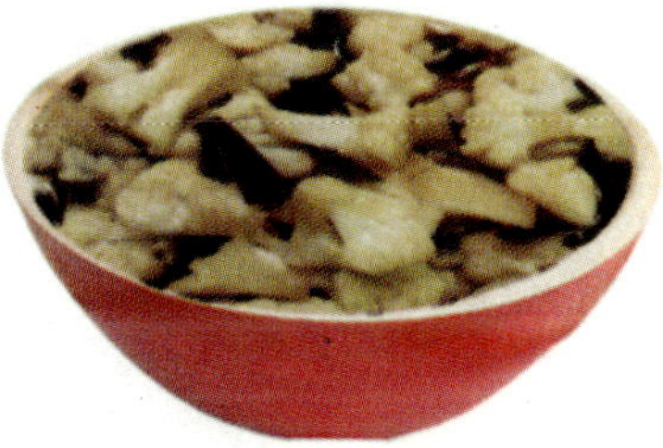

(c) In Alkaline pH

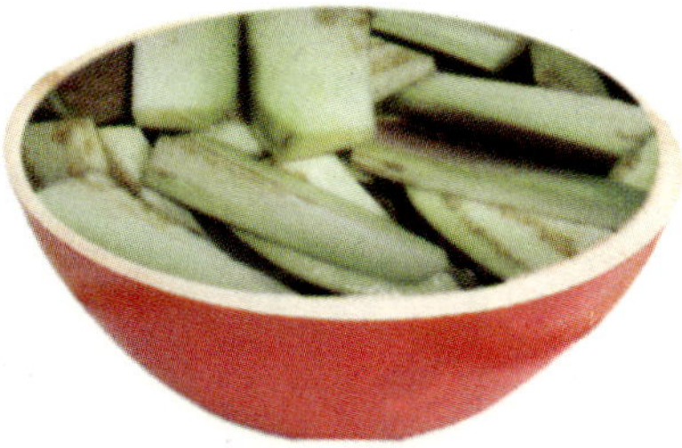

(a) Brinjal Uncooked

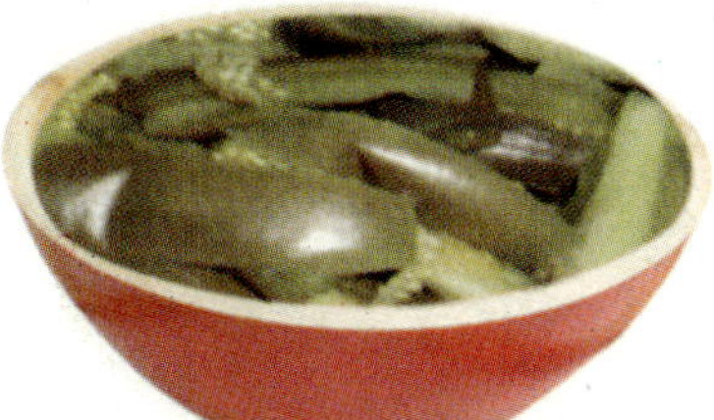

(b) In Acid pH

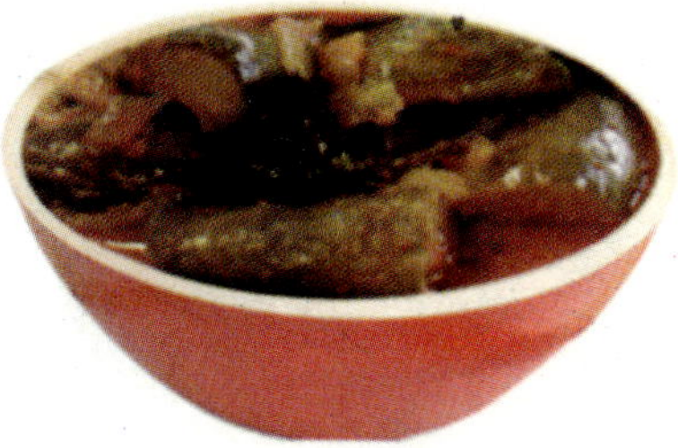

(c) In Alkaline pH

Plate VII-B: Effect of pH

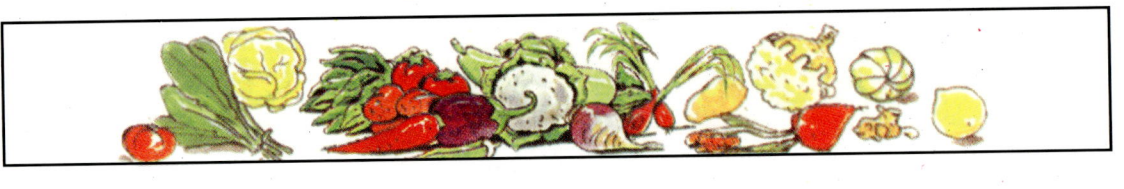

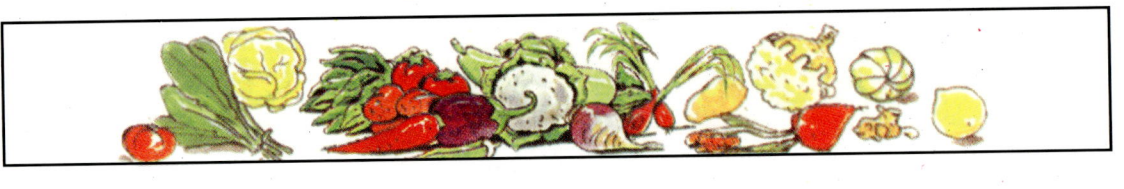

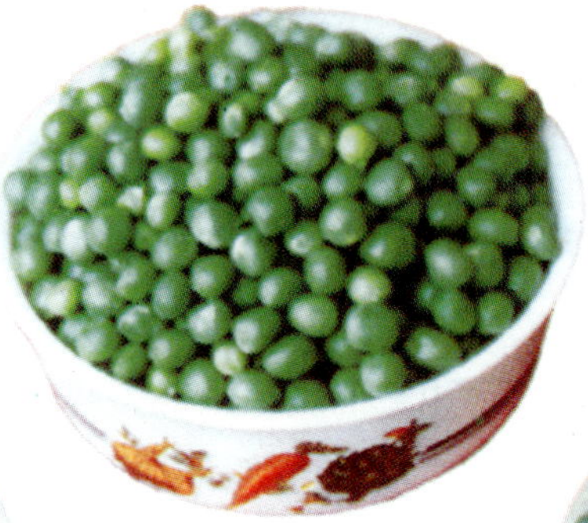

(a) Peas Uncooked

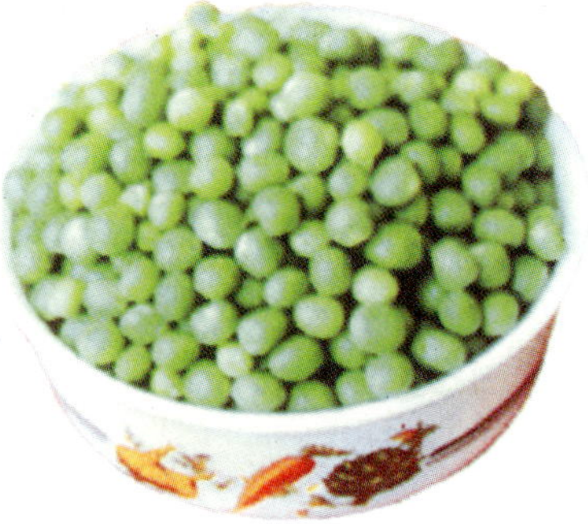

(b) In Acid pH

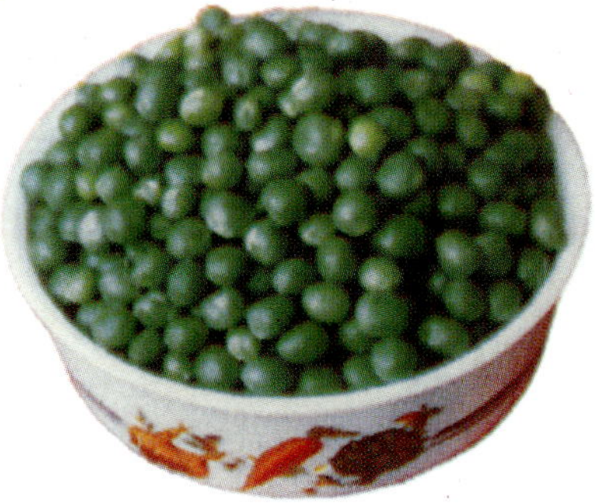

(c) In Alkaline pH

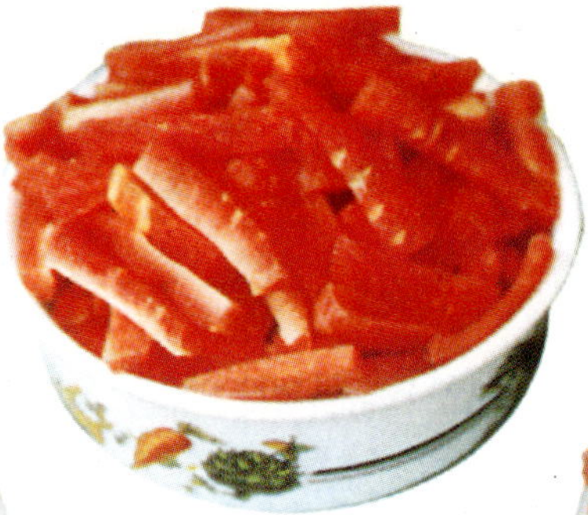

(a) Carrots Uncooked

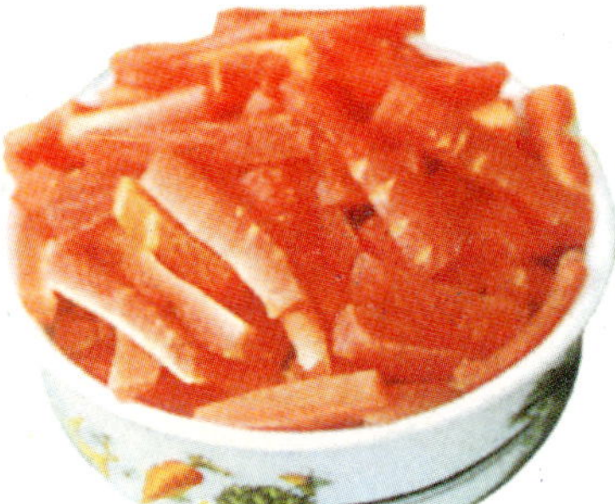

(b) In Acid pH

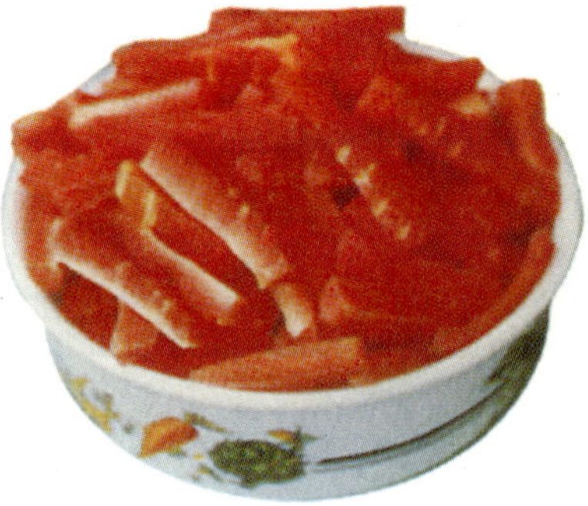

(c) In Alkaline pH

Plate VII-A: Effect of pH

Label all the samples carefully for the different variables and evaluate their sensory qualities and applicability for food preparation.

Other variations can be planned by varying the cooking method, like covering the pan fully or partially to observe the effect on the sensory qualities of the vegetable.

Observations

Record your observations with respect to pH, time of cooking, colour, texture, taste, and drainage, as per the format indicated in Table 4.2 for each vegetable studied.

Table 4.2 Effect of pH on cooking vegetables

Veg.	Liquid	Vegetable			Taste	Drainage		Time
	pH	Colour	Texture	Flavour		ml	pH	min
A. Spinach								
(a)								
(b)								
(c)								
(d)								
(e)								
(f)								
B. Carrot								
(a)								
*								
*								
(f)								
C. Beetroot								
(a)								
*								
*								
(f)								
D. Cauliflower								
(a)								
*								
*								
(f)								

Discuss the results obtained and draw inferences with respect to the best method of cooking each type of vegetable.

Precautions

1. While doing the experiments the conditions for each variable being studied should remain constant for comparable results.

2. Vegetables should be cut into uniform pieces for every experiment.
3. Weights and volumes of materials used for cooking should be the same in all experiments.
4. To evaluate the effect of the variables on the pigments a sample of the uncooked vegetable should be kept for comparison.

Practice Exercises

1. Prepare carrot kheer and comment on the colour, texture, taste and other sensory qualities when a vegetable is cooked in milk and sugar added.
2. Make a raita using carrot and differentiate its sensory qualities from that of carrot kheer prepared. Give reasons for the differences.
3. Make a list of vegetables and fruits in the cooking of which acid is used. What are the special characteristics of the preparations which were desired by adding the acid.

APPLICATIONS OF CARBOHYDRATES

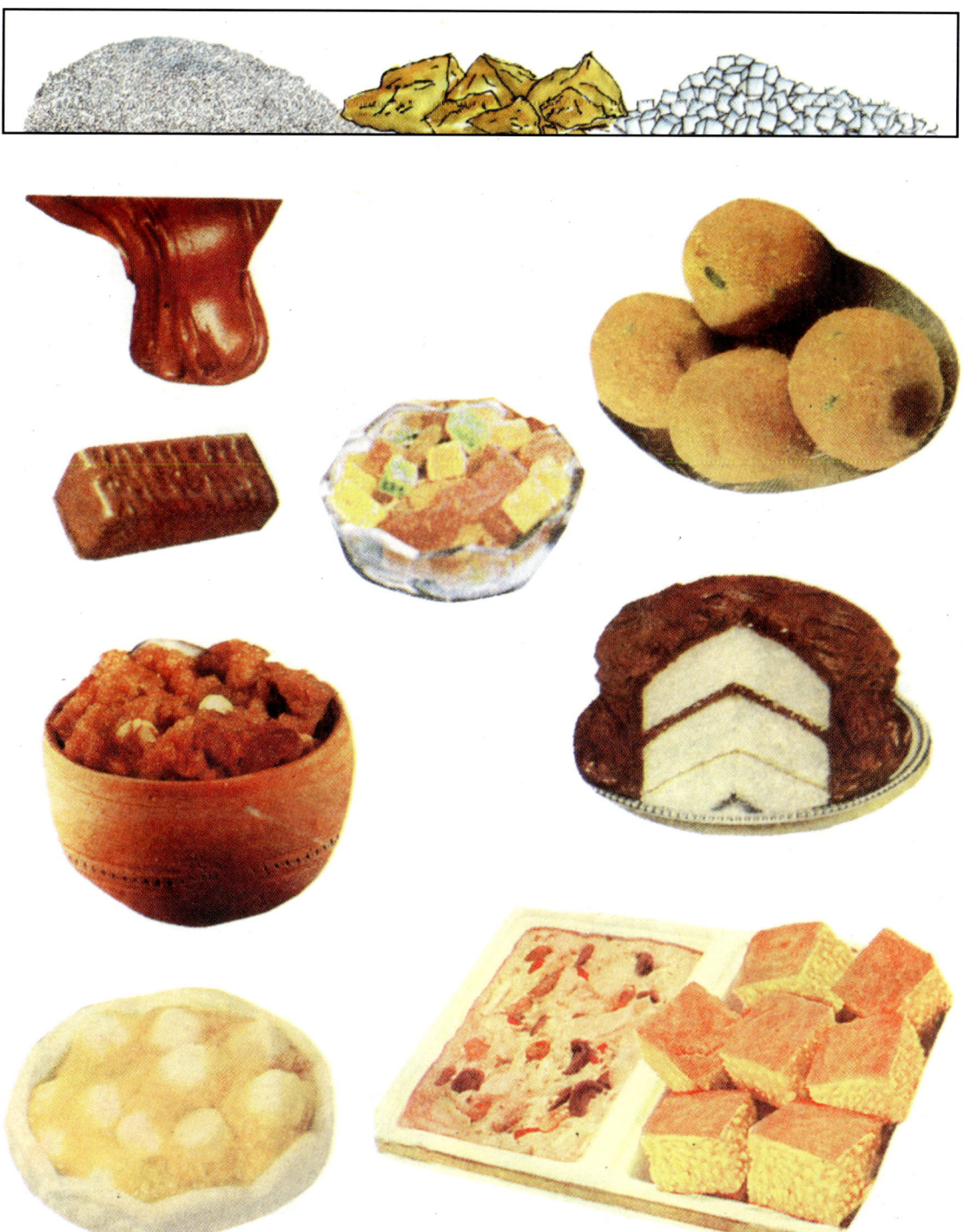

Plate VIII-A: Food products using sugars

APPLICATIONS OF CARBOHYDRATES

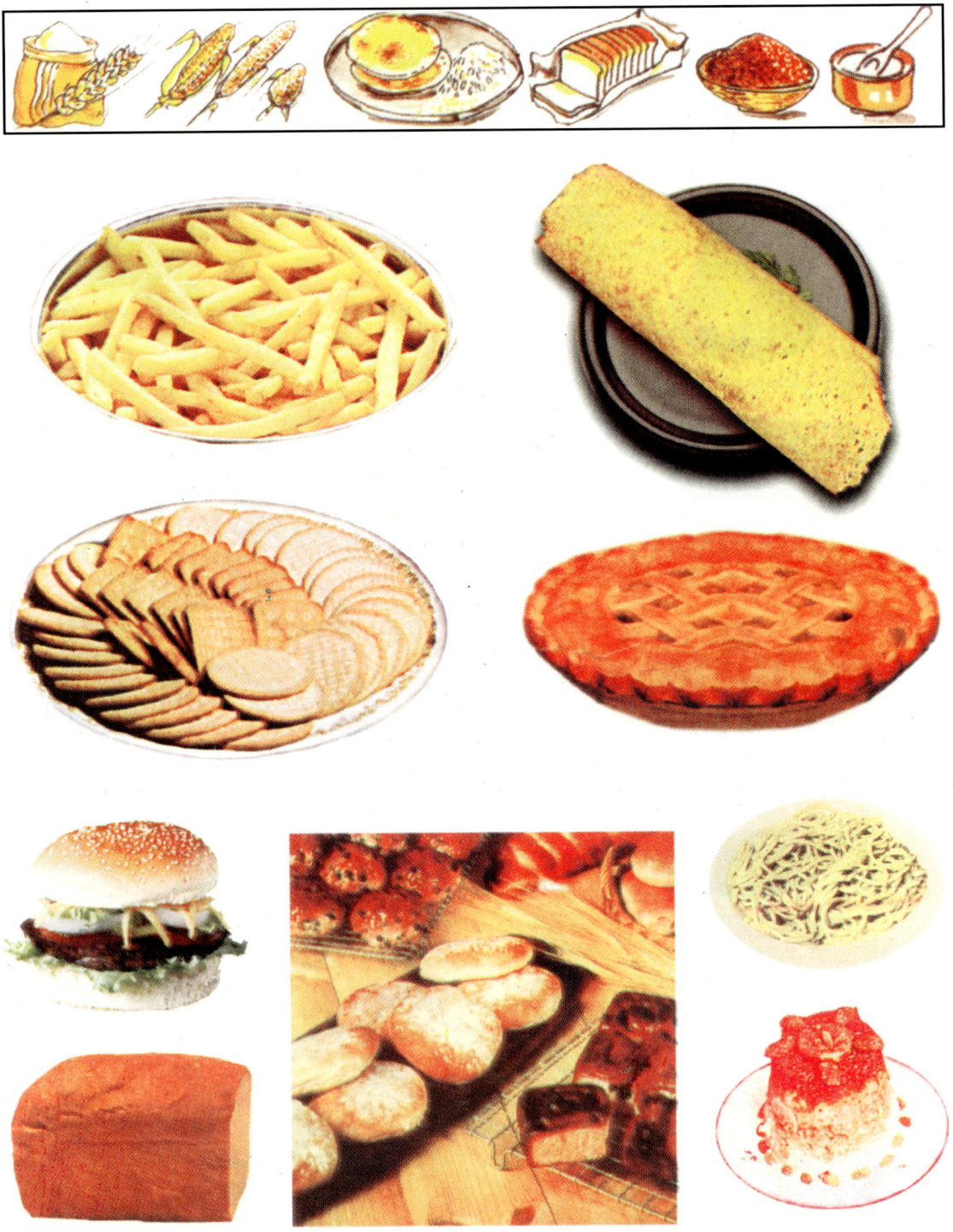

Plate VIII-B: Starchy preparations

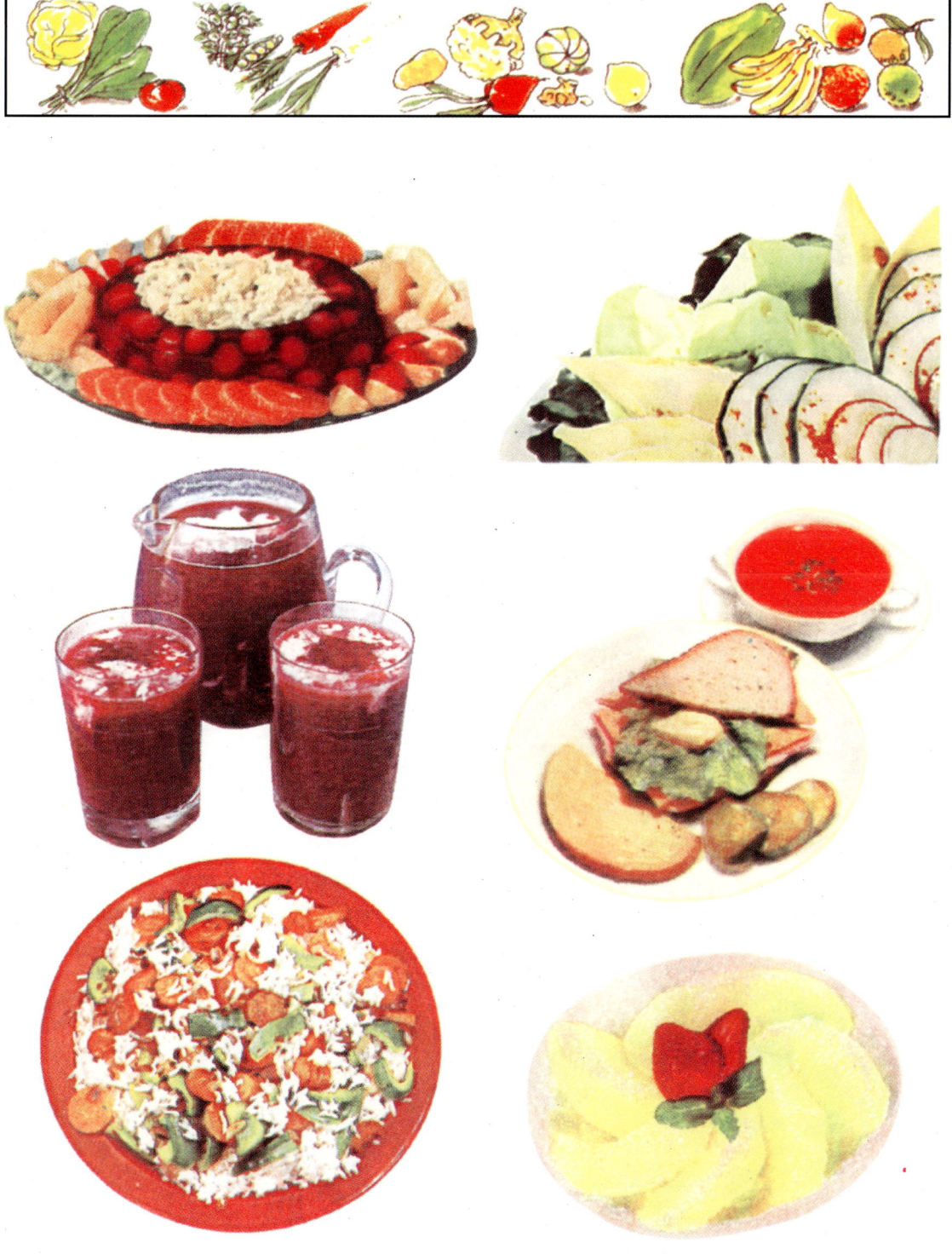

Plate VIII-C: Fruits and Vegetable Dishes

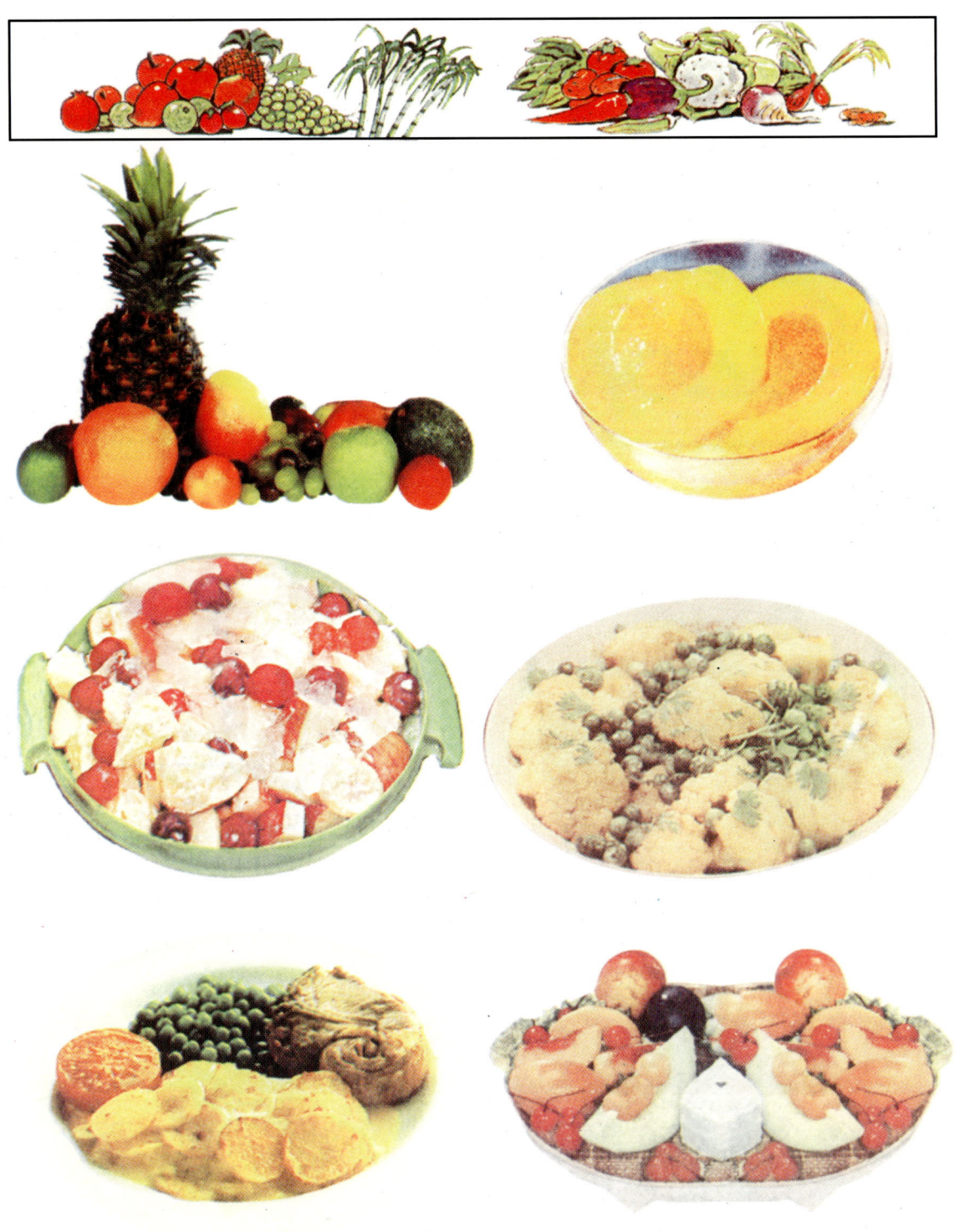

Plate VIII-D: Fruits and Vegetable preparations

EXPERIMENT 17

Aim

To determine the best method of preparing cream of tomato soup.

Equipment

Cooking pans, steel knife, thermometer, measuring cylinder, pH paper.

Materials

Tomatoes, beetroot, onion, butter, cornflour, refined flour(maida), milk, bayleaf, peppercorn, citric acid, cooking soda and salt to taste.

Principle

The sensory qualities of cream soups such as colour, flavour, viscosity, temperature and taste are of utmost importance in their acceptability. The principle involved in the preparation of a good cream of tomato soup is to balance the low pH of tomato juice with the near neutral pH of milk or cream, to give it a flavour, consistency and taste that is neither milky or sharply acidic. Since the isoelectric point of milk proteins is 4.5, that is the pH at which they remain in solution or stable dispersion, any shift from this pH will bring about their curdling making the soup unacceptable. Cooking procedures therefore need to be established that will enable foods to be mixed or gradually neutralized to prevent the denaturation or coagulation of proteins.

Procedure

The procedure involves three stages one, the preparation of tomato juice or puree from the tomatoes and two, the preparation of white sauce which enables the tomato juice to acquire a creamy consistency and milky flavour and three, mixing the two to prepare the soup.

A. (1). *Preparation of tomato juice*

  (*i*) Heat one teaspoon of butter in a pan and add 20g chopped onion, 150g sliced tomatoes, lbayleaf and a peppercorn. Stir fry for one minute.

  (*ii*) Add enough water to cover and simmer at 98°C for 30 minutes.

  (*iii*) Cool slightly and blend the contents and strain the juice or puree.

  (*iv*) Measure the volume, which should be approximately 150 ml, and the pH using a pH paper. Keep till required.

(2). *Preparation of white sauce*

  (*i*) Heat 1T butter in a saucepan and stir in lT *maida* stirring for about 1 minute till it is of grainy consistency and the butter leaves the sides of the pan.

  (*ii*) Remove from heat and gradually stir in 80ml milk at room temperature or warmed, with constant stirring to avoid lumping.

  (*iii*) Return to heat and cook to boiling with constant stirring till the sauce coats the back of the spoon.

(3). *Preparation of soup*

    (*i*) Reheat the tomato puree and using a whisk mix it into the white sauce gradually. Note the pH of the finished soup.

    (*ii*) Heat to serving temperature but do not boil. Add salt to taste and serve.

B. Repeat the above procedure varying the method of preparation of the soup to see the differences in the end product. The variations to use are:

I. Method of addition of the ingredients

    (*i*) Add hot tomato juice or puree to hot white sauce.

    (*ii*) Add cold juice to hot sauce.

    (*iii*) Add cold juice to cold sauce.

    (*iv*) Add hot juice to cold sauce.

Note: Cold refers to room temperature and not refrigerated.

    Place each of the soup samples in separate bowls in a hot water bath after mixing by the different methods to maintain the soup at serving temperature.

    Keep for evaluation and record your observations.

C. Effect of pH

Lower or raise the pH of the juice by adding a pinch of citric acid or soda and keep all other factors constant. Choose the method of addition used in Experiment A. Follow procedure B after soup samples are ready and labelled for pH.

D. Effect of adding beetroot

In the preparation of tomato juice vary the amounts of beetroot added to at least 3 samples. Follow experiment as for C. Compare with products for A, such as temperature, time of cooking, volume etc.

Observations

Tabulate your observations with respect to volume of juices and sauce obtained and their initial and final pH, temperature along with the sensory qualities of the end products. Draw inferences from the observations tabulated and identify the best method of making cream of tomato soup.

Precautions

    1. While doing the experiments the conditions for each variable being studied should remain constant for comparable results.

    2. The experimental conditions such as pH, temperature of cooking, size of pans and other factors are kept controlled using only the variations listed in B (i-iv).

    3. Use a steel knife for cutting tomatoes and onions so as not to alter the colour of the soup.

    4. Weight and volume of ingredients should be measured accurately for all experiments.

    5. Direct heat should be avoided after the soup is ready.

    6. Warming of milk while adding to flour for white sauce is only necessary if environmental temperature of lab is low.

Practice Exercises

1. Prepare cream of mushroom soup and see the effect of differences in pH on the sensory quality of the products.
2. Prepare mixed vegetable and mushroom soups and observe the differences in their sensory qualities. Try and explain why they occurred.
3. See how you can use a cream soup, if left over, to prepare another dish for lunch or dinner. Give examples.

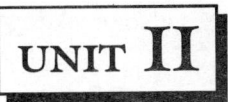

PROTEINS

Proteins are the structural components of all body cells and fluids, and form an integral part of hormones, enzymes and other vital compounds necessary for building up the structure of plant and animal foods. They are made up of amino acids which bond together as peptide linkages. Due to the bonding angles the molecules of many proteins tend to coil like a spring called the *helix*.

Proteins are nitrogenous compounds each differing in its structure and complexity depending on its source, molecular weight and structural arrangement. Proteins can be basically classified into simple, conjugated and derived all of which exhibit different properties with respect to solubility and their behaviour when subjected to heat, acid and alkali. Unlike carbohydrates some of which can be eaten in their natural forms, all protein foods need to be cooked or processed before consumption. Figure 5.0 shows the important food source of proteins along with their simple classification.

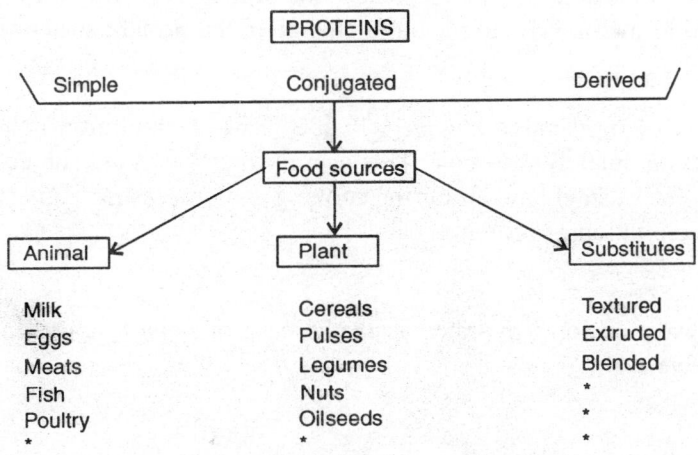

Fig. 5.0. Classification of Food Proteins.

Structure of Proteins

The main unit of linkage of the amino acids in proteins is through peptide bonds resulting from the

77

reaction of the α-carboxyl group of one amino acid with the α-amino group of another. However proteins do not all have a simple chain structure. The peptide bonds further link together through the carboxyl and amide groups of the peptide chain by means of hydrogen sulphide bonds. Many proteins thus, have a coiled, spherical or network arrangement in their structure, which keeps on changing as the bonding breaks down or continues as the case may be under different cooking or processing conditions. Proteolytic enzymes also breakdown protein structures as in the process of digestion of protein rich foods.

Simple Proteins

These yield only amino acids or their derivatives on hydrolysis, and include the proteins of eggs, peanuts, wheat, maize and fish such as salmon.

Conjugated Proteins

These include a group of proteins which are bonded with nucleic acid, carbohydrates or their derivatives, phosphorus, haem and lipids.

Derived Proteins

Those proteins which bond with the compounds remaining after acid, alkaline or enzyme hydrolysis of proteins.

Properties of Food Proteins

The properties of proteins vary for each food type depending on their structure and other molecules present. Specific proteins are discussed under the relevant chapters in this unit, dealing with foods rich in proteins, but some basic properties are common:

Denaturation

This is a process by which soluble proteins lose some of their solubility through exposure to heat, mild radiation, acid or alkali, bringing about a change in the protein structure.

Coagulation

This is a permanent or irreversible change which follows denaturation if heating is continued, making the proteins completely insoluble. This occurs when foods are subjected to high temperatures, acids, alkalis and other chemicals during cooking and processing. Agitation and freezing also bring about the precipitation of proteins.

Hydration

Proteins swell in water to form hydrates as in the case of gelatin, glutenin and gliadin. When warmed they dissolve.

Hydrolysis

This refers to breakdown of proteins into peptides and amino acids, the process being also known as proteolysis. Hydrolysis takes place due to the presence of acids, alkalis or enzymes in foods during preparation and cooking. Protein hydrolysates are present in meats and yeast extracts and therefore *marination* is often used to tenderize food made from them. The extracts also contain flavouring substances and amino acids which are products of hydrolysis.

These properties form the basis of textural effects that can be produced during cooking and processing of high protein foods.

Uses of Proteins

The main uses of proteins are their ability to provide the material necessary for body building, but, when required they can also be used as sources of energy in the body. Protein rich foods also provide satiety value to diets and nutrition as they contain other essential elements as well. The protein content of foods varies from 0.2-80 g per 100 g, but all foods do contain some protein as their building material.

Proteins undergo changes to create a variety of textures, flavours and palatability characteristics through formation of emulsions, foams and gels. Colours get enhanced through browning reactions when sugars and amino acids interact as seen in roasting. The reactions may be enzymatic or non-enzymatic in nature.

Proteins are now being used in the processing industry to manufacture edible packaging materials in the form of films and capsules for enhancing flavour of packaged foods as soon as they are opened for consumption. Encapsulation is useful not only for enhancement of aesthetic and nutrient quality but is also ecofriendly.

This Unit comprises of 5 chapters covering foods rich in their protein content such as milk and milk products, eggs, meats and meat substitutes, cereals, pulses and legumes, nuts and oilseeds. In each chapter, experiments have been designed to help to understand the effect of cooking and processing on the proteins in these foods.

5

Milk and Milk Products

Milk is the first natural food of all off-springs and therefore has an important place in the diet throughout life. It is for, this reason that food science research has focussed on it to a very great extent and today there are a number of products available in the market to add variety to our meals, as well as provide increasing convenience to the user. Being very versatile, milk is available in both fresh and processed forms, the former being sold as liquid milk drawn from the udder of the animal or after collection and pasteurization to make it safe for human consumption. Milk has been used at both household and industry levels after various treatments which decrease its perishability and that of its products, consequently increasing their shelf life.

In India, the most common milk used has been cow's milk although the milk of other mammals is also used in regions where cow's milk is not easily available. Even dairy milk which is the most popular form of milk consumed today, is comparable to the composition of cow's milk, although several types are now available which compare with buffalo and milk of other mammals. The latest trend in many developed countries today is goat's milk often recommended as a health food, which in fact is the poor man's milk in rural India where all people cannot afford to maintain cows or buffaloes.

Composition

Milk is a complex mixture of emulsified fat and a colloidal dispersion of a number of macro and micro-elements in the form of nutrients, organic and inorganic compounds, enzymes and pigments. These elements impart certain physical and chemical properties that are often utilized to produce desirable characteristics in food. A number of products may be prepared entirely from milk or the latter may be used as an ingredient in food preparation.

Macroelements

The macroelements present in milk are proteins, carbohydrates, fats and water, the latter forming the liquid base in which the other elements are dissolved or dispersed providing a transluscent liquid with characteristic refractive and flow properties.

Proteins

The main proteins present in milk are casein, lactalbumin, lactoglobulin and proteose-peptone.

Casein does not bind water readily and therefore destabilizes when acid or rennin is added to it and forms a gel. When this structure is altered in the process of cooking, the protein is said to be *denatured,* as is the case with most globular proteins. This property is used for curd or yoghurt preparation but is undesirable in cream soups. The lactoglobulin however precipitates only on heating. When milk clots the liquid which separates out is *whey* and on pressing it out, the clot sets to form cottage cheese. A large proportion of lactalbumins occur as β-lactoglobulins and are responsible for low levels of fermentation in foods. Some proteins in whey are enzymes. The milk globulins (whey proteins) promote the clustering of the creaming phenomenon, the extent depending on temperature, pH and fat present (see fats).

Carbohydrates

This is present in the form of lactose that is soluble in water and responsible for the mild sweetness of natural milk. The lactose content of human milk is higher than in cow's milk and therefore sugar has to be added to the latter to increase its calorie value. To most processed milks lactose is added through a mixture of cane sugar and starch as it is better tolerated than sucrose (sugar) alone.

In some people especially children the conversion of lactose to galactose cannot take place normally due to an inborn error of metabolism, and an intermediate product, galactone phosphate accumulates. This interferes with a number of processes essential for the normal function of the brain, liver and eyes. To avoid permanent damage milk substitutes are advised for people suffering from *lactose intolerance.*

Fats

These are present as fine globules dispersed in water along with small amounts of phospholipids like lecithin, sterols, fat soluble vitamins, carotenes and xanthophyll. Fat droplets are prevented from coalescing by a thin coating of phospholipids and lecithin which act as emulsifiers, keeping them dispersed. The lipid content consists of about 60% saturated fat and 7% Poly-Unsaturated Fatty Acids (PUFA) with small amounts of cholesterol. The unsaturated fatty acids are prone to air oxidation and easily lead to off-flavours in milk and its products. The fat content of raw milk is greater than that of boiled milk because most of the fat gets deposited in the scum which is usually removed, unless the procedure adopted for boiling prevents this change.

Organic Compounds

Some minor organic compounds like citric acid and nitrogenous substances are also present in milk.

Water

The amount of water in milk varies depending on the breed of the mammal, with only slight seasonal variations brought about by the feed composition. The approximate composition of milk is indicated in Fig. 5.1.

Microelements

The microelements present in milk are in the form of vitamins, mineral elements, pigments, enzymes, antibacterial metabolites and dissolved oxygen.

Vitamins

Milk has long been called a perfect food for health, but this is a misnomer as far as its vitamin content is concerned. Barring human milk which meets all infant requirements for 3-4 months, other forms of milk are deficient in vitamins C and D although it is rich in most B-vitamins. The content of riboflavin however, is significant but gets gradually lost on exposure to fluorescent light even at safe storage temperature of 4.4 °C, if milk is packed in transparent containers. The loss is less in paper or tinted plastics (Singh et al, 1975).

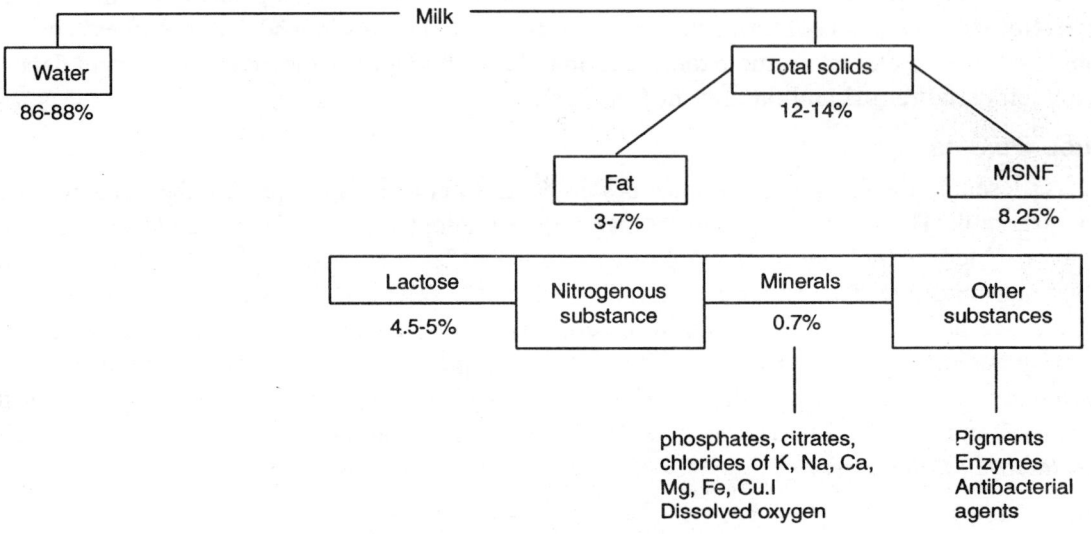

Fig. 5.1. Approximate composition of milk.

Mineral matter

This consists of sodium, potassium calcium, magnesium, chlorine and iron the latter being low in milk and hence needs to be supplemented through other foods in the diet.

Pigments

Carotene is found dissolved in fat globules of milk which gives the creamy colur to it. The intensity of the pigment varies with the feed of animals. It is this pigment which is responsible for the yellowish colour of clarified butter or *ghee*. However, the characteristic milky opaque colour of milk is due to the dispersion of proteins and calcium salts while the green-blue tinge results from the presence of riboflavin.

Enzymes

Some of the whey proteins of milk are enzymes. The enzyme phosphatase and lipase are present in milk. They get inactivated during pasteurization and hydrolytic rancidity is prevented. If freshly drawn milk is used as an ingredient for doughs, they acquire a sticky or slimy texture on storage due to the presence of enzymes.

Metabolites

Nicin present naturally in cow's milk is an active antibacterial metabolite *of Streptococcus lactis*. It is nontoxic and has much potential as a thermal aid for preservation of food (Singh et. al., 1987). It has been used successfully in the manufacture of cheese, pasteurized whole milk, flavoured milk drinks, sterilized milk, reconstituted and recombined milk products, canned milk puddings and the like (Eapen et. al., 1983).

Dissolved oxygen

This causes oxidative changes in milk products involving autoxidation of lipids, destruction of water soluble vitamins thereby affecting the bacterial quality of milk (Shekar and Bhat, 1984).

Properties of Milk Proteins

The properties exhibited by milk proteins during cooking form the basis of its versatility which gives rise to the various forms in which milk is available for consumption and incorporation into diets. The effect of changes in temperature, pH, and presence of other substances in milk or added to it during cooking and processing result in the great variety of tastes, textures, colours and flavours that milk products impart to meals.

Effect of heat milk

Ordinary heating of milk in food preparation does not bring about change. In fact, warming it up to 90°C beforehand improves its resistance to it.

Denaturation

When milk is subjected to direct heat, the denatured proteins settle at the bottom along with the precipitated calcium phosphate which results in scorching.

Coagulation

It has been reported that 12% of the albumin and globulin coagulate at 63°C, 83% at 80°C whereas heating at 100°C for 12 hours, 135°C for 1 hour or 150°C for 3 minutes can bring about total coagulation,. The clot or coagulum separates out from the liquid whey. However, on overheating the coagulation shrinks and becomes dry and leathery. Although, even mild heat inactivates the enzymes phosphatase and lipase and prevents hydrolytic rancidity as is evident in the process of pasteurization.

Skin formation

When milk is heated uncovered a skin forms on the surface due to evaporation of water and the concentration of surface proteins along with coalescence of mineral salts. The skin thus formed indicates partial coagulation of casein by heat. When milk is heated near boiling point the titrable acidity first decreases due to the formation of acids form milk constituents. The surface tension of milk decreases as the temperature increases, being 55-60 times greater per cm at 20°C and 42-45 times at 40°C. If the skin is removed from boiled milk 13% of the milk solids are lost which amount to losses of 3/4 of the albumin, 1/4 fat, 1/8 protein and 1/6 ash. The skin also entraps steam which if left undisturbed makes the milk boil over, while occasional stirring leads to the formation of a foam on the surface that prevents skin formation.

Scum Formation

Glasstone (1976) describes the phenomenon of scum formation on the basis of the theory of surface tension and energy release, stating that:

A molecule on the interior of a liquid is completely surrounded by other molecules and therefore on an average it is attracted equally in all directions. On a surface molecule however, the attraction is inwards because the number of molecules per unit volume is greater in the bulk of the liquid than in the vapour. Because of this inward pull, the surface tends to contract to the smallest possible area. Thus, drops of liquid seen as bubbles become spherical and start adhering to the inner surface of the skin and form a thick scum.

Colour and flavour

These are affected by long heating or high temperature treatments. The slightly cream brown colour that results from the reaction between sugar and amino groups of proteins is due to the *Maillard reaction.* Hydrogen and methyl sulphides from lactoglobulins contribute to the typical flavour of heated milk.

Milk fat when heated produces a compound called d-decalactone which lends the buttery flavour to foods cooked in it.

Effect of pH

Every protein has a pH at which it remains stable, known as the *iso-electric point.* This when disturbed by acid or akali resulting form reaction during cooking or processing results in destabilization causing the emulsion to break. Depending on the hydrogen ion concentration molecules may carry surplus negative or positive charges due to the —COO^- and NH_3^+ groups respectively. When these charges balance each other the protein is said to be at its iso-electric point. The pH of fresh milk is around 6.6, at which the proteins are cglloidally dispersed. If this pH is disturbed as when milk is kept in a warm place for a few hours, the pH gets lowered due to the accumulation of acid because of the action of *Lactobacillus casei,* which converts the lactose of milk to lactic acid. This disrupts the stability of the proteins causing denaturation followed by coagulation and precipitation of calcium. Any acid added to milk above 65°C brings about coagulation. Further reduction of pH by addition of excess acid however, breaks up the coagulum into smaller clots which do not bond together because of dehydration.

Effect of phenolic compounds

Milk tends to curdle when cooked with foods containing appreciable quantities of these compounds such as tannins. The precipitation is due to the dehydration of proteins as seen in cream of asparagus soup, or in foods baked in milk sauces containing salt.

Effect of enzymes

If milk is heated above 60°C any enzyme present gets inactivated. It is for this reason that when cultured products are to be prepared the milk is heated to 40°C or warm and then enzymes like rennin added. The casein of milk gets easily destabilized in the presence of rennin (chymosin).

The enzyme acts in two stages. At first the enzyme brings about clotting of the milk, and when the whey is removed these clots unite through hydrophobic bonding to form a 3-dimensional network which traps the remaining liquid. Unlike acid the enzyme does not remove the calcium from the micelles so the curd formed is calcium caseinate.

The effects of the various factors on milk have been used for making a variety of milks and their products traditionally, and by the foods processing industry.

Forms of Milk

Milk is available in different forms for use in food preparation and processing, each providing certain advantages in terms of shelf life and convenience to the user, while still being a source of nutrients required for all ages. The creativity with which the different forms of milk are used, depend on the users and the sensory qualities desired in the end products prepared.

Liquid milks

As the name suggests this is available in fluid form and usually called fresh milk. In effect however, it is not drawn fresh from the cow or other animals as it used to be in India many decades ago. This practice is still prevalent in some rural areas but in general the developments in the dairy industry have brought about changes in the way milk is treated and consumed as a nourishing fluid. Today, milk from different sources are now collected at centres eannaked in different states and then transported to processing plants where the wholesomeness is ascertained against certain minimum standards and the milk accepted or rejected as the case may be. If accepted it is treated through a process of heating under strictly controlled conditions to maintain the quality till it reaches the consumer. Dairy milk is available as full cream, toned and double toned depending on the fat contents of each type. Liquid milk marketed in various forms are:

Boiled

Fresh milk drawn from the animals is boiled in homes in India before consumption. This product usually results in losses of milk solids in the form of the skin and deposits which form on the top and bottom of the pan. The losses may amount to about 14% of calcium and protein, 20% fat and depending on the time for which it is boiled some labile vitamins. Traditionally however the top layer of fat is used to prepare butter or *ghee* and used in meals.

Pasteurized

This is prepared by heating milk below the boiling point using a number of methods, each employing different temperatures and holding times as indicated below.

- (*a*) Heating milk at 61-65°C for not less than 30 minutes. (Holder method)
- (*b*) Heating at 71-73°C for not less than 15 seconds. (High temperature short time or HTST method)
- (*c*) Heating at 85°C for a fraction of a second. (Flash process)

   Other modifications for time and temperature may be used for pasteurization as well.

Sterilized

This involves the destruction of all pathogenic bacteria. And requires vigorous heat treatment. Whole milk is first homogenized at 63-71°C to prevent separation of fat, then bottled, sealed and heated at 104-112°C for 20 minutes to one hour.

Ultra High Temperature (UHT)

In this milk is heated through a continuous process at 135-150°C for a few seconds before packaging for sale. In this method sterilization is total and the shelf life increases by 2-3 weeks, without adversely affecting the flavour of the milk. This is also called *Long Life* milk. *Amul Taaza* long life milk has a shelf life of 80 days at room temperature, and contains 8% fat and 8.5% SNF. It is homogenised to prevent cream formation.

Standard

This term is used for milk in which the fat content is between 2-3% but other constituents remain the same as in natural whole milk.

Toned

Toned as defined by the FAO (1959) involves the addition of reconstituted skimmed milk to locally produced milk in order to reduce its fat content to predetermined levels while maintaining or increasing the other milk solids. Double toned milk is also available and contains only 0.1-0.5% lipids.

Recombined

This is reconstituted skim milk to which butter oil or fat is suitably added to produce milk with the desired composition.

Separated

This is milk from which most of the fat has been removed, by skimming off the layer of fat. The product contains about 0.05-0.1% fat the globules therefore do not form a distinct cream line. Its other milk solids are however proportionately increased on a dry weight basis.

Homogenized

In this fat globules in whole or standard milk are mechanically broken to make them small enough to prevent the formation of the cream layer. The milk is heated to 57-60°C and forced under high pressure through tiny orifices, then pasteurized to destroy the enzyme lipase and prolong the shelf life of the product.

Acidulated

Liquid milk is also available in the form of buttermilk which is the liquid leftover after extraction of cream or butter from milk. See also under cultured products.

Flavoured

Any type of liquid milk can be flavoured with natural, processed or synthetic flavouring substances. Some types flavoured with coffee, chocolate, fruits essences are processed.

Processed forms of milk

Milk has been processed to provide a number of milk products in the form of concentrated, cultured and dried products, to be reconstituted into milk as required or mixed with other recipe ingredients to provide mixes for quick cooking, solids such as cheeses of various flavours and hues, and in condensed or evaporated forms for convenient transportation and longer shelf life.

Concentrated products

These constitute forms of milk from which water has been partially removed by various methods to make them bacteriologically safe and stable such as evaporated, condensed and others traditionally used in every country.

Evaporated

In preparation of the product, milk is heated to about 95°C for 10 minutes and then concentrated in vacuum pans 50-55°C, homogenizing the product. It is then packed and sterilized in an autoclave at 115°C for at least 15 minutes. Today. HTST methods are also used in which the milk is heated to 120°C for 3 minutes only or the UHT treatment for liquid milk is used. The ratio of milk solids is usually 2-2.5:1 in evaporated milk, colour is white to cream and has lower viscosity.

Condensed

In this product stability and safety are achieved by the bacteriostatic action of surose. The milk is heated for 15 minutes at 80°C before or after the addition of sugar and then condensed as for evaporated milk under reduced pressure. It is the then cooled to crystallize the lactose into non-gritty fine crystals and sealed in cans. The concentration of sugar varies from 40-45 percent and the milk keeps well at room temperatures without change in vitamins A or riboflavin. However there is constant loss of thiamine and vitamin C, with other nutrients deteriorating with time (storage). Condensed milk contains 31% total solids of which 9% are lipids. The product has 60% of the water removed.

Traditional products

Concentrated milk products commonly prepared in India are khoa, kheer and rabri. The concentrated top cream layer of skin from whole milk, called *malai* is also used for various purposes (see glossary).

Cultured products

These have been developed by culturing milk with *Lactobacillus casei and acidophilus, Pediococcus acidilactis,* and other strains of bacteria (Sarkar and Mishra, 1996). Various cultured milk products have been recommended for infant feeding due to their enhanced nutritional and therapeutic value. Products like *Kefir,* and *Biolakton* have already been developed for infant feeding and others prepared from whey water in liquid and powdered forms.

Buttermilk

This is liquid milk innocultated by acidifying bacteria usually of the lactobacillus strain. Other firms are soured and fermented milk preparations made from whole or skimmed milk.

Yoghurt or curd

These are processed forms which result in a set texture after being subjected to bacterial or enzymatic action for a few hours under controlled conditions of temperature and humidity. Sweet, sour and fruity preparations are now available. Deodhar, 1984 reported that yoghurt and related products are capable of restoring normal lactic intestinal flora and inhibiting proteolytic action.

Cheese

A variety of processed cheeses are now available for use in cooking or for direct consumption such as cottage cheese, cheddars, cream cheese and cheese spreads. They enhance the taste, flavour and texture of meals while also improving their protein quality.

Whey

This is the liquid which remains after separation of curd used in cheese making. Whey from acid curd contains more calcium and other minerals than that from renneted cheese manufacture. The composition of cheddar cheese whey is 93% water 0.9% protein 4.7% lactose 0.6% minerals. The vitamins present are thiamine 40 μg, riboflavin 80μg, pantothenic acid 350μg, vitamin B_6 20μg, biotin 1.51ag, vitamin B_{12}, 0.5 µg, nicotinic acid 70 µg, and vitamin C 1.5 mg per 100 ml of whey (Kon, 1959).

Whey is used in India as a beverage or ingredient in acidulated beverages like *lassi,* in curry preparation and for fermenting doughs and batters. Commercially, whey cheese is made in many countries such as *ziger* in Germany, *ricotta* and *broccia* in Italy and *skuta* in Yugoslavia.

Dried milks

These forms have very long shelf life as all the water is removed by processing methods like roller, spray and freeze drying. In freeze drying the water is removed by sublimation of the ice crystals from the deep frozen product at low temperature in high vacuum conditions. This also helps to maintain the original flavour of the milk on reconstitution.

Filled or imitated milk

These include products in which the fat of milk is replaced partially or wholly by fat or oils from plants sources. Other products are non dairy whiteners which are made with sodium caseinate or soy protein and vegetable oil.

Milk substitutes

These includes milk and beverages processed from plant sources such as groundnut, soybean, coconut or malted grains. These are available as liquid milk or dried products to be reconstituted with water. Some examples are soy, coconut and groundnut milks, horlicks and lactose free weaning formulae.

Soya milk

As early as 1909 soya milk used to be fed to babies who were intolerant to cow's milk. The formulae are based on soy-protein isolate supplemented with L-methionine, taurine and carnitine (MacDonald, 2000). The globulin fraction of soyabean is the major protein component (90%) composed mainly of the glycoprotein β-conglycin and glycine.

The physical, chemical and nutritional qualities of milk have thus been creatively used in producing variety in meal preparation and food processing. Experiments 18 to 22 have been designed to understand the use of milk and its applications in food preparation.

EXPERIMENT 18

Aim

To determine the relative density of milk at different temperatures.

Equipment

Lactometer (graduated 1.0-1.4), pyrex beakers, thermometer, gauze, burner and refrigerator.

Materials

Whole or full cream milk, homogenized, toned and double toned milk, chocolate milk, coconut milk.

Principle

Relative density is the weight of known volume of a substance divided by the weight of the same volume of water. It shows the number of times a substance is heavier or lighter than water. Relative density (R.D.) measurements help to determine the quality of food being bought. The R.D. of cow's milk is 1.03, and those of other milks can be determined as standards when measured at 20°C or at room temperature. Any adulteration with water can be detected by reading off the calibration on the stem of a lactometer, and comparing the R.D. with the standard for each milk.

Procedure

The experiment has two parts A and B.

A. (*i*) Take 200 ml of each type of milk in a beaker along with separate beakers for distilled and drinking water. Label all the beakers and keep in a row on a flat surface.

(*ii*) Allow the lactometer to float in each beaker one at a time. The depth to which it sinks is read off from the calibrated stem.

(*iii*) Note the R.D. of the water and the different milks at 20°C or room temperature, reading the lower meniscus of the water level and the upper meniscus of the milks.

B. (*i*) Place a set of samples in the refrigerator for 1 hour. Note the temperature and the R.D.s

(*ii*) Repeat the steps in A but measure the R.D.s after heating the samples to 40°C, 60°C, and 80°C. Note the effect of temperature on the R.D.s of the samples in (*i*) and (*ii*).

Observations

Record the results obtained according to the sample format in Table 5.1.

Table 5.1 Relative density of milk

Milk		RELATIVE DENSITY AT					
	Room Temp	5°C	20°C	40°C	60°C	80°C	
Whole							
Homogenized Toned							
Double toned Chocolate							
Coconut							
*							
*							

Note the effect of temperature on the R.D. of the milk samples. Represent the results graphically.

Precautions

1. Keep the lactometer suspended vertically and take the readings from the stem at eye level with the liquid.
2. The lower meniscus should be read in all transparent samples.
3. The bulb of the lactometer should not touch the bottom of the beaker.
4. R.D.s should be compared keeping the room temperature values as the standard for each sample.
5. Vegetable milks should be either commercially processed or made in the laboratory using distilled water only.

Practice Exercises

1. Describe the uses to which a lactometer can be put. Can a lactometer show the R.D. *jal jeera, nimbu pani* and juice. Comment.
2. Measure the R.D. of milk after dilution with water and compare the reading with that of the original sample. How can R.D. measurements be used to detect adulteration of milk sample.
3. Determine the R.D. of salted and sweet *lassi* prepared in the home.

EXPERIMENT 19

Aim

To study the effect of heat on milk.

Equipment

Lactometer, burner, beakers, stirrer, holder, thermometer and refrigerator.

Materials

Whole milk, homogenized milk, toned and double toned milk.

Principle

When milk is heated a number of changes take place. Most of them are exhibited by the different proteins present especially casein. These changes are skin formation, precipitation of salts at the bottom of beaker, changes in colour, flavour and viscosity.

The skin formed is thin and mobile at first then gradually becomes thick as the albumin and globulins coagulate and rise to the surface to form the scum or sink to the bottom as a precipitate. Removal of the scum may lead to losses of 10-13% of the milk solids. The casein is however, relatively stable to heat, and when it does get denatured to form visible curds the reaction is endothermic in nature accompanied by the precipitation of calcium and magnesium salts.

Increase in temperatures reduces the surface tension giving rise to a foam, which holds the steam formed and the milk tends to *boil-over.* The foam is however; less stable at lower temperatures. When milk is heated to near or above boiling point the titrable acidity first decreases because of loss of CO_2 and then increases due to formation of acid from the constituents of milk.

In fresh milk the fat in emulsified and dispersed as fine droplets, which are prevented from coalescing by a thin coating of emulsifier around them at the liquid-fat interface. When milk is cooled or heated and cooled the emulsion breaks making the fat globules rise to the surface as a creamy layer, the phenomenon being promoted chiefly by the globulins or whey proteins. The degree of changes observed however, depend on the heating time and temperature and the fat content.

Procedure

A. (*i*) Take 240 ml of each kind of milk and refrigerate for few hours. Note the cream layer on the top and compare the layers for colour and texture.

  (*ii*) Heat the samples without stirring to 60, 80 and 100°C and record the temperature of boiling-over of the samples. Note the differences in the samples and the time taken to reach boiling-over point.

 (*iii*) Cool to room temperature and record the R.D.s as learnt.

 (*iv*) Refrigerate till surface layer becomes firm. Remove the cream layers and compare their sensory characteristics.

  (*v*) Again measure the R.D.s

B. (*i*) Take another set of milk samples and heat as in A (*ii*) stirring occasionally during heating and observe the differences in the boiling-over point and the creaming properties.

(*ii*) Pour the milk out of the beakers and examine the precipitates at the bottom for colour, texture and flavour.

Observations

Record your observations as indicated in Table 5.2

Table 5.2 Effect of the heat on milk

Milk	Temp °C	Time Min	Colour	Texture	Flavour	R.D.	Precipitate		
							Colour	Texture	Flavour
Whole									
Homogenized									
Toned									
*									
*									

Draw your inferences and indicate how the changes can be prevented or used fruitfully in cooking and processing to provide variety.

Precautions

1. The volume of the samples should be measured accurately.
2. Thermometer bulb should not touch the bottom or sides of the beakers and be fixed vertically for taking temperature.
3. All beakers should be of the same size and have enough head space for milk to rise without spilling when beginning to boil-over.
4. The temperature should be taken when the milk has been taken off the burner.

Practice Exercises

1. Take whole milk and heat to reduce its volume to half. Observe the changes in sensory qualities. Note the time taken.
2. Prepare *rabri* and note the time taken to completely dry off the moisture. Comment on its colour, texture and flavour. Record the temperature at which the cooking was done.
3. Repeat 1 and 2 using other milks and describe the differences observed.

EXPERIMENT 20

Aim

Effect of heat and acid on the proteins of milk.

Equipment

Burner, 500 ml beakers, holder, thermometer, measuring jar or cup, standard spoons, strainer and muslin cloth, pH paper.

Materials

Milk, lemon juice.

Principle

The protein casein which constitutes 80% of the proteins in milk does not bind water readily. It is easily destabilized in the presence of acid and curdles to form a gel. This is undesirable in the preparation of most food products such as soups and vegetables although well used in the preparation of cottage cheese for which casein can be precipitated by acidification at 20°C and pH 4.6 which is its isoelectric point at which casein is least soluble. If the pH is lowered further, casein salts of chloride and lactate are formed, and the casein goes back into solution. Very low or high pH values, reduce the amounts of sulphides liberated from milk proteins. The greater the time and temperature of heating the greater is the release of these compounds which are responsible for the cooked flavour of milk.

When milk is heated in the presence of acid, the lactose also gets hydrolysed to lactic acid which removes the calcium of milk as salts from the casein micelles. Lactoglobulin and lactalbumin are coagulated by heat. The natural sugar lactose starts to caramelize at a very low temperature.

Procedure

A. Temperature variation

1. (*i*) Heat 200 ml of milk in a beaker to 60°C and add 2t of lemon juice.
   (*ii*) Continue heating only till the milk splits and the whey separates from the milk solids.
   (*iii*) Strain through muslin to remove the whey. Measure the volume of the whey and the weight of the coagulum.
   (*iv*) Observe both the fractions for colour, volume, weight, texture and taste.
2. Heat milk to 100°C and then add 2t of lemon juice. Repeat A (*ii-iv*).
3. Bring the milk to bubbling boil. Note the temperature and repeat A (*ii-iv*).

B. Acid or pH variation

1. (*i*) Heat 200ml of milk and repeat A (*ii-iii*) using 4 teaspoons of lemon juice, but keeping the volume of milk and the temperature at 60°C constant.
   (*ii*) Record the pH of the milk and the whey using pH paper. Evaluate for sensory characteristics.

2. Repeat the experiment with milk volume and temperature constant at 60°C using 1 t of cooking soda instead of lemon juice. Record the pH as in B (*ii*).

More experiments can be planned with variations in the type of milk, acids and temperatures used.

Observations

Record your observations in tabular format as learnt, and comment on the ideal method of preparing cottage cheese or *paneer*.

Precautions

1. Heat milk in a double boiler to prevent scorching of proteins at the bottom of the pan.
2. Measure all ingredients accurately using standard measuring equipment.
3. Do not over heat the milk after it splits.

Practice Exercises

1. Make cottage cheese using other types of milk and compare the sensory attributes with those of cheese made from cow's milk.
2. Cook green beans in milk from different sources. Note the differences in the products. Which do you like best and why?
3. What qualities does milk impart to a food product cooked in it. Discuss.

EXPERIMENT 21

Aim

Effect of added substances on the stability of milk.

Equipment

Cooking pans, stirrer, standard cup and spoons, ladle beaker, pan, holder and burner.

Materials

Milk raw and homogenized, sugar, salt, vegetables, fat and refined wheat flour.

Principle

The effects of added substances to milk during cooking depend on the nature of the substances and their constituents. When sugar is added the lactose caramelizes, the *Maillard* reaction takes place between the amino group of milk proteins and the sugar, thus imparting a creamy or brown colour to the milk depending on the temperature and time of heating. The flavour also changes due to the release of the hydrogen and methyl sulphides from the protein 13-lactoglobulin.

When salt is added as in the cooking of vegetables in milk, the latter foams and the phenolic compounds present in vegetables hasten the coagulation process. If the cooking is done quickly at high temperatures the coagulum gets dehydrated and becomes tough and rubbery appearing as fine white specs in the vegetable.

Cooking vegetables in milk softens them quickly because of the action of milk enzymes especially in low temperature slow cooking. The rate of lipase activity increases with decrease in temperature.

When refined flour and milk are combined to make white sauce as used in baked dishes, denaturation slows down or can be totally prevented, unless high acid foods such as tomatoes are used. This is because the flour binds the free liquid and prevents precipitation and separation of the milk proteins.

On addition of fat, the fat globules become so large that the surface tension is disturbed, destabilizing the natural milk emulsion.

Addition of substances to milk can easily be detected by measuring its relative density. The manner in which the substances are added and the resultant ionic charge, plays an important role in precipitation of milk proteins. The proteins are most sensitive between pH 5.2-5.4 and 6.2-6.4.

Procedure

This experiment is performed in 5 parts A, B and C, D and E each demonstrating the effects of the particular added substances on the behaviour of milk components during cooking. Variations in concentration of added substances are used to demonstrate the behaviour or milk under different cooking conditions.

A. Addition of sugar

(*i*) Take 250ml milk in a pan and heat till the volume in reduced to half stirring occasionally. Pour the contents in a 2 bowls and keep one at (R.T.) and one in the fridge (F.T.) to cool for one hour.

(*ii*) Dissolve log sugar in 250ml milk. Repeat (*i*)

(*iii*) Dissolve 25g sugar in 250ml milk and repeat (*i*).

(*iv*) Place all the samples together and evaluate for colour texture and flavour both at room temperature and after cooling in a refrigerator for 1 hour.

B. Addition of salt

(*i*) Wash and cut 100g green beans and cook in a pan on high heat at first, then add 100ml milk, cover and cook on low heat till vegetable is tender. Remove the sample and keep aside.

(*ii*) Repeat (*i*) with 1/2 teaspoon salt. Keep aside.

(*iii*) Repeat (*i*) with 1 teaspoon salt. Keep aside.

Note the time taken to tenderize the vegetable in each case and the time taken for milk to foam, form skin and finally coagulate.

C. Addition of vegetables

(*i*) Wash, peel and cut 100g carrots and cook in a pan as in B (*i*) with 100 ml water till tender. Drain any liquid and keep vegetable and liquid aside for observation.

(*ii*) Repeat with 100ml milk instead of water and cook till vegetable is tender. Proceed as in (*i*)

(*iii*) Repeat (*ii*) using 100 spinach instead of carrots.

Note the time taken to tenderize the vegetables and observe their sensory qualities. Compare the volume and pH of the liquid from each sample.

D. Addition of fruits

(*i*) Add 100ml milk to a cup of mixed fruits. Keep aside for 1/2 and hour to cool.

(*ii*) Repeat (*i*) and keep in the fridge for 1/2 an hour.

(*iii*) Add 100ml cream and repeat as in (*ii*).

Note the sensory and palatability characteristics of the samples.

E. Addition of refined flour and fat

(*i*) Take 1 teaspoon butter and 1 tablespoon flour and saute on low fire till grainy in texture. Remove from source of heat.

(*ii*) Take 100 ml milk separately and warm it.

(*iii*) Add little at time to the flour mixture to make a smooth paste.

(*iv*) Add the rest of the milk and restart heating, stirring constantly till the mixture coats the back of the ladle or spoon. The white sauce is now ready.

(*v*) Add any chopped vegetable to this sauce and cook for a few minutes till tender.

(*vi*) Pour the mixture into a baking dish and bake at 200°C till the dish is brown on the top and set.

(*vii*) Cool for 2 minutes. Scoop out a portion with a spoon and evaluate for colour, texture, taste and flavour.

Variations in white sauce preparation may be studied using cornflour or arrowroot to replace refined wheat flour in the experiment and the results compared.

Observations

Tabulate your observations as indicated in Table 5.3 and show how the difference in sensory qualities observed can be applied effectively in food preparation and processing.

Table 5.3 Effect of added substances to milk in food preparation

Added Substance	Temperature		Cooking time	Amt.		Colour		Flavour		Texture	
	Room	Frig		Wt.	Vol.	P.	L.	P.	L.	MP.	L.M.
Sugar (i)											
*											
*											
Salt (i)											
*											
*											
Vegetables											
(i)											
*											
*											
Fruits (i)											
*											
*											
Flour and Fat											
*											
*											

P. = Product ; L. = Liquid; L.M. = Liquid Milk ; M.P. = Milk Product

Comment on the role of added substances in cooking milk and its products. How can palatability be enhanced with the knowledge gained. Comment on the applications of the products in food preparation.

Precautions

1. Milk should be brought to room temperature before using for cooking.
2. When cooking with milk the pan should be kept uncovered initially to prevent boiling over.
3. Keep enough space to allow for foaming and boiling-over of contents.
4. Cook at medium heat.
5. Stir occasionally to prevent scorching of the precipitated proteins.
6. Do not cook for long time after coagulation takes place as the coagulum will become rubbery and indigestible.

Practice Exercises

1. List 5 dishes prepared commonly in the home in which milk or its products are used as the main ingredient.

2. Prepare white sauce as learnt and thicken tomato juice with it to make cream of tomato soup. Make observations about the soup and comment on the behavior of milk proteins.
3. Prepare rice *kheer* and *phirni*. Explain the differences in sensory qualities of the preparations inspite of ingredients being the same.
4. Prepare spinach in milk by baking and sauteing. Comment on the sensory qualities of the products prepared by the two methods.

EXPERIMENT 22

Aim
Effect of fermentation on milk proteins.

Equipment
Beakers, standard spoons, cooking thermometer, incubator, refrigerator, gas burner and pH paper.

Materials
Milk samples whole, homogenized, skimmed and toned milk, soya milk peanut milk and coconut milk, 50g bacterial culture of preset curd.

Principle
The normal microbial flora associated with foods can produce a wide range of breakdown products. Depending on the major food substrates attacked, these microorganisms can be designated as proteolytic, lipolytic or fermentative. In milk the sugar lactose is fermented by *Streptococcus lactis* bacteria which curdle the milk. The organism is gradually inhibited from further growth by its own acidity. *Lactobacillus* bacteria which are commonly responsible for curdling in milk are more acid tolerant than *S. lactics* bacteria. If however the fermentation process is continued for an unduly long time the acid tolerant yeasts and molds take over and the curds starts to get digested. As a result a gaseous complex is formed which gives an off-odour characteristic of putrefaction. Therefore optimum time and temperature are important for the formation of ideal curds.

Procedure

A. Effect of temperature on milk fermentation.
  (*i*) Record the room temperature
  (*ii*) Take 100 ml each of the milk samples in 250 ml beakers.
  (*iii*) Leave them at room temperature for air fermentation for 24 hours.
  (*iv*) Observe for sensory attributes.

B. Setting of curd.
  (*i*) Take 100 ml of each milk sample and heat to 60°C.
  (*ii*) Add 1t of culture and leave overnight to set at room temperature.
  (*iii*) Take 100 ml of each milk sample from the refrigerator and note the temperature.
  (*iv*) Inoculate with the culture and keep in the refrigerator overnight.
  (*v*) Repeat (*iii*)-(*iv*) but keep the samples at 37°C in an incubator overnight.

Compare the products of A and B fermentations.

Observations
Note the temperature, and pH of each sample at the end of the fermentation. Tabulate the results observed as learnt and comment on the sensory qualities as well as the nature of the curds set, indicating the best method of preparation. Write about the applications of each kind of fermented

milk with respect to food preparation and processing, stating examples of foods for which each can be used effectively.

Precautions

1. Measurement of ingredients in all the sample should be the same.
2. The beakers should be of the same size.
3. Temperature and pH of the milk should be recorded accurately before and after the fermentation.

Practice Exercises

1. Name 5 products in which fermentation of milk is done using air, bacilli or enzymes in food preparation or processing.
2. Prepare some products in which each of the methods of fermentation is used. Comment of their texture, taste, flavour and acceptability. How can new products be developed in the light of your knowledge of fermention methods.

6

Eggs

In food preparation the eggs of hen are widely used, although those of other birds too, may form part of dietaries in some countries. Eggs can be prepared in many ways, but as ingredients for the preparation of other food products, they perform a number of useful functions. Eggs have been preserved too, in the form of powders and in frozen form to be used when required.

Structure and Composition

Eggs are structurally divided into two distinct compartments, the white and the yolk, each with a characteristic composition exhibiting different physical, chemical and nutritional properties. The

Table 6.1 Composition of egg as compared to milk (%)

Element	Whole			Milk			
	White	egg	yolk	Cow's	Dairy*	Soyamilk**	Coconut
Water (%)	88	68	48	87.5	84-88	8.1	42.8
Protein (g)	11	28.5	17.5	3.3	3-3.5	6.4	3.4
Fat (g)	0.2	32.7	32.5	4.1	1.5-6.0	3.2	41.0
Minerals (g)	0.8	2.8	2.0	0.8	0.7-0.75	4.6	0.9
Vitamin A (I.U.)	zero	1.200	1200	174	150 + 200***	...	...
Carotene (µg)	...	600	...	6	...	426	zero
Thiamin (mg)	zero	0.10	0.1	0.05	0.04	0.73	0.08
Riboflavin (mg)	0.1	0.40	0.26	0.19	0.17	0.39	0.04
Vitamin B12 (µg)	0.2	0.64	0.44	0.14	...	zero	zero
Folic Acid (pg)	...	70.3	...	5.6	...	8.65	...
Lactose (%)	zero	zero	zero	4.70	4.70	zero	zero
Carbohydrate (%)	0.9	1.9	1.0	4.4	...	3.6	11.9
Cholesterol (g)						0.0	
Dietary fiber (g)						2.0	

*Refers to values provided for *Mother Dairy* milk. A range is given to cover values for toned and whole milk.
** Different brands of milk carry printed nutritional values which may be referred to when used in packaged forms. Values indicated are for a 200 ml pack of *Sofit*.
*** The value stands for fortified amount present. Where no values are given they were not available.
Source: NIN-ICMR. *Nutritive Values of Indian Foods.* Reprint 1999. Kilgour, *Complete Catering Science.* Heinemann, London. 1986.

approximate composition of the yolk and white are indicated in Table 6.1 Along with values for cows's and dairy milk for comparison.

Table 6.1 shows that eggs are high in moisture, protein, fat, rich in B-complex vitamins, provide a fair amount of minerals, but contain only traces of carbohydrates, except for cow's milk. However, the amount of energy provided by the yolk and white is approximately 1500 and 195 KJ per 100g respectively. Vitamin B12 is only present in traces in those products which are of animal origin. However folic acid is widely distributed in plant foods as well, milk and its products are a good source. Egg yolk however, has the highest amount of folic acid being 70.3 µg/100 g. The other nutrients are briefly discussed below.

Proteins

The proteins of egg are of high quality and therefore easily assimilated in the body. The main proteins of egg white are *ovalbumin* (over 50%), *conalbumin* (14%) and *ovomucoid* (12%). In addition there are three glycoproteins the globulins (7%) including *lysozyme, ovomucin* (less than 12%) and small amounts of *avidin*. The globulins lysozyme and avidin impart antimicrobial properties to eggs by dissolving the cell walls of bacteria, whereas ovomucin and avidin are responsible for the thickness of egg white. The riboflavin present in egg white is also bound to a protein.

Proteins form 1/3 of the egg yolk solids of which the main protein is a lipoprotein complex called *vitellin*, which along with phosphoprotein, *phosvitin* and a sulphur containing protein *livetin* are dispersed in the water phase.

Fats

Fats constitute 2/3 of the solids in the yolk, and comprise of triglycerides, phospholipids and cholesterol. The triglycerides contain the fatty acids oleic, palmitic, stearic and linoleic and are present as a microemulsion of micelles in which are suspended. Very little if any, free fat is present. The main phospholipid is *lecithin* (Phosphatidyl choline) with small amounts of P. ethanolamine and P.serine.

Particles of fat and protein are suspended in the acqueous phase of the yolk appearing as micelles to which the functional properties of egg yolk in baking are attributed. Some of the fat is also in emulsified form and as granules of cholesterol. The functional properties of the yolk are mainly attributed to the micelles as seen in baking.

Vitamins

Eggs are rich in vitamins of the B group and vitamin A but most carotenoids present in yolk have no vitamin A value. Eggs are also deficient in Vitamin C.

Minerals

The main minerals are calcium, phosphorus and iron in yolk.

Enzymes

In addition to proteins, vitamins and minerals, eggs also contain the enzyme alpha-amylase which is higher in the yolk than in the white.

Pigments

Carotenoid pigments are mainly present in egg yolk and impart the yellow colour to it. The depth of the colour however, does not necessarily indicate higher Vitamin A content, because all the carotenoids are not precursors of the vitamin.

Egg Quality

Many factors determine egg quality. The quality of eggs begins to deteriorate as soon as they are laid and can affect the wholesomeness of eggs as well as the food products prepared from them. A few simple methods of testing egg quality are:

Bloom

The dull waxy sheen on the shell of fresh eggs is referred to as bloom. It forms a barrier to the entry of extraneous substances including microorganisms into the egg, at the same time inhibiting the escape of moisture and gases from the egg contents, leading to changes in its properties.

Candling

This is a process of viewing an egg held vertically with apex down, against a candle or light source. It enables the viewer to see the size and position of the air cell, transparency of the white, position and spread of the yolk without actually breaking the shell. Candling is used in food service and processing operations where large quantities of eggs are used.

Position of yolk

The fresh egg yolk is usually centered in the thick egg white. After it is laid the contents shrink more than the shell, and an air space gets formed between the membranes of the yolk and the white. This cell is usually found at the wider end of the egg.

Height of yolk

The height of yolk can be objectively measured as it stands upright in a fine membrane in the fresh egg. The lower the height the less fresh the egg, and when broken if the yolk spreads out the egg is positively stale. The *egg freshness index* can be measured by dividing the yolk height by its diameter. A high index indicates freshness.

White-yolk ratio

The fresh egg has a high proportion of white to yolk, the latter being centrally held. With time, the membrane surrounding the yolk loses its elasticity and the yolk spreads disturbing this ratio.

Size of air cell

As eggs remain in storage the air cell enlarges because of moisture loss through the pores of the shell. In addition some CO_2 is also lost resulting in the white becoming more alkaline.

pH of egg white

The pH of fresh egg white is 7.6 but may increase to over 9.0 depending on the degree of CO_2 loss.

   Viscosity: Ovomucin contributes to the viscosity of egg white. The resistance of the white to spread can be measured with a micrometer on random samples before using for processing. At household level however, viscosity is usually judged through sensory perception when eggs are broken onto a plate or the white separated from the yolk in the course of food preparation. Thick whites indicate freshness in contrast to free flowing ones in which the yolk tends to mix while separating them.

Handling: While eggs are endowed with natural defenses against spoilage they require careful handling to prevent the shell from cracking, as it is delicate and porous. Further, the contents need to be guarded against contamination to retain their wholesomeness and shelf life.

Storage: Eggs once laid have to be cooled immediately from 40°C to 4.4°C to maintain quality and then held at that temperature till required for use. If they need to be stored for long periods they are thermostabilized by dipping in a warm solution of mineral oil to block the pores.

Properties of Eggs

Besides being a storehouse of health giving elements eggs exhibit a number of useful properties which add variety to food products and meals. Due to their characteristic physical and chemical structure and behaviour, when subjected to different treatments, eggs perform a number of functions in food preparation and processing, which are briefly enumerated.

Solubility

Both soluble and insoluble proteins are present in eggs, but since these are normally eaten cooked, the proteins become insoluble on denaturation at low temperatures. However they are easily miscible with other ingredients and dispersed easily as foams or emulsions providing smooth textures to foods when desired.

Denaturation and coagulation

Egg white proteins readily get denatured even by brisk whisking or beating. On heating they coagulate and at very high temperatures or long cooking become tough and rubbery. Eggs therefore, should not be cooked for a long time, reheated or held hot.

Gelling

Eggs have the unique property of forming gels as in the preparation of egg custards or in thickening of soups. By changing the temperature, time and method of cooking, the proteins can be coagulated to make them set as in the preparation of moulded puddings or in thickening batters.

Emulsification

Eggs contain some natural emulsifiers in the form of *lecithin* and *phospholipids,* and are therefore important ingredients in the preparation or permanent food emulsions like mayonnaise, salad creams, spreads and dips.

Foaming

When eggs are beaten they tend to foam, the white giving better volume and stability to the foam than the yolk, due to the presence of globulins, ovomucin and conalbumin. With rapid initial beating the foam acquires a larger volume because the shearing action forms uniform coils of ovomucin which appear as fibrous hollow tubes. When the ovomucin spreads in layers at the interface between the air and the liquid films around it, uncoiling takes place exposing reactive R-groups of the protein thereby stabilizing the foam.

Excessive beating gives an inelastic foam in which the proteins get denatured and liquid is released or drained out from the foam as indicated in Fig.6.1. The liquid contains low concentration of ovomucin along with lysozyme, conalbumin and globulins. Lysozyme may influence foaming quality, but higher levels yield foams of lower volume (Sauter and Montocore, 1972). A number of other factors affect the foaming ability of eggs such as shape and size of bowl to type of beater, egg freshness, separation of egg white, pH, temperature, and added substances.

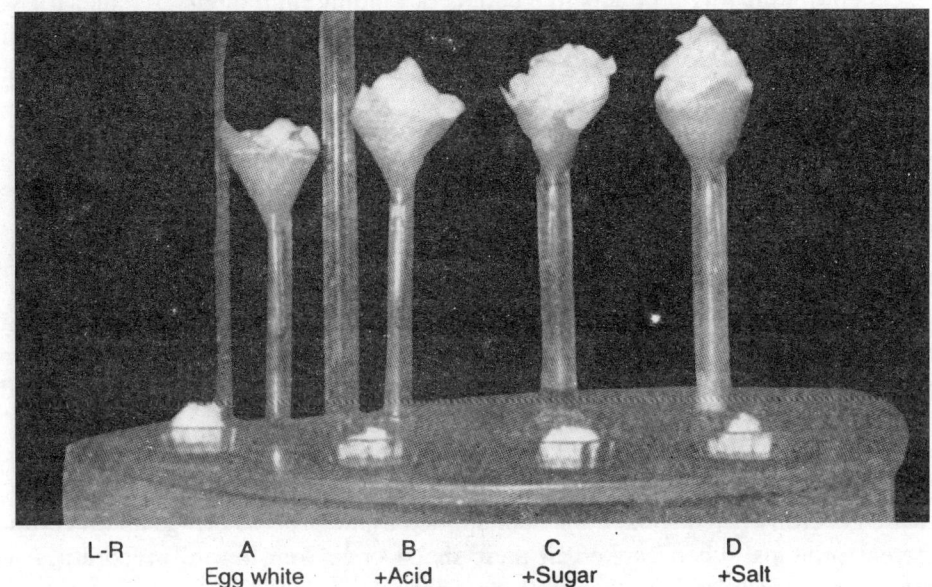

L-R	A	B	C	D
	Egg white	+Acid	+Sugar	+Salt

Fig. 6.1. Egg white foams.

Leavening

This refers to the property of aerating foods to give a light and soft texture to products like cakes, meringues and batter products because of the excellent foaming properties of egg white.

Shortening

The property of adding softness and crispness to foods is called shortening. The texture is achieved because of the high content of fat in the egg yolk.

Antimicrobial action

Freshly laid eggs are coated with mucin which prevents bacterial invasion When this seal is broken by washing, the egg becomes vulnerable to entry by microbes and moisture. The second line of defense are the shell membranes which act as a physical barrier to entry of microbes. In case pathogenic microorganisms penetrate the cell membranes, they multiply very rapidly in the egg white to cause food poisoning. Therefore, if the egg breaks it gets quickly contaminated and even the natural antimicrobials present are unable to cope with the influx, making eggs highly perishable.

The natural antimicrobial agents in egg white are *lysozyme, avidin* and *conalbumin*. The *lysozyme* dissolves the cell membranes of some bacteria, and is an effective germicidal agent. The lower the pH the greater is its effectiveness, which is an added reason for the prevention of CO_2 loss from eggs. The *avidin* acts by binding biotin, a nutrient needed by some microorganisms and thus inhibits their growth. Lastly, the *conalbumin* unites with iron and makes it unavailable for the growth of microbes.

Coating, binding and glazing

Eggs are excellent for coating products like cutlets or binding ingredients together for kebabs and other foods. The property of forming thin films on foods is due to the coagulation of egg proteins. If a product is brushed with egg and then baked or fried it gives *a glaze,* a crisp texture and golden brown colour, while at the same time sealing-in its flavour and the moisture.

Providing structure

Eggs give structure to food products because of its coagulation and leavening properties as seen in cakes, biscuits and desserts.

Nutrition

Eggs are an excellent source of proteins of high biological value, in addition to providing vitamins and micronutrients essential to health. As far as energy is concerned the yolk provides more kcals than the white, being richer in its fat content. The white is higher in its protein content and provides mainly riboflavin.

Effect of Heat on Egg Proteins

Since eggs are generally eaten cooked the heat applied in the process brings about certain changes in the different proteins, when cooked in their shells or broken before preparation. Egg white proteins are more sensitive to heat than yolk proteins.

On heating denaturation takes place followed by coagulation. The white starts destabilizing at 60°C converting the fluid white to a non-flowing gel. The yolk coagulates at 68°C but if beaten together they coagulate between 63- 65°C. The ovalbumin of egg white is readily denatured while ovomucoid is not affected. The denaturation of the *ovomucin-lysozyme* complex however, precedes the coagulation of the egg white, the latter changing from a thick transparent fluid to an opaque white coagulum. If heating is continued the proteins shrink and the texture becomes leathery and indigestible. When other substances like sugar and milk are added to egg in the preparation of custards the temperatures of coagulation increase.

Since most of the usefulness of eggs in cooking and food processing revolve around the main properties of coagulation, emulsification and foam formation, it is imperative to include a discussion on food emulsions and foams.

EMULSIONS

Emulsions are heterogenous systems consisting basically of two immiscible liquids, one dispersed in the other. Emulsions exhibit the characteristics of colloidal systems, the particles of the dispersed phase being about O.lum. The liquid in which the dispersion takes place is called the continuous phase.

Types of Emulsions

Emulsions are basically of two types, the *oil in water emulsions* in which the water is the continuous phase, while the oil forms the dispersed phase, and the *water in oil* type in which the phases are reversed. Examples of the former are mayonnaise and other salad dressings, milk etc., whereas the latter include butter, cream and so on. It may be noted however, that water may be replaced in an emulsion by any liquid or its mixtures, and therefore it is perfectly right to call it an *oil in liquid emulsion* or vice versa.

Classification of Emulsions

Whatever be the nature of the phases in an emulsion, all emulsions are not stable and tend to separate out on standing. Such products are called temporary emulsions as against the permanent ones which do not separate out at room temperatures. On the basis of their stability they can be classified into three categories, temporary, semi-permanent and permanent emulsions.

Temporary emulsions

These require rigorous shaking just before they are used as they separate out easily on storage as seen in French and Italian dressings. Such emulsions flow readily when mixed and exhibit a low viscosity. On standing the two liquid layers separate easily and any dry spices added tend to settle at the bottom of the jar. The physical act of shaking breaks the oil into small droplets which then distribute themselves uniformly.

Semi-permanent emulsions

Such emulsions have the viscosity of thick cream, and therefore tend to be more stable. Salad dressings containing syrups, honey, condensed soups or commercial stabilizers such as gums or pectins are examples of this category.

Permanent emulsions

These are characterized by a very high viscosity and therefore greatest stability. Maintenance of the stability during transportation and storage depends on both internal and external factors, such as the composition of the product, packaging, temperature and physical impact. The most permanent emulsions can break with time if certain materials are not present to hold them together. Such compounds are called emulsifiers.

Stability of Emulsions

A number of factors affect the stability of emulsions such as the type and amounts of ingredients added, and use of the product and so on. These are briefly enumerated below.

Degree of dispersion

This is important because the degree of dispersion depends largely on the particle size of the dispersed phase. The smaller the particle size the greater is the stability of the emulsion.

Amount of emulsifier present

Every emulsifier has a polar and a nonpolar end, each attaching themselves to the water and the oil phases respectively. They thus form a protective covering around each droplet preventing them from coalescing and destabilizing an emulsion. The concentration of the emulsifier is also important to enable all the droplets in an emulsion to be protected and kept dispersed.

Nature of the emulsifying agents

Some foods contain emulsifiers in their natural forms such as, lecithin in egg yolk, soya bean, peanut and maize, phospholipids and proteins in milk and milk products and so on, while other foods depend on added compounds to maintain them in emulsified form.

Nature of the oil

This refers to the structure and composition of the oil used in making the emulsion. Oils which have mono and diglycerides and their derivatives are used in making salad dressings because of their viscosity and clarity. Olive and other salad oils impart a smoothness, lightness and sheen to emulsified products, besides imparting a rich, smooth mouthfeel.

Addition of ingredients

The proportions of the two phases of an emulsion and the order of addition of the ingredients affects the stability and mouthfeel of the product.

Viscosity of the dispersion medium

This is important for stability since the droplets of the dispersed phase are already positioned by interstitial forces.

Emulsifiers

Emulsifiers are part of a group of chemicals commonly known as surface active agents, because they exert their effects mainly at surfaces. These substances are used in industry to stabilize oil-in-water, water-in-oil, and gas-liquid and solid mixtures. Plant sources which are commonly used as surface active agents are gum acacia, guar gum, extract of Irish moss, pectin, cellulose gum (carboxymethyl cellulose or CMC) which is used commercially in the preparation of ice-creams.

Emulsifiers are bipolar in nature and act as a result of their electrically charged polar and non charged nonpolar ends exhibiting hydrophilic as well as hydrophobic properties respectively. This enables the emulsifier to attach itself to the water and oil or fat component of an emulsion, preventing the two liquids from separating out.

Thus, for emulsions to form it is necessary to create new surfaces or interfaces. An emulsifier reduces interfacial tension and therefore less effort is required to create these surfaces. Emulsifiers also help the formation of small droplets and reduce the chances of their coalescing and disturbing stability of the emulsion. After an emulsion is formed, the emulsifier arranges itself at the phase interface forming electrical barriers, which limit movement of the droplets and stabilizes the product.

For oil-in-water emulsions like mayonnaise, the emulsifiers to choose are those which have a greater water solubility and some oil solubility. Conversely the water-in-oil emulsions are best stabilized by emulsifiers which possess a higher oil solubility as compared to its water solubility. In other words, the former type of emulsion has a greater number of positive electrical charges as against the latter which has fewer polar ends compared to the non charged nonpolar ends.

Types of Emulsifiers

There two basic types of emulsifiers–natural and synthetic, the former appearing naturally in foods, while the latter may be simulated in structure and activity from synthetic materials, being put together in the laboratory or factory.

Some examples of natural emulsifiers are phospholipids and lecithin in egg yolk, which are responsible for the natural stability of mayonnaise and other products. Lecithins are similar in their structure to fats but in addition contain phosphoric acid, and therefore possess positively and negatively charged polar and nonpolar ends.

Synthetic

These are chemicals prepared in laboratories which are used to stabilize food products during their manufacture, and help to prolong their shelf life. Examples are mono and diglycerides and their derivatives, certain fatty acids and their derivatives. In the body bile acids are the emulsifiers that help in the digestion and absorption of fats.

Food Emulsions

Foods that exist as emulsions or can be made into them may be placed in 7 distinct categories as discussed briefly below:

Butter and margarines

These exist as water in oil emulsions having a plastic continuous phase. In butter the continuous phase is milk fat whereas in margarines a number if oils and fats from both plant and animal sources may be used. These foods have only 20% water finely dispersed in semisolid fat. Their stability being attributed to the semisolid consistency of the continuous phase rather than to perfect emulsification (Kalab, 1985).

Gravies, sauces and cream soups

This group of food emulsions are stabilized using flour, and therefore generally have a higher percentage of water than oil for stability. There are however some sauces and soups which are prepared using egg yolk during cooking to thicken the product, but the temperatures are controlled between 66-74°C and whisking or stirring is continuous for a smooth texture. The liquid phase may consist of water and lemon juice or vinegar or any other food extract.

Egg yolk acts as an efficient emulsifier because it contains about 30% fat in dispersed form, in addition to phospholipids of which 79% are found as lecithins which are responsible for the emulsifying properties of egg yolk.

In milk only 1-3% fat is dispersed in a liquid phase, the stabilizing agents being the phospholipids, proteins and salts.

Salad dressings and dips

These are emulsions usually containing oil, egg yolk and acidifying ingredients but can also be prepared without eggs, using ingredients like milk with starches, cooked together to bind free water as in the preparation of white sauce. This is then used as a base for the preparation of mayonnaise or other salad dressings. Dips of various kinds can also be prepared using a variety of ingredients to promote taste, texture, nutrition and special-function foods.

Salad Dressings

Dressings add colour and flavour to salads, besides improving their appearance, palatability, and ingestibility, through helping to combine ingredients for better textural properties. There are four basic types of salad dressings:

- Temporary emulsions

- Stable emulsions
- Cooked dressings
- Milk based preparations.

Temporary Emulsions

These usually consist of a mixture of oil, spices and acid as in the case of French dressing. These tend to coat salads well as they are of pouring consistency. They are light to digest, but on keeping separate out into liquid and oil or spice layers.

Stable Emulsions

These do not separate out when stored and can be spooned out of a jar when required. A good example is mayonnaise or salad creams.

Cooked Dressings

These are ingredient mixtures usually thickened with egg and flour, or different starches and milk.

Many types of dips are made these days using cooked, soaked or sprouted cereals and pulses or green and other vegetables and nuts as base. Dips help the user to make dishes and snacks less spicy so that individual levels of spicing can be done through the accompaniments to enhance taste and flavour.

Milk Dressings

As the name suggests the basic ingredient is milk, a little butter or oil is thickened generally with a flour or starch, by cooking. A milk dressing can also use yoghurt, curd or cream cheese as the base, with other ingredients whipped in or added for variety. Such preparations do not require cooking.

All dressings can be varied for flavour by changing ingredients added such as chopped onions, grated cabbage, capsicum, tomato, fruits, different spices or nuts and so on. *Low calorie dressings* are usually made with juices or purees of fruits and vegetables or skimmed milk as their base. These may replace part or all of the oil generally used. Soft margarines and curds or yoghurts are good substitutes for cream or oil.

Dips

This term may be used synonymously with the traditional *chutney* or sauce, commonly used in India as an accompaniment to snacks and meals. There is a wide variety that can be made and consists of mixing or grinding ingredients together in fresh forms and then spicing to suit requirements of the dish it is served with. Europeans use the term *dip* because a piece of salad vegetable or snack is dipped in the sauce before eating. Many types of dips are made these days using cooked, soaked or sprouted cereals and pulses or green and other vegetables and nuts as base. Dips help the user to make dishes and snacks less spicy so that individual levels of spicing can be done through the accompaniments to enhance taste and flavour.

Choux pastry

This is the base for a number of bakery products and is basically an emulsion of water, shortening or fat, flour, salt and eggs. Heat is used to boil the water and melt the fat before the flour is added. The emulsification is brought about due to the addition of egg. If egg is used in insufficient quantities the emulsion does not form properly and the baked product exhibits low volume.

Chocolate

This is an emulsion of cocoa and fat, although other ingredients such as milk, nuts and flavourings may be added for variety. Emulsifiers are used in the manufacture of chocolates in order to provide stability and control the *bloom* thus preventing surface change that may otherwise occur during storage.

Emulsifiers such as lecithin and monosodium phosphate derivatives of mono- and diglycerides are used to, decrease the chewiness of caramels and prevent them from sticking to their wrappers. The emulsifiers also help to disperse water insoluble essential oils and flavours in candies and beverages. Thus helping to maintain their sensory characteristics.

Batters and doughs

Fat is present in emulsified form in batters and doughs used for preparing a number of food products, such as griddle cakes, souffles, muffins and other products. The batters are usually oil-in-water emulsions, whereas the fat in a cake batter may be wholly or partly emulsified. Emulsifying agents in baked products serve two purposes. In doughs they improve the intimate mixing of the ingredients, and thereby the quality of the final product, in which staling is retarded. In cake batters they permit baking of cakes containing a high ratio of sugar to flour, thereby enhancing flavour with no loss of volume.

Food emulsions therefore include cream pastes, dips, sauces, cream soups etc. Some foods have only some to their fat emulsified as in meat products, batters and doughs, icecreams and other desserts. The term *meat emulsion is* sometimes commonly used for pork products made out of ground meat mixed with spices and shaped as desired. This is a misnomer, because the particles of the fat in such products is not of colloidal size to classify them as emulsions. A meat batter is therefore more adequately described as a gel filled with emulsified fat and coagulated protein as in the manufacture of sausages. The meat proteins stabilize the fat and prevent coalescence.

Uses of Emulsions

Emulsions provide many useful functions in food preparation and processing.

(*i*) They act as vehicles for adding flavour to foods.
(*ii*) Dilute ingredients.
(*iii*) Hide objectionable odours or tastes.
(*iv*) Provide variety in food preparation.
(*v*) Control agglomeration of fat globules in food products.
(*vi*) Modify the rheological properties of doughs, by reacting with gluten proteins.
(*vii*) Improve wettability and dispensability of dehydrated products.
(*viii*) Modify crystals in candies.
(*ix*) Dissolve flavours and essential oils in micelles of aqueous systems.

FOAMS

Foams differ from emulsions in that they are dispersions of gas or air bubbles in a continuous liquid or semisolid phase containing a soluble surface active agent. The liquid films separating the air bubbles in a foam are colloidal in size and nature. A good foaming agent is also a good emulsifying agent, although in general foams are less stable than emulsions.

Foaming Agents

Egg white is used extensively as a foaming agent. Although creams, edible gums and gels, food proteins and their hydrolyzed derivatives are also employed in food manufacture. When a liquid sol is agitated or repeatedly cut by mechanical action gas may be introduced into foods to make them foamy or light and fluffy in texture.

Methods of Foam Formation

There are two basic methods used in the formation of foams whipping and condensation, involving processes that produce dispersions of gas or air in liquid. All foams require air to be incorporated in foods for making them light in texture. This can be done in a number of ways such as beating, folding and rolling, creaming or sifting dry ingredients together.

Whipping

Whipping describes the action involved in the process for which different types of equipment are used. This is the most common method used as it forms bubbles by cutting the surface and introducing air into the liquid. Repeated action makes the bubbles progressively smaller and creates a fine dispersion which is foamy and light and even in texture.

Condensation

In this method a pressurized solution is suddenly released to expand the number of gas bubbles which then rise through the liquid. In this method the size of the bubbles become larger with time and cannot form an even textured foam.

Factors Affecting Foam formation

There are a number of factors that affect foam formation and its stability such as age, temperature, food qulity and pH. For example, fresh eggs do not form good foams, while ageing tenderizes its proteins which become more extensible for foaming. Whites foam better than the yolks, which separate best at room temperature (25-28°C). Each protein has different foaming abilities, ovalbumin forming the strongest foam, with structures that support many times their weight of other ingredients. Eggs foam best at 27°C. pH is important to egg foaming, the best foam being formed between 3.7-4.0 pH. Albumins however, require a slightly acidic or alkaline pH, around 6.5 being best for eggs. Other factors affecting foam quality are briefly described.

Surface tension

Solutes that lower the surface tension of the air-water interface form better foams. Limited heat treatment of proteins decreases surface tension. High viscosity and greater **hydrophobicity** increase the capacity of mixtures to foam. (Phillips, 1981).

Iso-electric point

Iso-electric point is that pH at which proteins remain dispersed in the continuous phase. At their isoelectric point, the effect of electrical or ionic charges in the dispersion is weakest, and therefore solutions or mixtures generally exhibit good foaming properties (Kinsella,1981).

Solubility of surfactant

Solubility, movement and molecular flexibility of surfactant are necessary for foam formation.

Most protein and polysaccharide foams have enough gas to enable the liquid phase to exist between any adjacent bubbles (Richert,1979) .

Low vapour pressure

A low vapour pressure of the liquid ensures that the liquid phase does not evaporate too quickly and affect foam formation.

The volume of a foam increases when new air or gas cells form and the rate of formation is greater than the rate of collapse by denaturation of the proteins in a mixture. Increased reduction of the surface area of some bubbles or a break in the protein structure due to over whipping can lead to *clump* formation. Examples of this phenomenon are seen when churning out butter from cream, or over whipping egg whites beyond the stiff peak stage (Brooker,1985).

The time taken for a foam to form its volume depends largely on the whipping agent, composition of the liquids and the speed with which the whipping is done.

Foam Stability

The stability of a foam can be determined by the degree of drainage from the foam and the bubble size produced through air incorporation by beating or whipping rhythmically.

Drainage

The volume of the liquid drained due to gravitational forces when a foam is left to stand for 20-30 minutes indicates the stability of the foam. The greater the drainage the less stable is the foam.

Bubble size

The larger the size of the bubbles in a foam the greater is the instability, because it indicates rupture of the lamellae separating the gas bubbles and their diffusion to form larger ones. The size can easily be detected by the naked eye. In low density foams the bubbles are easily deformed.

Bubble surfaces in most foods are elastic due to presence of proteins, which have a high molecular weight. Factors which affect foam formation are pH, presence of salts, sugar and fat. Oilseed proteins have been reported to have the greatest foam stability at their isoelectric points (Bowers, 1992).

Factors Affecting Stability of Foams

A number of factors such as presence of sugar, salt, acid, size and type of bowl used, temperature, contaminants and protein concentration affect foam stability.

Sugar

Addition of sugar affects the stability of foams adversely if added to a mixture before the foaming atarts, but once the foam starts to form its addition in small quantities during beating results in a stable foam. This foam also has a characteristic whiteness and sheen, although the time taken for foaming is prolonged.

Salt

Addition of salt decreases the stability of a foam because of its hygroscopic nature, the salt having the ability to attract moisture from the food mixture and disturbing the whipping quality of the solids present.

Acid

Lowering of pH brings about greater stability therefore good foams do not form if mixtures are even slightly alkaline.

Size and type of bowl

A bowl should be large enough to allow vigorous and free whisking, while being non absorbent as far as oils and fats are concerned. Suitable materials are glass, porcelain or metals, which are conducive to better foam formation than plastics, to which oils adhere easily forming a thin almost invisible layer. The best material is unlined copper, which in traces reacts with the mixture to strengthen the walls surrounding the air bubbles formed on whisking. This gives rise to a more stable foam even if the mixture contains other added substances. The inner surface of the bowl used should be hemispherical, to enable the blades of the whisk or beater to move through the liquid freely enough to shear the contents. A flat surface however will obstruct the smoothness of the whisking action. A balloon whisk is ideal for foam formation as its wire loops quickly forcing air into the mixture.

Temperature

Temperature as the temperature increases the surface tension is lowered easing the ability of the liquid to form a stable foam. Therefore egg whites at room temperature form better foams than those which are used straight from the fridge.

Presence of yolk

If egg white gets slightly mixed with the yolk during the separation process, foam formation is adversely affected, because of the presence of fat from the yolk. Besides the volume of the foam decreasing, the colour too becomes pale instead of being white.

Concentration of protein

The addition of water or other liquid to egg whites or yolk increases initial foam volume, but has a noticeable negative effect on stability because of decrease in the protein concentration of the mixture.

Food Foams

A number of foods possess good foaming properties on account of the proteins they contain that can provide the stability to products and impart characteristic qualities to foods. Of these foods eggs provide an excellent example.

Egg foam formation

When egg is whipped or beaten air gets entrapped in the liquid present, and an interfacial tension is established between the air-liquid interface. The three main proteins helpful in the foaming process are globulins, ovalbumin and ovomucin which are basically egg white proteins. The ovomucin is also responsible for the thickening of the egg white. On beating, this protein gets sheared to form hollow tubes about 300-400μ in length, which is optimum for good foam formation. The foam is further helped by some protein coagulation at the air-water interface, started by the frictional heat produced during the beating process.

Egg white proteins thus, have excellent foaming qualities because of their low surface tension and vapour pressure. With very little effort, egg contents can be stretched out into thin fibrils or strands which encompass air to form high volume foams. The foam volume desired can be controlled by the degree of mechanical whipping of the egg or mixture. A stable egg white foam stands in rigid peaks even when the beater is removed. If beating is continued beyond this point, the foam becomes flaky, the rigid structure breaks forming flocs which do not blend easily into any food mixture. This is often called the dry stage at which the foam becomes brittle and looses the sheen normally seen in egg white foams.

Egg foams at their different stages of formation have many applications in food preparation and processing. Foamy eggs or whites are usually used for:

(*i*) Clarifying soups and consumes
(*ii*) Coating foods
(*iii*) Mixing with batters and doughs to bind ingredients, seal-in flavours and provide softness and crispness especially in products such as french toast, fluffy omelettes, angel cakes, sponge cakes, meringue, souffles and the like.
(*iv*) Soft peaks are used for a number of baked products such as cakes meringues, souffles.
(*vi*) The stiff peak stage of a foam is needed for hard meringues and chiffon cakes, as well as sponges and souffles.
(*v*) The dry stage is reached when the foam is whisked beyond the stiff peak and attains a crumbly appearance. This is also referred to as the flocculent stage. Used for preparing products in which egg white is generally folded into a mixture or in egg preparations with a firm texture. A higher proportion of egg is required to provide enough structure to prevent a drop in volume on cooling as in the case of baked or steamed custards.

Gelatin foam

A gelatin sol may be beaten when it has thickened but not quite set. Such beating increases the volume of the gel 2-3 fold imparting to it a light and spongy texture. The stage at which to start beating is when the dispersion resembles whipping cream, as the mixture is elastic at this point. The beating needs to be continuous until the point of stiffness to prevent layers of liquid separating out.

Eggs and gelatin are extensively used as ingredients in many foods to impart a soft and spongy yet firm texture to products, although some dairy products such as cream and evaporated milk may also be used. Examples of some food foams are icecreams, leavened breads, sponge cakes and the like, which gain their stability from the proteins present. The foams form because the protein containing liquid has a relatively low surface tension, which allows the liquid to increase its surface area around the gas bubble without squeezing out the air too quickly. To add to this the low vapour pressure prevents the evaporation of the liquid from the food.

Some food products based on foam development during cooking or in processing are briefly discussed below.

Icecream: This is a frozen foam in which the incorporated air bubbles are held together partly by the emulsified fat and partly by a network of colloidally dispersed ice crystals in a sugar solution.

Batters and Doughs: Numerous baked products are made when flour is combined with liquid in such ratios as to form either a batter or dough. These are foams in which the liquid acts as the continuous phase, in which the egg proteins are colloidally and flour particles coarsely dispersed. The air enclosed in the matrix is done mechanically by creaming, or whipping mixtures or kneading as in doughs. Similarly breads, cakes or other products prepared from batters and doughs entraps gas or air bubbles which on proofing and cooking expand and escape to give a foam-like light structure to the product. Examples are cream puffs, muffins, cakes and breads. While cream puffs, sponge and angel cakes and muffins are prepared from drop batters, the yeast breads, *kulcha, naan, bhatura* are leavened by CO_2 formed in the process of fermentation by microorganisms. Sponge and angel cakes are therefore some-times referred to as *foam cakes*.

The experiments 23-32 have been designed to enable a study of the effect of temperature, other ingredients and methods of adding them on the qualities of natural and prepared emulsions and foams.

EXPERIMENT 23

Aim

To study the effect of cooking time on the colour, texture and acceptability of whole egg.

Equipment

Heavy bottomed steel pan, spoon, burner, microwave oven, thermometer, stop watch, measuring cup.

Materials

Water, whole eggs.

Principle

The proteins of egg white are more sensitive to heat than those of the yolk. Coagulation begins near 60°C and is completed at 65°C, while the yolk loses its fluidity around 70°C. The denaturation of the ovomucin-lysozyme complex may be the first step in the coagulation but it is the ovalbumin which is mainly denatured. Overcooking egg makes the contents tough and more hydrogen sulphide is liberated.

Procedure

A. (*i*) Warm 200 ml water in a pan heated to 60°C and slide a whole egg into it, when the water starts boiling lower the heat or flame, cover and cook for 12 minutes.

  (*ii*) Remove from heat and cool immediately under running tap water. Note the time taken for egg to cool to handling temperature.

 (*iii*) Remove the shell of the egg and observe whether the shell comes off' easily.

 (*iv*) Cut the egg vertically and note the position of the yolk, white, their spread and acceptability.

B. (*i*) Take another egg and cook as in A (*i*) for 10 minutes.

 (*ii*) Repeat as in A (*i-iv*).

C. (*i*) Take another egg and cook as in A (*i*) for 20 minutes.

 (*ii*) Repeat A (*i-iv*).

    Experiments may be designed with other variations in which cooking time can be kept constant but the method of cooling changed. Some ideas are presented in the practice exercises drawn up.

D. (*i*) Heat water to boiling, then add the egg.
     Cook for 8-10 mins.

 (*ii*) Repeat A (*ii-iv*).

Observations

Tabulate your observations as learnt and draw your inferences on the best method of boiling eggs. Show how each of the results obtained from A-D can be creatively used in food preparation.

Precautions

1. Avoid high temperatures and very rapid cooking.

2. Do not over cook.
3. The egg should be cooled enough to be handled with ease.

Practice Exercises

1. Boil eggs for a fixed time but cool in air, and in the pan in which it is cooked, then shell and comment on the sensory qualities, and their applications in food preparation.
2. List 5 dishes in which boiled eggs are used. Describe how they are cut for particular purposes and why.
3. Take a fresh egg, and a week old one, cook and observe the differences. Are there any signs in the cooked egg which indicate freshness and staleness. Describe them.

EXPERIMENT 24

Aim
To observe the effect of method of cooking on the coagulation property of eggs.

Equipment
Gas burner or hot-plate, frying fan, saucers, microwave dish, fork and spatula.

Materials
Cooking oil, water, eggs.

Principle
Egg proteins respond differently in terms of time and temperature of coagulation according to the method of cooking used. The products obtained by the different moist and dry heat methods are also different.

Procedure
A. (*i*) Break an egg by striking the blunt edge of a table knife in the centre of the egg held horizontally above a saucer, and let the contents slide into it without disturbing the position of the yolk.

(*ii*) Heat 1 T oil in a frying pan and slide the egg into the hot oil. Note the time taken for the white and yolk to coagulate.

(*iii*) Remove the egg from the oil with the spatula and keep aside in a fresh saucer for evaluation.

B. (*i*) Repeat A (*i*).

(*ii*) Repeat A (*ii*) but this time reduce the flame after adding the egg to the hot pan, and cover to cook. Note the time taken.

(*iii*) As in A (*iii*).

C. (*i*) Wipe the pan dry and put 200 ml water in it. Heat till it starts to simmer or reaches 95-97°C.

(*ii*) Slide an egg from a saucer into the simmering water. Cook till it coagulates.

(*iii*) As in A (*iii*).

D. (*i*) Break an egg in a microwave dish.

(*ii*) Prick the yolk with a fork without disturbing its position in the white.

(*iii*) Cook in the microwave oven for 30 seconds. Remove from oven and keep for evaluation.

Observations
Place all the cooked samples from A-D together for evaluation, and tabulate your results with respect to position of yolk, rigidity of white and yolk, time taken for the coagulation, colour, texture flavour and mouthfeel. Draw your inferences regarding the appropriate method to be used for cooking eggs for different end uses in food preparation, indicating suitable applications with examples.

Precautions
1. Eggs should never be cooked at boiling temperatures.

2. Overcooking needs to be avoided, to get maximum value from eggs.
3. Egg preparations need to be watched carefully and removed from heat as soon as they are ready.
4. They need to be served immediately for best sensory qualities.

This experiment may be used as a demonstration class to show the properties of egg coagulation by frying, poaching, scrambling, microwave cooking or preparing omelettes both plain and foamy.

Practice Exercises

1. Prepare a poached egg as learnt, by using 1 teaspoon of white vinegar or salt in the water used for cooking. Note the difference between the sample you prepared with water alone and comment on the differences observed.
2. Prepare a fried egg as learnt. Note the time and temperature required for the gelation in Exercise 1 and 2. Evaluate both the preparations for their sensory qualities.
3. List 5 dishes in which the properties of gelation, coagulation, hydration and aeration are used in food preparation. Explain why the methods of cooking used are suitable for each dish.

EXPERIMENT 25

Aim
To study the effect of different factors on the gelation temperature and consistency of egg custard.

Equipment
Gas burner or hot plate, heavy bottomed steel pan, weighing scale, measuring cups and spoons, cooking thermometer, stirrer or wooden spoon and double boiler, bowls.

Materials
Eggs, milk, sugar, salt and essence (optional).

Principle
In an egg custard, molecules of proteins mainly ovalbumin get denatured by heat, and unite to form a network which enmeshes the fluid milk to form a gel. Gelation begins at 65°C and is completed at 70°C. A soft custard is formed when a thick velvety coating is visible on the back of the spoon with which the mixture is constantly stirred to prevent coagulation. If overcooked curdling takes place as the proteins begin to coagulate. Therefore gentle, preferably indirect moist heat is necessary for a smooth product. Addition of salt produces a firmer gel, whereas adding sugar increases the temperature of gelation and retards the process of denaturation.

Procedure
A (i) Scald 150 ml of milk in a double boiler placed on direct heat.
  (ii) Beat 1 egg lightly till bubbles appear and yolk and white is well blended.
  (iii) Add 2 teaspoon sugar and blend into egg.
  (iv) Remove the milk from the double boiler and gradually blend it into the egg mixture while stirring.
  (v) Return the mixture to the double boiler, fix the thermometer to dip vertically in the mixture, and cook over simmering water, stirring constantly with a wooden spoon. Ensure that the temperature rises not more than 1°C every 3 minutes.
  (vi) When the custard coats the back of the spoon, note the time taken and the temperature of the custard.
  (vii) Remove into two bowls and keep aside to cool covering one of the bowls and leaving the other to air cool.

B. Repeat A (i-vii) but add a pinch of salt in addition.

C. Repeat A (i-vii) but without adding sugar or salt.

D. Repeat A (i-vii) using $1^1/_2$ t custard powder instead of egg.

Observations
Compare the results of products from A and C and tabulate them to show the differences in colour, consistency, texture, taste and applicability in food preparation Indicate the time and temperatures noted during the experiment.

Precautions

1. Custards should be prepared using only indirect heat.
2. The temperature of the water in the double boiler should be at simmering temperature.
3. The right proportion of eggs and milk or liquid is important for proper consistency Too few eggs will not cause gelation.
4. The custard should be stirred constantly to enable even heating and prevention of coagulation.
5. Store covered to prevent skin formation due to the presence of milk in the product.
6. Avoid over heating. If curdling occurs cool and whisk till smooth.

Practice Exercises

1. Prepare custards by substituting 2 egg, 2 yolks and 2 whites for 1 egg. Comment of the 3 products formed with respect to their sensory qualities, time taken for preparation and their applicability in food preparation.
2. Prepare the original custard mixture with one egg, pour into a baking dish and place in a tray of hot water in a preheated oven. Bake at 177°C for 20 minutes or until set. Remove, cool and evaluate. Record the difference in texture, and other sensory qualities between a stirred and a baked custard.
3. Cut some fruit and mix with cooled custard. Place in the refrigerator for one hour. Record your observation and explain what happens.

Further experiments may be planned by using different methods of cooking custards or using different proportions and kinds of ingredients. Samples of the custard may be removed from the boiler at different temperatures (65, 72, 76, 80, 82°C) and the temperature at which the custard curdles recorded. Evaluation of the samples for sensory attributes and applicability may also be conducted.

EXPERIMENT 26

Aim

To study the effect of temperature on stability of a natural emulsion.

Equipment

Cooking pan, heating element or gas burner, thermometer, clamp, measuring cylinder pH paper, stop watch, slides and microscope.

Materials

Milk.

Principle

Milk is a liquid food obtained from natural sources and is a fine example of a stable emulsion in which milk solids are dispersed in water. Being high in protein molecules and containing about 20 amino acids these arrange themselves in formations called R-Groups that play an important role in the way proteins behave as colloids. (Charley, 1982). Such dispersions are also called *sols*. A number of changes are visible when milk is heated to different temperatures as its various components react differently. This alters the structure of the colloidal solution and stability of the emulsion.

Procedure

A. (*i*) Take 250 ml of milk in a cooking pan and note its temperature.

(*ii*) Prepare a slide and observe the emulsion under the microscope.

(*iii*) Place on medium heat and observe the milk at 60, 70, 80, 90, 100 and 110°C. Note any changes that occur in colour, transluscency, consistency, foaming and so on.

(*iv*) Prepare slides of the emulsion at each of the above temperatures and observe under the micro-scope. Note the temperature at which the emulsion starts to change in structure and or destabilisers.

Note the time taken to reach each temperature and the pH of the milk at each stage.

Observations

Tabulate your observations as learnt and draw inferences with respect to the temperatures at which milk remains a stable emulsion.

Precautions

1. Use only medium heat throughout the experiment.
2. Switch off the heat as soon as the required temperature is reached and make your observations. Then again switch on the burner for the next temperature.
3. Remove a drop of the milk on prearranged and labelled slides at the right temperature.
4. The-thermometer should dip in the milk and not touch the bottom or sides of the pan.
5. Do not stir the milk during heating.

Practice Exercises

1. Perform the experiment learnt using direct heat. Comment on the custard formed.
2. Repeat the experiment using different kinds of milk available in the market, such as cow's and buffalo milk, dairy milks such as pasteurized, homogenized, toned and double toned and compare the observations.
3. Add water to milk and observe what happens to its stability and other sensory qualities.

EXPERIMENT 27

Aim

To study the effect of adding sugar and acid on the stability of a natural emulsion.

Materials

Acid, sugar, milk.

Principle

When the pH of milk is changed the proteins lose their equilibrium and tend to denature causing the emulsion to destabilise depending on the nature and quantity of the added substances. Every protein has a specific iso-electric point which if disturbed causes proteins to precipitate out. The iso-electric pH of casein the main protein of milk is 6.6. It is only when this pH goes below 5.2 that the colloidal dispersion of calcium phosphocaseinate is converted to a gel of neutral casein. On further reduction of pH the protein forms clots seen as specs when milk or white sauce is added to hot tomato or spinach soup or in baked dishes.

Procedure

A. Addition of sugar

   (*i*) Take 250 ml milk in each of 4 pans, and note the pH and temperature of the milk.

   (*ii*) Add 5, 10, 15 and 20g sugar in each of the pans and heat as in experiment 24 at all the different temperatures. Note the changes and record observations as learnt.

   (*iii*) Compare your results with those obtained in experiment 22 for egg coagulation.

B. (*i*) Repeat steps A (*i-iii*) above by replacing the sugar with 1/2, 1, $1^1/_2$ and 2T of glacial acetic acid.

   (*ii*) Measure the pH at which the emulsions destabilize.

Observations

Record your observations and draw inferences with respect to stability of the natural milk emulsion.

Precautions

As in experiment 26.

Practice Exercises

   1. Use jaggery and honey or corn syrup instead of crystalline sugar in the experiment and record the differences in effects on the stability.

   2. Use lemon juice, vinegar or any other acid substance commonly used in cooking and note the differences in stability.

   3. List five dishes in which sugar or acid is used with milk and their effects are utilized to advantage in food preparation and processing.

> **EXPERIMENT 28**

Aim

To determine the best method of preparing a stable emulsion like mayonnaise.

Equipment

Rotary beater or whisk, blender, bowl, standard cups and spoons.

Materials

2 Eggs, 1 cup refined oil, 1T vinegar, or 1T lemon juice, 1/2 teaspoon salt, 1/2 teaspoon sugar, 1/2 teaspoon mustard powder, pepper a pinch, 1/2 cup evaporated milk.

Principle

Mayonnaise is an emulsified salad dressing which requires ingredients in certain proportions to be mixed together to form a stable oil-in-liquid emulsion. The egg forming about 20% of the total weight, provides the emulsifying agent lecithin, present in the yolk. This helps in stabilizing the other ingredients in the mixture. While whole egg may be used in the preparation of the product, it is the yolks which have better stabilizing ability as they hold the moisture in dispersion. Therefore the ratio of other ingredients such as oil, vinegar and spices should not exceed 65:10:5 per cent of the weight of the egg contents, since the yolks have limited assimilating power. Continuous beating breaks up the oil into fine globules which get simultaneously dispersed in liquid to convert it into a semisolid stable product. Besides ingredients, temperature too plays an important role in the formation of an emulsion. As temperature rises the surface tension of the continuous phase gets reduced, and the oil also becomes more mobile and less viscous.

Procedure

The experiment is divided into three sections A, B and C to study the effect of variations on the end result and determine the most suitable method of preparing mayonnaise for different applications.

A. Method of Preparing Mayonnaise

(*i*) Separate yolks from the eggs and drop into a small bowl.

(*ii*) Add all the ingredients except vinegar and oil to the yolks.

(*iii*) Beat with a whisk or beater till ingredients are well blended.

(*iv*) Add the oil drop by drop alternating it with the vinegar while continuously beating the mixture. Continue beating till the mixture begins to thicken.

(*v*) Continue the process, gradually increasing the quantity of oil added at one time, till all the ingredients have been used up and the resultant product is spoonable into a jar.

(*vi*) Observe samples for microscopic structure, colour, consistency taste, flavour and applicability.

B. Effect of Varying the Method of Combining Ingredients

(*i*) Add seasonings and vinegar to the yolks and then start the whisking. Add oil as in 'A' and when ready, keep sample aside for assessment and proceed till A (*v*).

(*ii*) Beat the egg yolks first and then add the oil drop by drop till thickened, followed by spices and vinegar. Set a sample aside.

(*iii*) To the yolk, add seasoning, 1/3 vinegar and then oil drop by drop beating till thickened, followed by 1/3 vinegar again and then the rest of the oil and the last 1/3 vinegar to complete the product. Keep sample aside.

For quick and even continous beating an electrical blender may be used and the ingredients continuously added without much pause following the method in A(i-vi). With this method the time can be monitored for equal number of revolutions when variations are used.

C. Effect of Substituting Emulsifying Agents

(*i*) Make a starch gel with 1/2 T of cornstarch and 1/2 cup of water. Cool the gel. Take 2 T of this gel and add it to the egg yolks with all the other ingredients except oil, and mix together. Add oil as in A (*iv*) and follow procedure till A(*vi*). Keep sample aside.

(*ii*) Prepare a gel using 2T gelatin in 1/2 cup water and cool to room temperature. Use IT of gel to make the emulsion as in (*i*) above. Keep sample aside.

(*iii*) Substitute egg white for yolk and proceed as in A(*i-vi*) Keep sample aside.

(*iv*) Substitute whole egg for yolk and proceed as in A(*i-vi*) Keep sample aside.

D. Effect of Temperature of Ingredients on Formation of Emulsion

(*i*) Add vinegar and seasonings to egg yolk at room temperature, then mix and refrigerate till cold. Keep the oil for the same time in the frig too. Remove from fridge and note the temperature of the mixture and oil. Place bowl in ice and add cold oil as in experiment A till ready. Keep aside.

(*ii*) Heat oil and vinegar separately to 100°C. Combine the ingredients as in 'A' till ready. Keep aside for assessment.

E. Effect of Substituting Egg with Evaporated Milk

(*i*) Put mustard, sugar, salt and pepper in a bowl.

(*ii*) Add evaporated milk, mix and gradually beat in the oil, or use a blender.

(*iii*) Add vinegar, blend till smooth.

Observations

All the samples should be labelled correctly and assessed for appearance, consistency, taste, mouthfeel and application in food preparation and service. The results may be tabulated as depicted in Table 6.2.

Table 6.2 Sensory quality of mayonnaise for different variations

Variation	Appearance	Stability	Taste	Mouthfeel	Application
A.					
B. (i)					
(ii)					
(iii)					
(iv)					
C. (i)					
(ii)					
(iii)					
D. (i)					
(ii)					
(iii)					
E.					

The microscopic structure of the different samples may be observed and recorded as shown in Table 6.3. For each fresh sample as well as after one week.

Table 6.3 Microscopical structure of mayonnaise

Variation	Microscopic Fresh	Structure After 1 week	Observations
A.			
B. (i)			
(ii)			
(iii)			
(iv)			
C. (i)			
(ii)			
(iii)			
D. (i)			
(ii)			
E.			

The structures described in Table 6.3 have been presented through plates IX A-C.

Precautions

1. The oil should be added dropwise initially and then gradually as the emulsion forms.
2. Beating should be continuous while preparing the product.
3. Proportion of ingredients should be exactly controlled for all samples even when substitutes are used.

4. Proportion of ingredients should be strictly controlled for all samples even when substitutes are used.
5. Adding oil and vinegar alternately is essential for dispersion.
6. Temperature must be kept constant throughout the experiment.

Practice Exercises

1. Prepare mayonnaise and substitute the oil with melted butter, dalda, corn oil, groundnut oil and so on. Assess the products and see which one you prefer and for what use.
2. Prepare mayonnaise by varying the temperature of ingredients and see the effect on the product. Comment on its qualities and use. (You will need to use thermometer to note down the temperature of oil, and other ingredients).
3. Prepare kadhi using 40g bengal gram flour, seasonings to taste, 8g fat and 100ml water. Observe the sensory attributes of the preparation and study the microscopic structure of the emulsion.

EXPERIMENT 29

Aim

To study the effect of salt, acid, sugar, fat and other variables on the stability of egg white foam.

Equipment

Measuring cylinder, funnel, stopwatch, filter paper, beater.

Materials

Eggs, salt, sugar, cream of tartar, fat, distilled water.

Principle

Egg white is a viscous transparent liquid which may be converted into a foam by beating or whipping air bubbles into it. The ease with which egg can be whipped into a fine foam is attributed to the presence of globulin, ovamucin and ovalbumin. When egg white is beaten both colour and viscosity change and the foam forms soft peaks. Further beating denatures the protein film causing it to collapse at places resulting in the escape of some of the air and formation of flocs or lumps, with escape of liquid. Such a foam is said to be destabilized. Egg pH is important to foaming, the ovalbumin foaming best between 3.7–4.0 and albumin between 6.5 and 9.5 respectively.

Procedure

A. *Preparation of egg white foam.*
- (*i*) Separate the white from the yolk of egg.
- (*ii*) Beat egg white to stiff peak stage using a rotary beater or a whisk and note the time taken for foam formation.
- (*iii*) Transfer the prepared foam to a funnel lined with filter paper and placed over a measuring cylinder. Keep aside for 45 minutes and record the volume of the liquid drained.
- (*iv*) Use one egg white for each of the variations B-I below, following steps A (*i-iii*).

B. Add 1/8 teaspoon salt to egg white for preparing the foam.
C. Add 1/8t cream of tartar and then beat.
D. Add 1/4t of egg yolk and then beat to a foam.
E. Add 10 ml of water and then beat.
F. Add 2t of castor sugar and prepare the foam.
G. Add 10 ml distilled water and proceed.
H. Add 10 ml oil and beat.
I. Use a different type of beater.

After keeping the foams for 45 minutes, compare the results of the samples A-I with respect to time taken for foam formation, and sensory qualities, to determine the most stable foam.

Observations

Record the observations made as indicated in Table 6.4.

Table 6.4 Effect of added substances on foam formation

Variation	Time (min)	Colour Foam	Liq.	Texture Foam	Liq.	Gloss	Stability	Liquid Drained ml	Applications
Egg white									
A.									
B.									
C.									
*									
*									

Note: Measure height of each foam and see which variation gives the greatest volume.

From the above observations inferences may be drawn regarding the stability and suitability of various foams for food preparation and processing.

Precautions

1. Egg white should be separated carefully from the yolk so as not to mix even at trace of the yolk.
2. Beating should be done till the stiff peak stage only.
3. Added substances should be measured accurately.
4. Time should be noted when the stiff peak stage is reached.
5. All samples should be neatly labelled on completion and drained for exactly 45 minutes before observations are recorded.

Practice Exercises

1. Prepare a list of food products in the preparation of which foams are used.
2. Prepare egg white foam and add sugar to it gradually after it begins to peak. Drop over a toast and bake in a moderate oven. Comment on the product.

EXPERIMENT 30

Aim

To demonstrate the effect of foaming on the volume and texture of omelettes.

Equipment

Bowls rotary beater, burner, pan.

Materials

Eggs, salt.

Principle

By separating the whites and yolks of eggs and beating them separately, more air is incorporated in the mixture and when cooked it assumes a light foamy texture of souffle, while at the same time has body because of the coagulation of egg proteins on contact with heat during cooking.

Procedure

A. (i) Take eggs at room temperature.
   (ii) Separate the whites of two eggs from their yolks and put into separate bowls.
   (iii) Whisk one white to soft peak stage and blend in the yolk.
   (iv) Heat a pan with 1 t of oil, and pour in the egg mixture and then fold over to make an omelette.
   (v) Turn on to a plate, sprinkle with salt, pepper, chopped coriander and serve.

B. (i) Beat the 2nd egg white to stiff peak and proceed as in A(iii-v).
   (ii) Repeat the experiment with more eggs using the following variations :

C. Repeat A(iii-v) but add the spices before foaming, and prepare the omelette. D Add finely chopped tomatoes in addition and prepare the omelette.
D. Add finely chopped tomatoes in addition and prepare the omelette.
E. Foam the whole egg and spices together and prepare an omelette.
F. Foam whole egg, prepare omelette but spread the spices and tomatoes on the raw side before finally folding into omelette. Compare the omelettes with respect to colour, volume, texture, flavour, and other qualities.

Observations

Tabulate the observations made as learnt and draw inferences indicating clearly the applications to which the foaming qualities of eggs can be put.

Precautions

1. Egg whites should be carefully separated so as not to mix even a trace of the yolk in it.
2. The eggs should not be straight from the refrigerator, but brought to room temperature.
3. The yolk should be blended immediately after the foam is formed and with gentle strokes to prevent air incorporated from coming out of the foam.

4. The mixture should be cooked instantly after blending.
5. Spicing should be added just prior to, during or after cooking.

Practice Exercises

1. Prepare omelettes using different methods of cooking and comment on the qualities of the product.
2. Prepare an omelette and fold it differently for service. Comment on suitability of the preparations for different meals.
3. List food foams you can think of in which eggs have been substituted by other ingredients.

EXPERIMENT 31

Aim

To demonstrate the effect of foaming in the preparation of cold and hot souffles.

Equipment

Baking dish, souffle dish, frying pan, weighing scale, measuring cups, spoons, spatula, beater refrigerator, oven.

Materials

Eggs, cream, lemon or orange, castor sugar, gelatin, water, essence, butter paper.

Principle

Souffles are egg white foams which can be modified to prepare savoury or sweet dishes. These preparations usually involve beating of egg whites till they foam to peak stage and then folding them into a flavoured base of other ingredients. If served hot they are usually baked just before service so as to prevent the foam from collapsing on cooling. In such preparations the air entrapped in the mixture during foaming expands on heating to give volumes which may be 2—2 Y$_2$ times greater on cooking. This results in products having a light soft texture and mouthfeel. However, on keeping the product its volume decreases due to some of the entrapped air bubbles escaping where the protein fibres are weak, having lost their elasticity. A well made product shows only slight variations in the volume because the denatured surface proteins on foaming, provide enough elasticity to stabilize the product. When served cold they are refrigerated immediately after the mixture is ready so that the protein films formed around the air bubbles get set preventing their escape and maintaining the volume of the dessert.

Procedure

A. Preparation of a cold souffle.

   (*i*) Prepare a souffle dish as demonstrated in Fig. 6.2.

  (*ii*) Wash and dry a small lemon. Grate the rind, extract the juice and keep aside.

 (*iii*) Take one egg, separate the white from the yolk, putting the yolk in a bowl along with 3/4 of the lemon extract and 30g of sugar.

  (*iv*) Place the bowl containing the mixture in a double boiler in which the water is simmering at 97°C and beat or whisk until creamy.

   (*v*) Remove the bowl from the boiler and continue beating till the mixture is cool.

  (*vi*) Sprinkle 5g (1/2T) gelatin in 30 ml water and keep aside for 5 minutes to swell. Then stir to dissolve.

 (*vii*) Add the gelatin to the egg yolk mixture gradually and mix well. Place in the refrigerator to set.

(*viii*) Whip 80g cream, and beat egg whites till peak stage.

  (*ix*) Fold in the whipped cream and the stiff egg white into the slightly set yolk mixture.

(*x*) Pour the mixture into the prepared souffle dish and leave in the refrigerator till set. Gently remove the paper from the dish before serving.

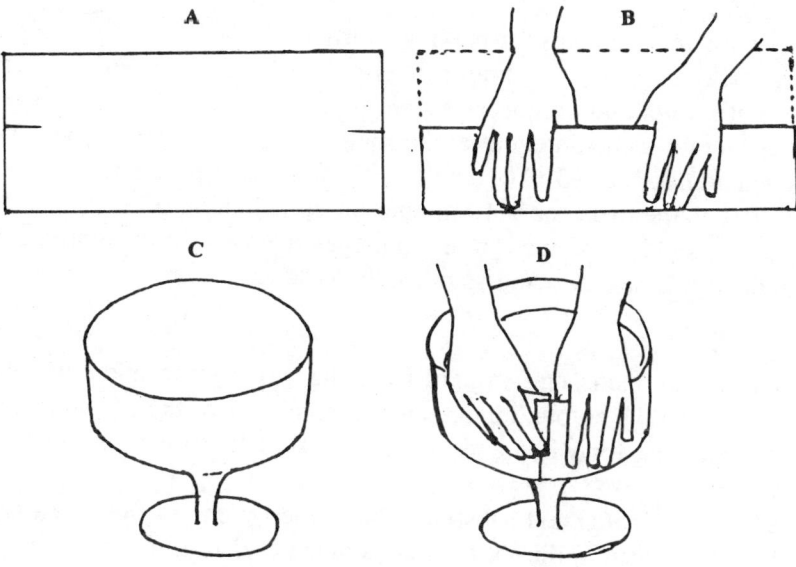

Fig. 6.2. Preparation of souffle dish.

(*a*) Size of paper   (*b*) Folding of grease proof paper   (*c*)   Souffle dish

(*d*) Securing the paper around the dish with double fold at bottom and standing 2" above the top edge of the dish.

B. Preparation of hot souffle.

(*i*) Melt 12g butter in a sauce pan stirring 12 g flour and stir cook for 1–2 minutes.

(*ii*) Gradually add 1/4 cup of scalded milk stirring continuously till it comes to a boil. Cook till the mixture coats the back of a spoon and remove from fire.

(*iii*) Prepare orange rind and extract juice of 1/2 orange. Stir the juice and 10 g of castor sugar into the sauce prepared in (*ii*).

(*iv*) Allow the mixture to cool and beat in $1\frac{1}{2}$ egg yolks.

(*v*) Whisk the egg whites to stiff peak stage and gently fold them into the prepared yolk mixture.

(*vi*) Spoon the mixture into a greased oven proof dish and bake at 177°C (350°F) for 20 minutes.

(*vii*) Serve hot decorated with orange rind.

C. Make variations in the souffle recipes A and B with regard to:

(*i*) The kind of beater used.

(*ii*) Improper yolk — white separation.

(*iii*) Amount of added ingredients.

Subject the samples to sensory evaluation.

Observations

Record the observations made through evaluation of A, B and C with respect to volume, % sag after

10 minutes at room temperature, texture, taste and acceptability. Indicate the applications of the foams as used in food preparation.

Precautions

1. Use dishes with vertical sides for making souffles.
2. To prevent sticking, coat the baking dish with butter and sugar. For cold souffles rinse out the dishes with water and do not wipe dry.
3. Bake or refrigerate immediately after the foam mixture is ready. Do not freeze.
4. Preheat oven an bake at 193°C to obtain a dry and stable product.
5. Leave souffles in the oven for 5–10 minutes after switching off.
6. To prevent their sudden collapse on serving, open the oven door slightly to enable temperature to gradually come down and stabilise the product.

Practice Exercises

1. Prepare souffles by using egg straight from the refrigerator, and comment on the effect temperature has on the colour, texture and acceptability of the product.
2. Substitute whole egg for white and prepare the souffle. Comment on the product and its suitability.
3. List some non-egg foams and substitute these one by one in the preparation of any food product. Discuss the suitability of the foams in the preparation of hot and cold souffles for making vegetarian meals.

EXPERIMENT 32

Aim

To study the effect of yolk contamination on the volume and texture of Angel Cake.

Equipment

Bowl, beater, oven, standard cups and spoons, weighing scale, baking dish, spatula, wooden spoon and butter paper.

Materials

Egg, cream of tartar, castor sugar refined flour (Maida), essence.

Principle

Angel cake are prepared from egg white foam stabilized with cream of tartar sugar and mixed gently with other cake ingredients. Since the foamy base entraps a large quantity of air, which expands on baking, the finished product is light, tender and airy in texture hence the name angel cake.

Procedure

A. *Basic Angel Cake*

   (*i*) Seive 1/2 cup flour and 6 tablespoons (T) of castor sugar into separate bowls.

  (*ii*) Separate 3 egg whites and whisk them to stiff peak stage.

 (*iii*) Fold in seived 1/4 t cream of tartar.

 (*iv*) Fold 1/2 the sugar in the egg whites followed by flour, essence and the rest of the sugar.

  (*v*) Put the cake mixture into an ungreased baking dish and bake at 168°C for 1 hour.

B. Repeat the procedure in A allowing a few drops of yolk to mix with whites.

C. Repeat the procedure in A using whole eggs instead of white only.
    Compare the results of the 3 procedures A, B and C.

Observations

Tabulate the observations made and study the effect of adding yolk in the preparation of angel cakes with respect to their colour, texture, volume, ease of removal from baking tin and general acceptability.

Precautions

  1. Separate egg whites carefully from the yolks.

  2. Adhere strictly to baking time and temperature.

  3. Let the cake cool after removal from the pan before evaluation.

Practice Exercises

  1. Prepare sponge cakes using whole egg and egg white only. Compare the colour, texture and applicability of the two products in food preparation.

2. Prepare idli batter and comment on the quality of the foam formed. What happens to the foam if the batter is kept for one day. Prepare idlis from both the batters and note down the differences in quality of the products.
3. Observe the foaming qualities of two brands of icecream. What makes you prefer one from the other. Explain the differences in the light of what you have learnt.

Microscopic structure of an emulsion as seen in the preparation of mayonnaise.

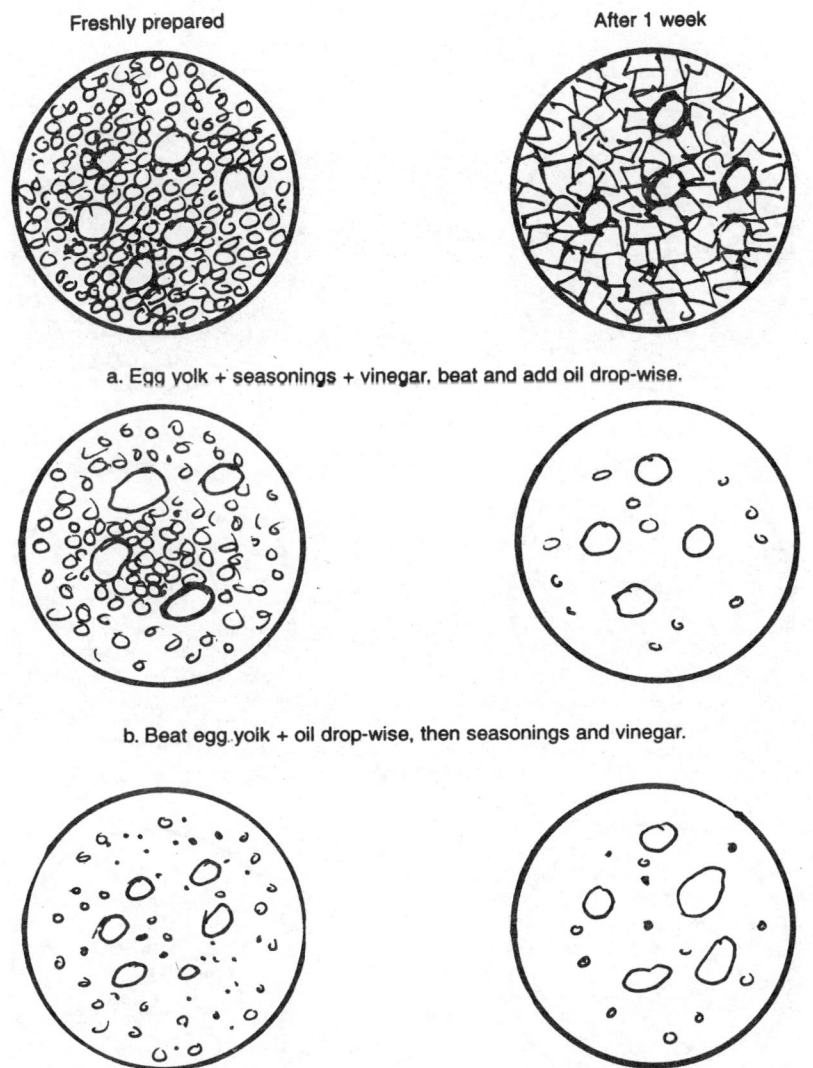

Freshly prepared   After 1 week

a. Egg yolk + seasonings + vinegar, beat and add oil drop-wise.

b. Beat egg yolk + oil drop-wise, then seasonings and vinegar.

c. Egg yolk + seasonings, + 1/3 vinegar and oil drop-wise alternately.

Plate IX: A. Effect of varying the method of combining ingredients on the formation of the emulsion.

The slides indicate that varying the method of combining ingredients affects the structure and thereby stability of emulsions.

Microscopic structure of an emulsion as seen in the preparation of mayonnaise.

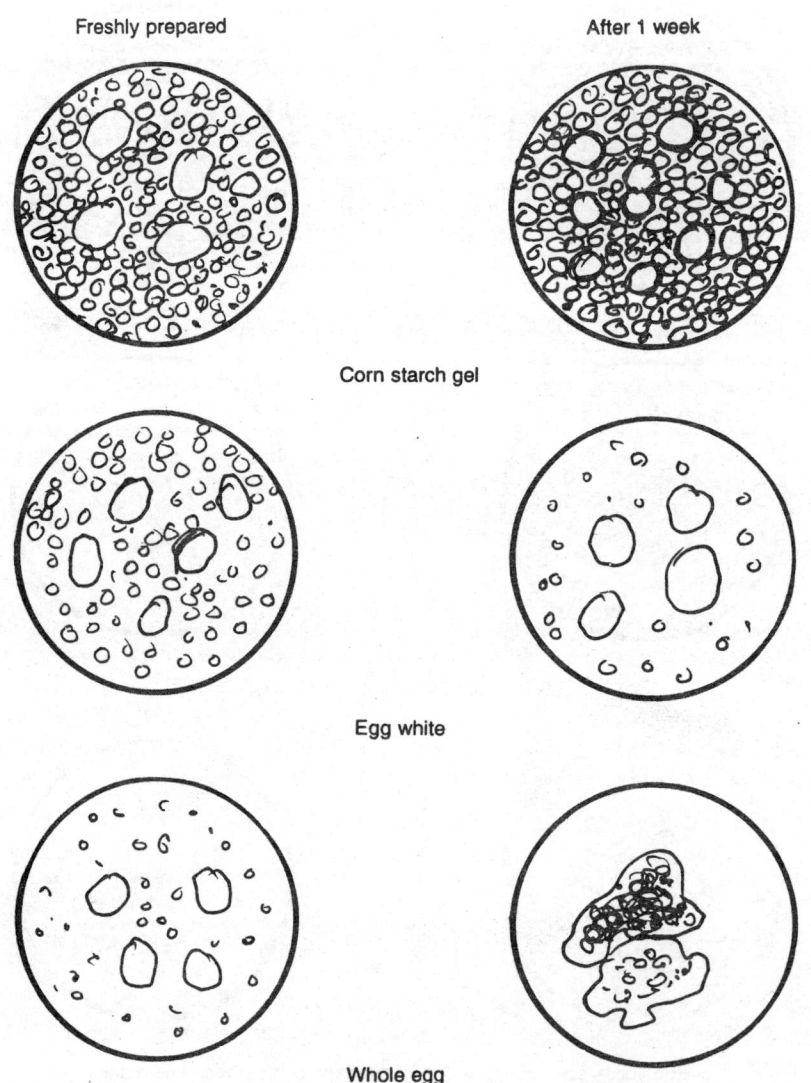

Freshly prepared · After 1 week

Corn starch gel

Egg white

Whole egg

Plate IX: B. Effect of using different emulsifying agents on emulsion formation.

It is apparent that different emulsifying agents affect emulsification and the network formed reflects stability.

Microscopic structure of an emulsion as seen in the preparation of mayonnaise.

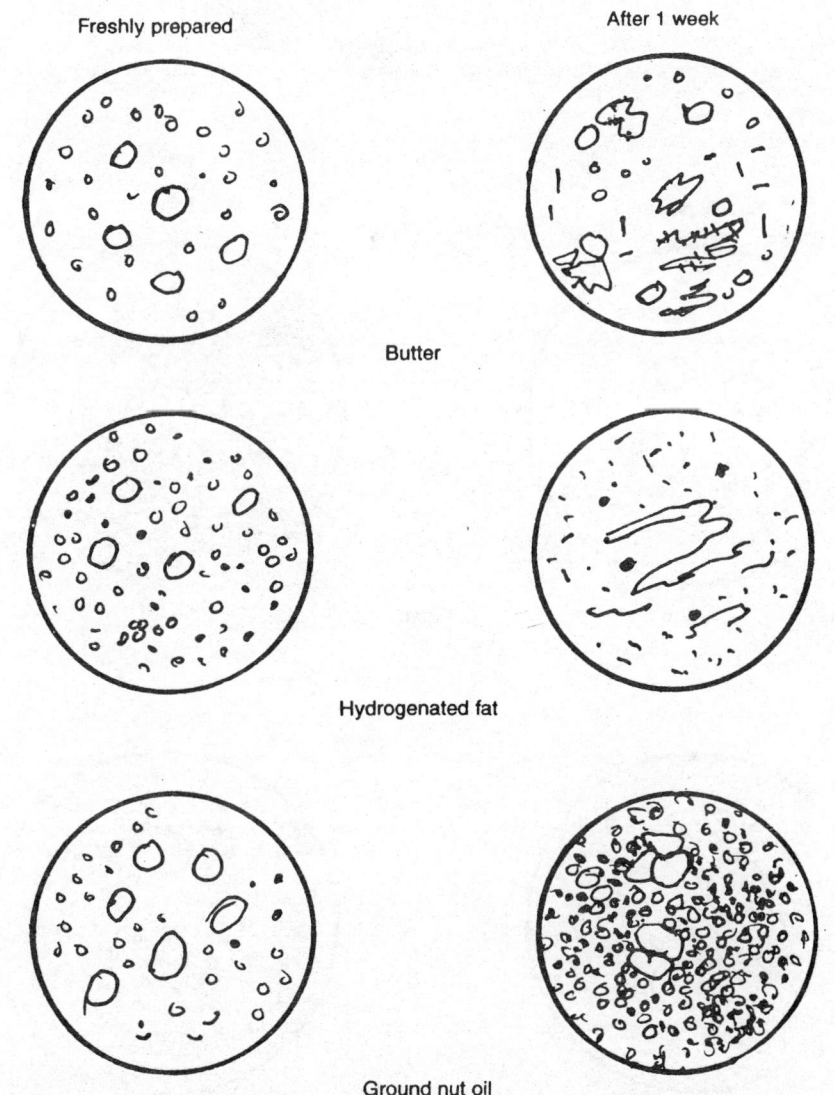

Freshly prepared

After 1 week

Butter

Hydrogenated fat

Ground nut oil

Plate IX: C. Effect of adding different fats relating to quality of emulsion.

It will be noticed that for freshly prepared samples the most even texture is obtained using butter, hydrogenated fat giving a denser product. After one week structures destabilize, the ground-nut oil providing a denser structure.

Microscopic structure of an emulsion as seen in the preparation of mayonnaise.

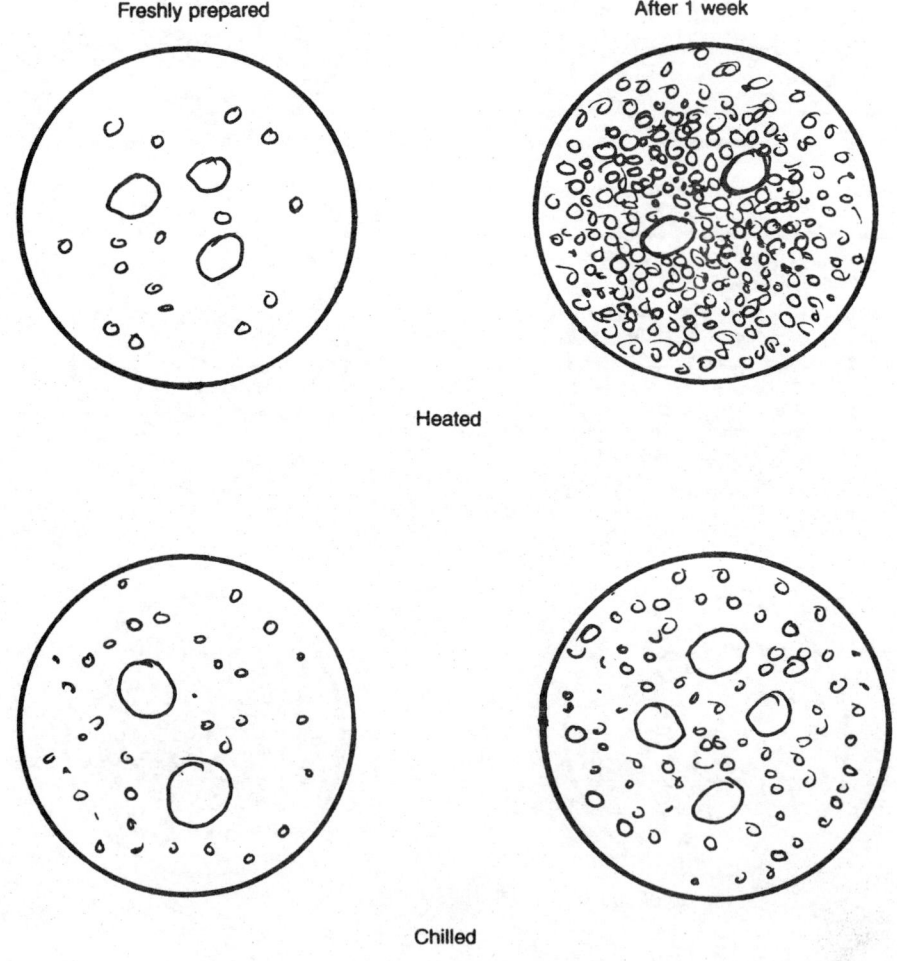

Plate IX: D. Effect of temperature of ingredients on emulsion formation.

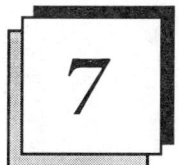

7

Meats and Meat Substitutes

The term *meat* signifies the edible part of animals, birds, fish and seafood, or insects eaten as food around the globe. Thus, all meats are rich sources of protein, fat and micro nutrients in the nonvegetarian diet. For people surviving on plant foods certain foods have been processed from plant sources which have equivalent nutrient composition to meat and are called *meat substitutes*.

Structure

Meat is made up of tube-like fibres tapered at both ends often seen when cooked meat or chicken is pulled apart during eating. Meats are usually valued for their protein content the structure of which varies widely according to the source of the meat and its composition. The proteins consist of amino acid units combined together through peptide linkages which may be globular or fibrous, the latter exhibiting elasticity to various extents, depending on the fibres in the muscle.

Globular Proteins

These proteins possess a 3-dimensional structure with the molecules scattered and arranged in a loose disorganised configuration. Such proteins therefore get easily dispersed to form colloids. Some examples are ovalbumin of egg whites, casein of milk, haemoglobin in animal tissues.

Fibrous Proteins

These are straighter and more organised in their structural arrangement the protein fibres being more closely packed together. Some fibres also have cross-linkages between adjacent amino acid chains which inhibit the penetration of water. Such proteins are therefore not water soluble as in the case of gluten of wheat. When wheat flour is kneaded into a dough the coiled fibres of gluten stretch but tend to return to ther original shape when the force is removed. Elastin of connective tissue also exhibits elasticity in contrast to collagen which has completely extended fibres that are nonelastic, as shown in Fig. 7.1.

During food preparation and processing the elastin structures undergo changes depending on the treatment they receive in the process.

The connective tissue of fish however, is made up entirely of collagen which is readily converted to soluble gelatin, while the muscle blocks readily separate out in the form of flakes.

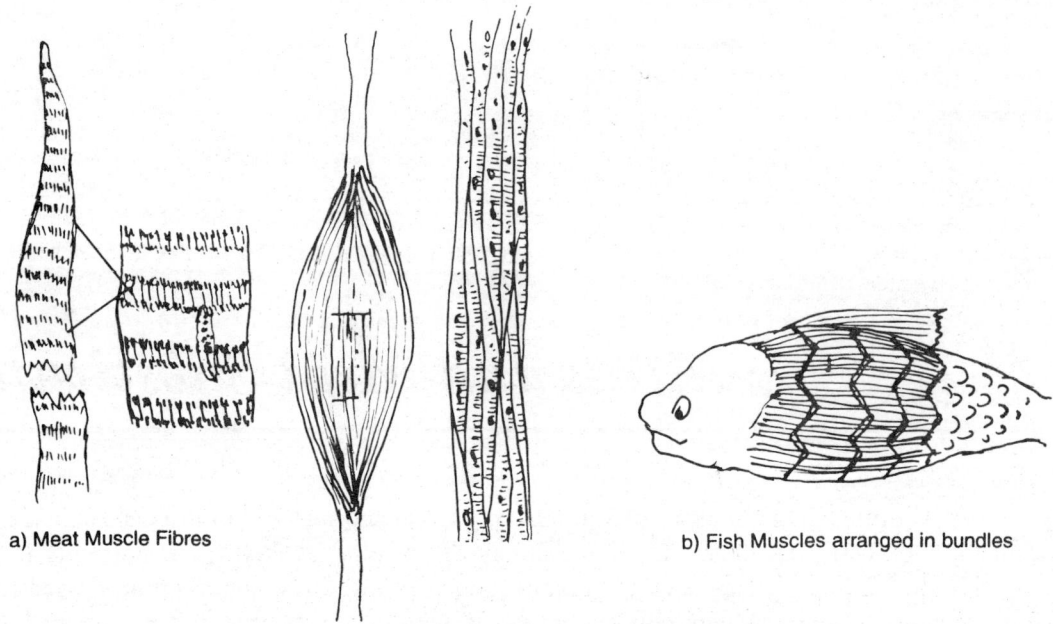

a) Meat Muscle Fibres   b) Fish Muscles arranged in bundles

Fig. 7.1. Structural arrangement of protein fibres.

Composition

Meats are important sources of proteins, fats, vitamins and minerals but relatively poor in carbo-hydrates. They form important components in dietaries of children and other vulnerable groups of the population. The approximate composition of meat muscle, fish, and poultry and seafood is presented in Table 7.1.

Table 7.1 Approximate composition of meats (%)

Meat	Water	CHO	Protein	Fat
Meat Muscle				
Lamb	65-75	1.0	10-25	3-10
Pork				45-50
Mutton				45-50
Organ meat	70-71	–	16-25	–
Liver	70-71	3.8	20-21	4-5
Poultry	51-68	–	16-20	11-32
Fish (white)	77-82	–	17-18	1-1.5
(oily)	57-73	–	19-25	11-12
Sea foods	72-87	0.1-3	6-18	1-3

Note: Fish is classified on the basis of the lipids present irrespective of its source.

Carbohydrates

As seen from Table 7.1 carbohydrates are present in very small amounts and mostly in storage form as glycogen which when required is converted into glucose, and circulates through the blood. The liver is the main storage organ for glycogen and usually has a higher percentage than that stored in the muscle. Glycogen is therefore often called *animal starch*. When an animal is slaughtered the glycogen is gradually converted to lactic acid. Fish however contain no carbohydrates.

Proteins

The proteins of muscle meat comprise of 55% myosin, 25% actin and 20% other proteins forming the different muscle fibres held together in a sheath. The different bundles are held together by connective tissue, made up of three distinct proteins, collagen, elastin and reticulin. Collagen forms tendons, cartilage and bone, while elastin largely forms the walls of arteries and other elastic ligaments which take the strain of movement. Reticulin is found in the muscle sheath mostly surrounding the liver, kidney and nerves, providing the tough stringy *gristle* in meat.

Meat from poultry and birds resembles meat of larger animals and undergoes similar changes during cooking. Fish meat also provides 14–20% proteins of high biological value (BV) providing all the essential amino acids, but being more delicate in its structure tends to cook quickly at lower temperatures.

Fats

Fats appear in meats in the form of true storage fat as well as lipids, about 50% of the fat being saturated. The amount of fat present in meat varies with age, breed and feed of the animal and the cut. For example lamb or goat's meat may contain from 3–10% lipids as against 40-50% in pork or other red meats.

Oily fish however, contain 10–21% fat mainly as polyunsaturated fatty acids (PUFA), but also provide cholesterol. Some fish and their oils are good sources of essential fatty acids containing the right proportions of n_3 : n_6 components, essential for health.

Vitamins

Meats are good sources of thiamine, riboflavin and nicotinic acid, but also contain a little vitamin E, A, D and C or ascorbic acid. Oily fish are excellent sources of vitamins A and D and provide some water soluble B-vitamins as well. Fish oils are therefore often recommended as supplements in deficiencies of fat soluble vitamins.

Minerals

Meats are rich sources of phosphorus, and iron which is present mainly in the liver and kidney. While calcium is also present it is mainly deposited in the bones which are not edible.

Pigments

The pigments present are *myoglobin* in the muscle and *haemoglobin* in blood, the former mainly responsible for the colour of muscle meat. When freshly cut meat is exposed to the air the myoglobin gets oxygenated to form *oxymyoglobin* which gives a bright red colour that slowly darkens. Meat of young animals is lighter in colour but when the muscles are exercised frequently they get darker.

Fish meat does not contain any pigment other than the hemoglobin in blood seen when cut afresh, and therefore the flesh does not change colour on cooking.

Water

As apparent from Table 7.1 meats contain a high percentage of water although it varies with the cut of meat, tenderness and amount of muscular development of the animal, bird or sea food. Water is the medium through which all other substances are transported in the body as required. Fish contains a higher proportion of water than most meats, with edible portions varying between 55–65% except in the case of small varieties consumed whole.

Properties of Meat Proteins

Meat proteins exhibit many important properties which account for the variety of products that are prepared by altering the cooking methods and conditions for pre-preparation and processing.

Solubility

The fibrous proteins are insoluble and therefore not largely affected during cooking or processing, as against globular proteins which disperse easily to form colloidal solutions and become reactive to the conditions of cooking.

Denaturation

Proteins undergo a process of denaturation in which their primary amino acid sequences remain the same while the shape of the molecule changes due to the breakdown of cross linkages in the structure of proteins. This phenomenon is irreversible and therefore affects the properties of the proteins. Denatured proteins are more easily acted upon by digestive enzymes and therefore cooked meats and other high protein foods are more easily digested.

Coagulation

This is a process through which proteins become insoluble because the unfolded molecules intertwine with each other to form clumps which on further manipulation or heating harden and set. It is for this reason that when meats are over-cooked they become hard and difficult to chew.

Shrinkage

Meat proteins coagulate at a higher temperature than egg, milk or plant proteins, therefore meat shrinks much more during cooking than other foods. The muscle proteins myosin and actin, denature at 40–50°C and shrink at 65°C. Well cooked meat reaches an internal temperature of 80°C.

On moist heating the collagen gets converted into soluble gelatin, while the elastin contracts causing shrinkage of the meat with consequent release of juices. Shrinkage is accompanied by tightening of meat fibres and therefore low temperature cooking gives best results.

Browning

Apart from shrinkage the pigments also get denatured to globin hemichrome which contributes to the greyish brown colour of meat. In addition, non enzymatic browning takes place during cooking as is seen when meats are roasted or grilled. This is referred to as *Maillard browning* and occurs due to the chemical reaction between a free amino group and carbonyl group in the food being cooked.

This browning makes the food attractive as well as imparts surface crispness which adds to the textural properties as well as seals in the juices and flavours. Tender cuts of meat are usually better cooked by dry heat methods such as roasting, grilling or microwave cooking.

Effect of Heat

Some of the effects of heat have already been described under the general properties of meat proteins, but, heating meat may either increase or decrease its tenderness depending on the amount and type of tissues in the cut, the temperatures to which they are subjected and the time for which they are heated. The time required for conversion of collagen to gelatin varies with the temperature and is best between 65-80°C. Cooking liquid from tough cuts which have been completely tenderized often gels on cooling due to this conversion.

The rate of heat penetration is an important determinant of tenderness, rather than only the temperature. It is therefore that, degree of doneness is judged by internal temperature of a cut. Various temperatures have been suggested in the literature according to the type of meat and the method of cooking used (Charley, 1982). The method which holds-in the moisture and reduces shrinkage is the most appropriate for cooking meats.

The temperature will vary with meat, poultry and fish, the fibres and connective tissues of the latter being far less tough than that of meat from large animals.

Effect of Acid

Acids used in cooking tend to toughen the meat and increase the cooking time. Therefore it is best to tenderize the meats as required before adding acid ingredients for taste. However, if meats are marinated in acidic foods like curd or in vinegar containing spices before cooking, the flavour, and tenderness improves and cooking time decreases. Moreover the strong odour of meats, fish or seafoods gets mellowed down enhancing the aroma of the cooked dishes.

Effect of Salt

Salt being hygroscopic in nature tends to draw out the moisture from the meat along with some of the juices responsible for flavour. This has an effect on heat penetration and tenderness. It is therefore recommended that meats be browned on the surface first to seal-in the moisture and flavours, and then salt and spices added. However, it depends on the final product desired, and if the juices are part of the dish as in curries and stews then salt may be added initially and simmered till ready.

Effect of Enzymes

Enzymes have a tenderizing effect on meats, as observed when meats are hung in cold storage. The protein splitting enzymes called *cathepsins* attack connective tissues separating the muscle fibres. This process called autolysis tenderizes the meat. The traditional practice of throwing a piece of raw papaya into the pan while cooking meat to tenderize it is based on the action of the enzyme *papain* present in papaya. Similarly, use of raw pineapple providing *bromelin* and figs supplying *ficin* are also used in different regions of the country.

In some countries, animals are injected with sterile papain solution before slaughter, or enzyme solutions or powders rubbed on to tough cuts of meat before packing in order to tenderize them by the time they are used for cooking.

Effect of Mechanical Action

This is a common method of separating the muscle fibres in meats by physical means, through the action of beating, pounding, cutting fine or mincing. Mechanical action is generally used to tenderize tough cuts of meat off or on the bone, before cooking. In India a large piece of broken porcelain was sometimes placed in the cooking pan, both for its mechanical action during heating as well as the leaching of ions during cooking which was believed to help in tenderizing the meat.

Commercially, electrical stimulation of carcasses is used following slaughter to bring about tenderization. This results in rapid muscle contractions which produce physical as well as biochemical effects.

Meat Quality

Meats from exercising animals or those struggling before slaughter are of poor quality and shelf life because of low glycogen reserves in the muscle and consequently less lactic acid.

Valuable water soluble vitamins are lost when moist cooking methods are used, unless the water is retained in the final preparation as in curries, soups and stews. The fat drippings from barbecued meats or other dry heat methods remove cholesterol, but along with it the fat soluble vitamins A, D, E, and K are also lost.

Freshly slaughtered meat is unsuitable for cooking due to the effects of rigor mortis. The quality improves on storage, when carcasses are suspended for 7–10 days before sale at cold storage temperatures, as this enables the conversion of glycogen to lactic acid which tenderizes the meats. Poultry meat undergoes similar changes.

Cooking Meat

Experience has shown that the best approach to cooking meats is to cook them at high temperature initially to coagulate the surface proteins and seal-in the moisture and flavours, then reduce the flame or source of heat for gradual heat penetration. This also makes the meat safer by destroying surface microorganisms. Cooking also affects colour, texture and flavour by bringing about changes in the water holding capacity of the tissues.

Cooking also influences the degree of tenderness of meats in three ways. The solid fat melts, collagen gets converted to soluble gelatin and the muscle fibres separate out to increase the tenderness, thereby increasing chewing properties and overall palatability. However, overcooking can also cause meats to become *rubbery* through excessive contraction of the muscle fibres leading to undue shrinkage, dryness and toughening.

Poultry, fish and seafood tend to soften more quickly as compared to meats, and therefore require less time to prepare. Reheating of meats in any form is not recommended as it toughens the fibres due to further shrinkage. Fish however, shrinks much less on cooking and due to the finely textured fibres and connective tissues, does not require cooking methods that involve long periods of heating. Good quality fish if cooked correctly should not have a strong fishy flavour.

Nutritionally, meats remain good sources of protein, fat, minerals and fat soluble vitamins. In addition, cooking increases the calcium content by partially dissolving out the mineral from the bones and making it available for consumption.

Colour of meat

Differences in the colour of meats can be attributed to the concentration of myoglobin in the muscles which represents 75% of the total pigment present. The rest is due to the haemoglobin of the blood. In the unoxygenated form myoglobin contains iron in its ferrous state which imparts a purplish red colour to the meat. When the meat is cut the surface gets exposed to the air and the pigment becomes oxygenated to oxymyoglobin which makes the meat look bright red. This is due to the conversion of the ferrous iron to its ferric form. This colour however, is not very stable and on prolonged exposure the myoglobin shifts to become metmyoglobin which gives the meat a brown colour.

Colour of meats has always been associated with its degree of doneness, the hues indicating the tenderness or dryness of the meat, which also corresponds with the amount of oxygmyoglobin present in the product after cooking.

Meats cured with nitrites remain red or pink even after cooking as nitrites combine with myoglobin to form nitric-oxide-myoglobin. On cooking this compound is converted to stable nitrosohemochrome which is red or pink in colour as seen in cooked ham or bacon.

Tenderness in Meat

Although tenderness of raw meat depends largely on age, breed, feed and environmental conditions in which the animals are reared, tough meats can also be tenderized in many ways before or during cooking. Some methods commonly used have been discussed under properties of meats (p.146).

Long slow methods of tenderizing are not necessary for fish, and seafood because their fibres are more delicate, connective tissue is finer and shrink much less on cooking than meat and poultry.

Flavour of Meat

Less tender cuts have more flavour compounds than cuts with muscles that have been less excercised. Lactones and sulphur containing compounds contribute to flavour in meats. Quick cooking methods like microwave or pressure cooking do not give the best flavour as compared to slow long time methods, by which a meaty flavour develops. Each type of meat has a characteristic aroma often referred to as a meaty, or fishy smell, which results from the heating of the fat present in the meat. Reheating cooked meat looses the characteristic aroma by which it is identified on first cooking. Such meats are susceptible to oxidative rancidity and acquire a warmed-over flavour.

Effect of Storage

Freshly slaughtered meat is unsuitable for cooking and has to be stored under suitable cold storage temperatures for at least 7–10 days to develop tenderness, keeping quality and flavour. During this period, surface bacteria grow because of the high moisture content therefore once marketed it should be cooked and used up within 3–4 days to prevent spoilage. Storage at low temperatures (–18°C) is important till used. Cooked meat too is highly perishable and preferably bought in small quantities for prompt use.

Advances in controlled atmosphere packaging have helped to increase the shelf life of meats to a large extent. The Central Institute of Fisheries Technology (CIFT) has developed a new technology for ready–to–serve fish curry which is packed in three layers of flexible pouches that ensure a shelf life or one year. (AFST (I), 1999). .

Meat Substitutes

Meat substitutes are high protein foods resembling meat in nutritional quality which can replace meats in vegetarian dietaries, or provide cheaper alternatives. Substitutes may be processed to appear and possess sensory qualities exactly similar to meat products, or cheaper cuts of meat may be combined with ingredients from plant sources to manufacture products that provide cheaper nutrition as required.

Fish meal prepared from species that are usually not eaten are used to manufacture meat substitutes by applying processing techniques that deodourize and detoxify it for incorporation into food products. The shrimp industry produces 30–40% of the potential recoverable proteinaceous by–products largely used for poultry feed. In addition to their protein contributions other seafoods are rich sources of carotenoids (Venugopal, 1995).

Traditional methods of preparing meat substitutes involved grinding foods rich in protein together, making a dough and passing it through metal sieves into hot oil, or shaping them by hand and cooking by different methods for using in meals and as snacks. Some examples are the preparation of koftas, vadas, kebabs and the like. Textured vegetable proteins in the form of dehydrated products are being processed. On rehydration and cooking they possess all the qualities of meat and choices of meat sized pieces or a granular texture resembling minced meat are available. These are extensively used as such or as ingredients in cooking.

Today meat substitutes are prepared or processed by blenderizing, texturizing and extrusion, using foods like soyabean, peanut, and defatted products as supplementing agents for improving the protein content of foods. *Mince Savour* is a granular textured protein product which is made by extrusion from defatted soya flour seasoned with herbs and spices for use with minced meat. It contains 40% protein, 30% carbohydrates, 6% fat and 24% moisture, fibre and ash and has a storage life of one year at room temperature.

Since meats are expensive, comminuted meat products are now being processed using low-cost non-meat extenders like shredded potatoes, wheat flour, riceflour and bread crumbs. A goat *tikka* has been developed, having unique textural properties and high acceptability (Sahoo and Verma, 1999).

Various cheese analogues or substitutes are also being processed from vegetable proteins and fats, the incentives being, enchancement of protein in diets at lower cost and ready availability without jeopardizing health.

Experiments 33-35 demonstrate the effects of some techniques on tenderization and cooking quality of meats and meat substitutes.

EXPERIMENT 33

Aim

To demonstrate the effects of pre-preparation techniques on meat tenderization.

Equipment

Weighing scales, cooking pans, bowls, knife, spoons, standard cups and spoons, stop watch oven.

Materials

Meats, lemon, curds, vinegar, raw papaya, ginger, garlic and salt.

Principle

Tenderization is the process by which a gradual breakdown of connective tissues takes place between muscle fibres of the meat. This is then followed by the action of proteolytic enzymes present to bring about the breakdown of the muscle fibres. Tenderization can be hastened by any of the methods already discussed (p. 146-149).

Salt solubilizes the proteins, whereas enzymes act till the meat reaches a temperature of 82°C after which they become inactivated. Mechanical and electrical stimulation methods work through providing ultrasonic vibrations.

Procedure

A. (*i*) Take five 50g portions of meat and wipe dry with a moist clean cloth or kitchen towel.
  (*ii*) Prick the pieces with a fork.
  (*iii*) Apply the following on the surface of the meat pieces rubbing in the ingredients gently and keeping each portion for 1/2 hour.

  (*a*) One teaspoon (1t) salt.
  (*b*) Two tablespoons (2T) raw papaya juice.
  (*c*) One tablespoon ginger-garlic paste.
  (*d*) 50g beaten curd.
  (*e*) 1t lemon juice or synthetic vinegar.

  (*iv*) Cook each portion separately in a covered pan on low to moderate heat till the required tenderness and flavour is obtained.
  (*v*) Carefully note the time taken to cook the meat, its degree of tenderness, initial and final weight, and the flavour obtained. Note down the % shrinkage that takes place.

B. Repeat experiment A using chicken instead of meat.

C. Repeat A using fish or prawns.

Observations

Tabulate your observations as learnt for A, B and C. Draw inferences as to which method gives the best colour, flavour, portion size and tenderness for each kind of meat used. Discuss the applications of each alternative used in the light of preparation of meat dishes or products.

Precautions

1. Do not wash meat pieces, only wipe well with moist cloth as it will lose its juices.
2. Prick the meat sufficiently before applying tenderizers to ensure uniform penetration.
3. Keep aside for at least 1/2 an hour before cooking.

Practice Exercises

1. Prepare meat, chicken and fish tikka without tenderizing the meat as learnt. Comment on the tenderness, juiciness, colour, texture and mouthfeel of the product. Compare with products prepared in the experiment.
2. Name other traditionally used tenderizing agents. Make a list of dishes for which they are used.
3. List meat dishes for the preparation of which mechanical methods of tenderization are used. Prepare one dish with and without tenderizing and evaluate its acceptability.

EXPERIMENT 34

Aim
To determine the effect of time and temperature on cooking of meats.

Equipment
Cooking pans, burners, ladles, oven, chopper, bowls and stop watch.

Materials
Deboned meat, chicken and fish fillets, salt and pepper to taste, water.

Principle
While meat, poultry and fish are governed by the same principles as learnt, they differ in the structure and elasticity of their muscle fibres. Each method of cooking therefore has effect on the outcome of the final product depending on the temperatures involved, and the time taken.

Procedure
A. (*i*) Add 10 one-inch cubes of meat in a litre of water and simmer for 1 hour. Remove one piece and keep aside in a bowl.

  (*ii*) Continue cooking nonstop removing one piece after every 15 minutes and keeping aside in bowls. Note the time when each piece was taken out of the pan, using a stop watch.

  (*iii*) Check the pieces for colour, flavour, texture, chewability and general acceptability by scoring on a 6–point scale representing 5 for excellent and 0 for poor or not acceptable. Total the scores for each quality characteristic.

B. (*i*) Repeat experiment as in A using chicken pieces instead.

  (*ii*) Remove the 1st piece when it is done, and note the time taken.

C. Repeat experiment B using fish or any seafood.

Observations
Observe the samples from A, B and C, tabulate results of sensory evaluation as learnt, giving the time, for which each sample was cooked and the temperature at which each sample was removed from the pan for evaluation temperature. Record the acceptability scores and comment on the applications of the samples in food preparation and processing. Comment on the best method of cooking each type of meat explaining why you think so.

Precautions
1. Temperature should be constant at simmering, throughout the experiment.
2. Pieces should all be the same size for all meats.
3. The size of the pans should be the same.

Practice Exercises

1. Cook nutrinuggets (meat substitute from soyabean) as learnt in (*i-iii*). How does this compare with the meat samples in the experiment.

2. Marinate the different meats as learnt in experiment 31 and cook using broiling, roasting and deep frying methods. Comment on the acceptability of the products.

3. How can meat products be cooked for best results. Give reasons for your choice.

EXPERIMENT 35

Aim

To test the acceptability of texturized food product as an alternative to meat.

Equipment

Gas burner, cooking pans, ladle, standard cups and measuring cylinder.

Materials

Nutrinuggets, ginger, garlic, onions, coriander seeds, curd, salt, red chilli powder, garam masala, green cardamom, cloves cinnamon, cumin seeds, turmeric powder, cooking oil and hot water.

Principle

Nutrinuggets are small pieces textured from soya protein and made to provide a meat-like texture, chewability and other sensory characteristics on reconstitution and cooking. The product contains 50–55% good quality protein and is rich in lysine, an essential amino acid. Defatted soyabean flour is also an important source of manufacture of other meat analogues, which are low in fat, cholesterol and sodium, that are present in appreciable amounts in fresh meats.

Procedure

A. (*i*) Soak 20g nutrinugget chunks for 1/2 an hour in sufficient water to allow them to swell.
  (*ii*) Prepare the marinade by mixing 75g curd, salt, chilli pd. and garam masala according to taste.
 (*iii*) Squeeze the water from the swollen chunks and add to the marinade prepared in (*ii*). Leave this mixture undisturbed for 1/2 an hour.
 (*iv*) Heat 2T oil in a cooking pan and fry 40g thinly sliced onions till they are golden brown.
  (*v*) Add the marinated chunks and stir fry till they are lightly coloured.
 (*vi*) Make a paste of ginger, garlic and the remaining spices, and add to the pan.
 (*vii*) Continue to cook till the fat separates out from the mixture.
(*viii*) Add one cup of hot water and cook on low heat till the spices are well blended and the chunks are cooked but tender.

B. (*i*) Follow experiment A (*i-viii*) using fresh bone less meat pieces instead of nutrinuggets.
 (*ii*) Compare the results of A and B in terms of colour, texture, flavour, chewability, taste, aroma and time of cooking.

Observation

Tabulate your observations for both the experiments A and B, and comment on the sensory characteristics of the products obtained. Draw your inferences with respect to their suitability and applicability for both home food preparation and food processing.

Precautions

1. Soak the nutrinuggest for at least 1/2 an hour before cooking.

2. Use constant moderate to low temperatures for cooking to avoid excessive shrinkage and toughening of the protein fibres.

Practice Exercises

1. Prepare nutrinugget keema using your own recipe and compare its organoleptic properties with those of mutton keema

2. Prepare paneer tikka using cottage cheese and soya paneer. Evaluate the sensory qualities of both and comment on their acceptability.

3. List the uses to which meat substitutes can be put in meal preparation. Compare the costs of the natural products with those of the textured alternatives used.

8

Cereals, Pulses and Legumes

Cereals, pulses and legumes are basic to vegetarian diets in India. It is virtually unthinkable to consume a cereal without a pulse or legume in traditional dietaries, and therefore they are being discussed together. There are 16 different types of cereals, 11 varieties of pulses or *dals* as they are commonly known and 4-6 types of legumes used in the country. These foods are good sources of macro-and micro-nutrients but individually lack in some essential amino acids. Together they tend to supplement each other to improve the nutritional contribution and protein availability from diets.

Structure

Being grain foods, the structure of cereals, pulses and legumes is basically similar in that, they contain a seed coat, an aleurone layer, endosperm and germ as indicated in Fig. 8.1. All grains are covered with a husk which is removed during harvesting. Each layer contributes different macro and micro-nutrients according to the composition of the extracted products and their use in food preparation and processing.

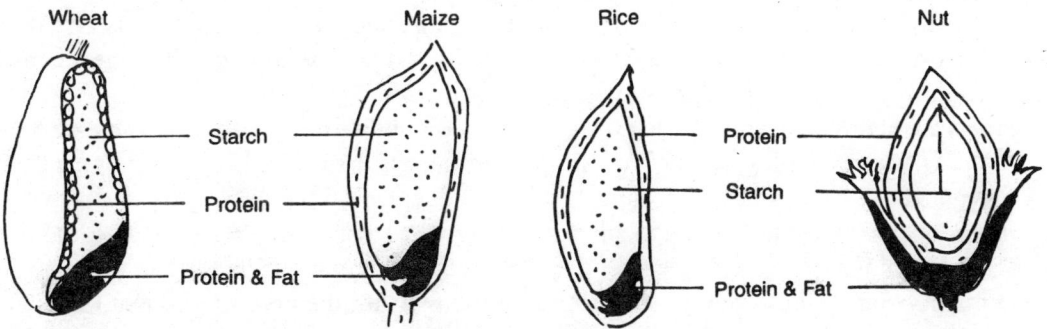

Fig. 8.1. Longitudinal section of grain foods.

Composition

Grain foods contain relatively low moisture content and are therefore classed as semiperishable foods as compared to their fresh counterparts. The endosperm layers are almost entirely made up of carbohydrates in the form of characteristic starches, by which they can be microscopically identified (See experiments in chapter 2). Proteins, vitamins, minerals and related substances are concentrated in the aleurone and germ whereas fat is present only in the germ along with fat soluble vitamins and lipids. The approximate composition is presented in Table 8.1.

Table 8.1 Composition of cereals, pulses and legumes (g per 100 g)

	Cereals	*Pulses*	*Legumes*
Moisture	9–15	10–13	9–12
Protein	6–12	17–28	22–43
Fat	1–7	0.3–5.6	2.5–4.6
ohydrate	60-79	50-70	20-60
Minerals	0.6-3.8	2-3	3-6

Source: Nutritive Value of Indian Foods National Institute of Nutrition, Hyderabad. India. ICMR. 2005.

Cereals

Cereals rank the highest in carbohydrates, the starch content of parboiled milled rice (*Oryza sativa*) being 97%. They also contain cellulose, most of which is lost in the process of refining. As seen from Table 8.1 cereals are poorer in their protein content than pulses and legumes although they provide an important dietary source because of the quantity in which they are consumed. The quality of proteins is however, of lower biological value (B.V.) than that of milk, eggs and meats. Cereal proteins are deficient in the amino acid lysine and have very little tryptopan and methionine.

Cereals also provide water soluble vitamins, minerals and fibre. They are fairly good sources of B-group vitamins especially thiamine and niacin, but their availability depends largely on the preparation methods used. Cereals also contain carotenes but are poor sources of vitamin C. The most commonly used cereals are wheat, rice and maize or corn although some minor cereals, like *bajra, jowar* and *ragi* among others are also used infrequently.

Most cereals are poor in minerals and micronutrients, except phosphorus (P), but unfortunately this is found in bound form as *phytin* and unavailable to the body. Phytin phosphorus also interferes with the absorption of dietary calcium and iron. Cereals contain calcium too although rice is a poor source. The millets *bajra and ragi* are good sources of iron.

Cereals are rarely consumed as harvested and need to be processed to different extents before being used as such or as ingredients for the preparation of dishes and incorporation into meals. They are generally used as flour ground to various degrees of fineness, grits and semolina for preparation of porridges, desserts and snacks. The nutrient contribution varies with the different stages of extraction of the cereals, coarser products providing more nutrients than finer ones which include mainly starch and some gluten forming proteins from the endosperm. (Sultan, 1972).

Wheat

There are mainly three varieties of wheat *Triticum vulgare, Triticum durum and Triticum aestivum* or bulgar wheat, mainly used for making flour suitable for breads, cakes and biscuits, and the latter for semolina and pastas. On milling the grains provide strong flours and products like semolina and wheat germ through the various extraction fractions.

Rice

Various kinds of rice are consumed in the different regions of India extending from raw, parboiled to refined. Unlike wheat, rice grains are usually cooked whole by various moist heat cooking methods like boiling, steaming, baking or sauteeing with spices and then boiling for preparation of *pulaos*. Boiled rice may be used as an ingredient in salads and puddings too. It is also prepared by dry heat methods and consumed as snack in the form of puffed rice. Other processed forms used are parched, flaked, ground as semolina and flours. Flours are commonly used to prepare doughs, batters and pastes of different consistencies to provide a variety of dishes and food products.

Parboiled rice contains significant amounts of thiamine, as the vitamin from the outer layers seeps into the inner parts of the grain during parboiling protecting it from loss during milling.

Rice bran produced in modern rice mills is mixed with rice germ and starch. The yield of bran depends on the degree of milling of brown rice which may vary from 5–10 per cent. Rice bran is a rich source of proteins, fats, minerals and micronutrients such as B-vitamins and trace elements. Rice bran also contains a high level of roughage and phytochemicals. Today, rice bran forms an important ingredient for processing of functional foods and health supplements (Narasinga Rao, 2000).

Corn

Corn is not so extensively used except in the North and that too as maize flour for making *roti* seasonally in winter eaten along with dark green leafy preparations, or when freshly harvested and roasted on the cob. Popped corn is a popular item especially with children. Cornflour however, is used as a thickening agent in baked dishes, soups and desserts. Yellow maize provides some β-carotene, but other varieties have little or no vitamin A activity or vitamin C.

Other Cereals

The other minor cereals also called coarse grains or millets are *bajra, jowar ragi* and others. These have gradually been replaced by refined less nutritious forms. If used, they are mixed with other cereal flours and used seasonally.

Bajra

Commonly known as pearl millet (*Pennisetum typhoideum*), it contains 12.4% moisture, 8.8—16.1% protein, 5% fat, 67% carbohydrate, 1.2% fibre and 2.7% minerals mainly calcium, phosphorus and iron. The digestibility of *bajra is* poor because of the presence of phytin. The main proteins are prolamine, globulin and albumins. The grain is high in the amino acid trytophan and fair amounts of lysine are present. The carbohydrates mostly starch comprises of 32% amylose and the rest amylopectin.

Jowar

After wheat and rice, *jowar or Sorghum (Sorghum vulgare)* is an important cereal and is processed and cooked whole as grits or used as flour. Sorghum has a higher protein content than maize and a lower fat content. The lipid consists of triglycerides which are rich in unsaturated fatty acids and phospholipids, mainly lectithin. The minerals (1.6%) are calcium, magnesium potassium and iron. It contains the same amounts of riboflavin and pyridoxine as maize but is richer in pantothenic acid, niacin and biotin, the niacin being in a freely available form. However, on germination it produces a cyanogenetic glucoside *dhurrin,* which releases hydrogen cyanide on hydrolysis leading to poisoning (Manay and Shadaksharaswamy, 1987).

Ragi

Also called finger millet (*Eleusine coracana*) is usually used as flour for various preparations *Ragi* is nutritionally better than rice and other cereals and contains 13.1% moisture, 7.1% protein, 1.3% fat, 76.3% carbohydrates and 2.2% minerals. It is a rich source of calcium, phosphorus and iron, but the phosphorus is in the form of phytin phosphorus. It is a poor source of riboflavin but contains other B-vitamins in fair amounts. The major proteins are prolamins and glutelins with an adequate supply of essential amino acids. *Ragi* is also malted for use in beverages.

Other cereals like barley (*Hordeum vulgare*) oats (*Avena saliva*) and rye (*Secale cereale*) are also used after malting for production of breakfast foods and in the brewery industry. The variety of oats cultivated in India is *A. byzantina* and provides 13.6% protein 7.6% fat and is a good source of B-vitamins. These cereals however get attacked by the fungus *ergot* which can cause toxicity. Many hybrid cereals are now being cultivated to get rid of toxic vulnerability, such as a cross between wheat and rye called *Triticale.*

Pulses

Pulses are used in many forms as whole, split and dehusked, to be further prepared as such or ground and used for batter, pastes and doughs before being subjected to different cooking and processing methods.

Pulses are good sources of proteins though they do not contain all the amino acids to the same extent as milk and eggs. However, they supplement the missing amino acids of cereals when eaten together with them or through cereal-pulse combinations, because pulses are rich in lysine. Red gram however, is deficient in tryptophan which cereals or other quality protein foods supplement. This helps to improve the protein availability from diets. Traditionally all diets in India are based on such combinations, or ones in which milk, meat or eggs may be combined with cereals and pulses in meals and snacks, the latter protein foods performing the supplemental function.

Legumes

Legumes are basically foods casually referred to as *beans,* and consumed in dry and fresh forms when in season. Among the legumes soybean has the highest protein and fat, and the lowest carbohydrate content of all the grains. It is therefore extensively used for manufacture of meat substitutes. The usual way of consuming legumes and pulses is to soak and boil them and when tender use them as such in salads, curries or in mixed vegetables.

Pulses and legumes are clubbed together in terms of supplemental effects on cereals. They however, cannot be considered good sources of minerals and micronutrients in the small amounts in which they are consumed.

Properties of Grain Foods

Cereals, legumes and pulses exhibit the combined properties of their components namely starches, proteins and fats. These are enumerated briefly as follows:

Gelation

When these foods are soaked they absorb water and swell, and form weak or strong gels on cooking

APPLICATIONS OF PROTEINS

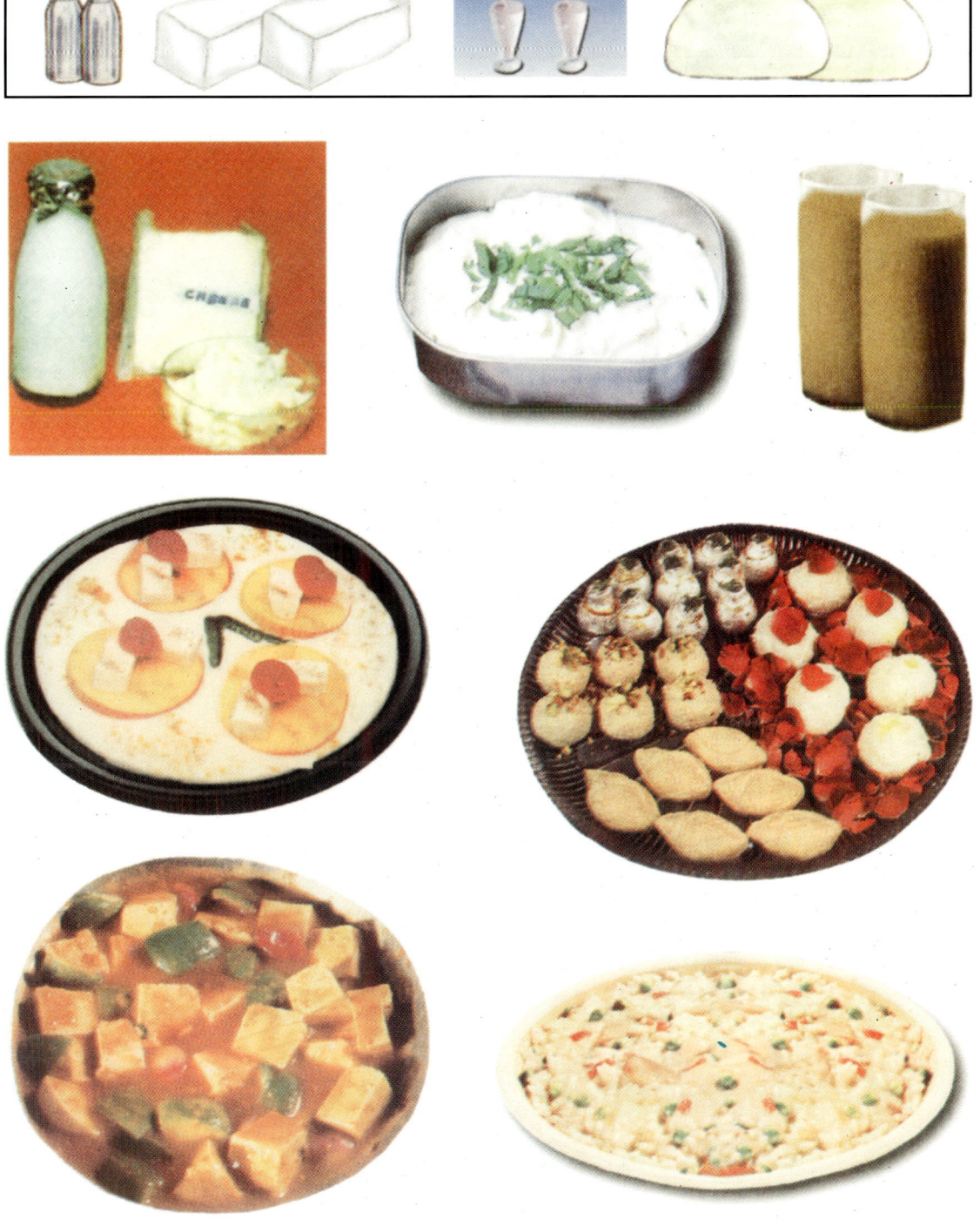

Plate X-A: Milk and Milk products

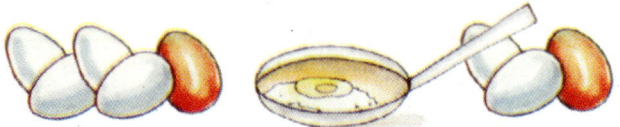

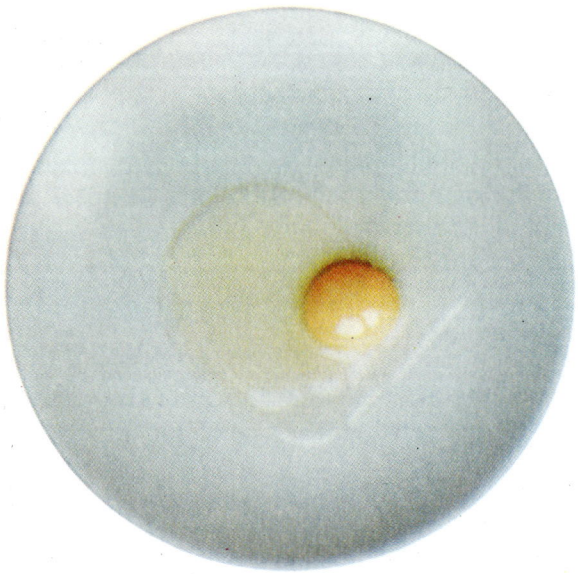

Fresh egg indicating the upright yolk and two distinct layers of white

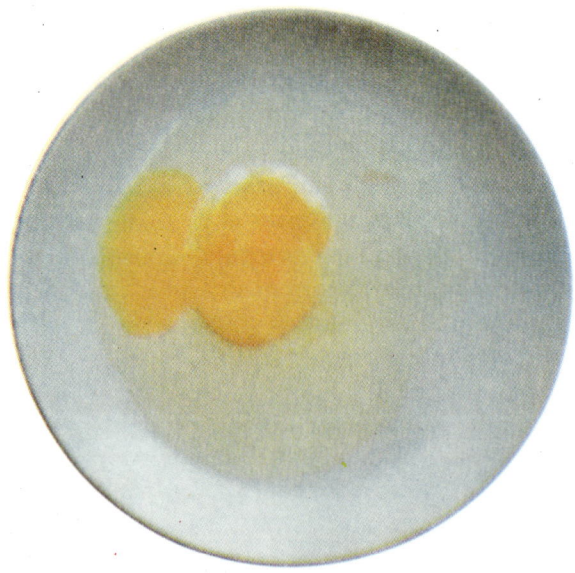

Stale egg with yolk spread out with increase in egg white volume

Plate X-B: Judging Egg Quality

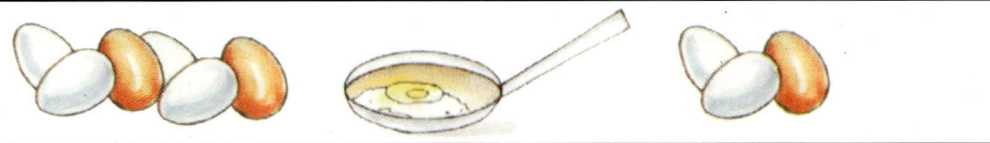

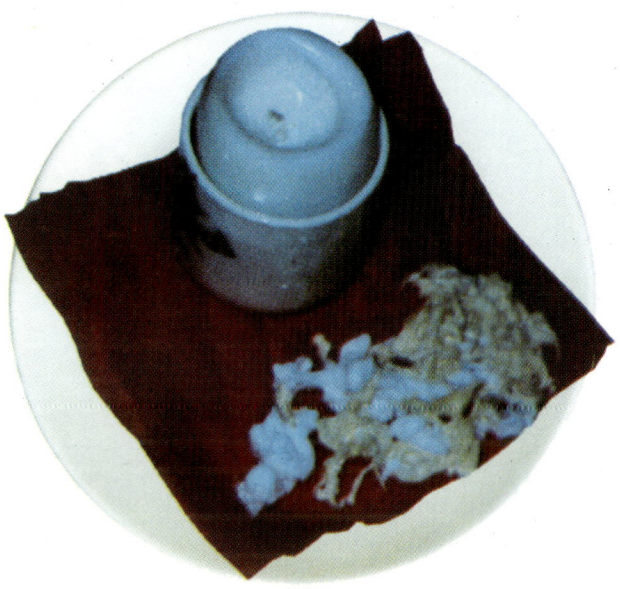

Boiled egg showing enlarged air space

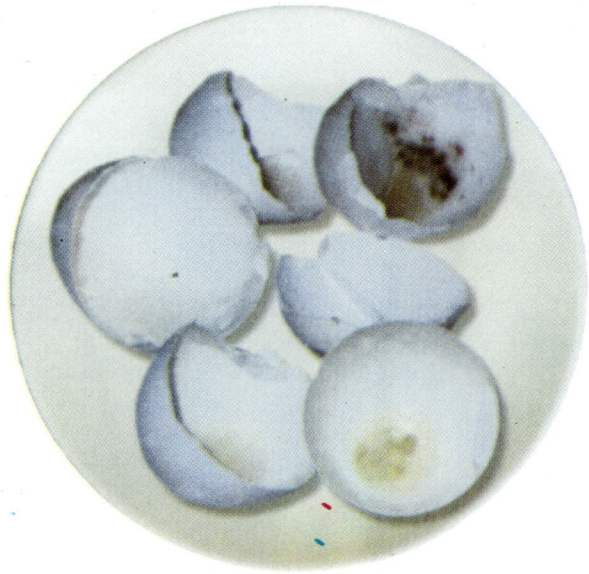

Cracked egg showing fungus in shell

Plate X-C: Judging Egg Quality

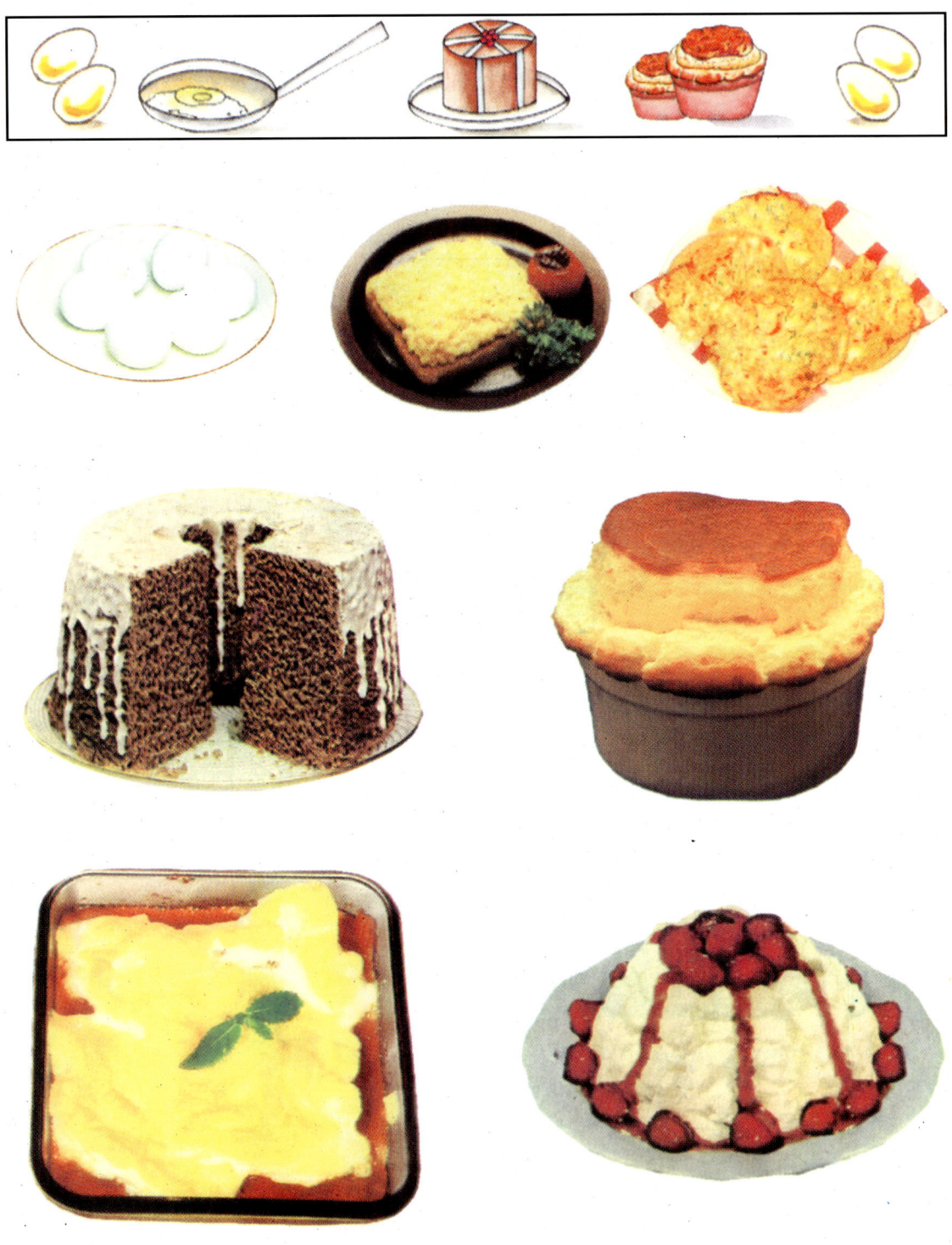

Plate X-D: Egg preparations

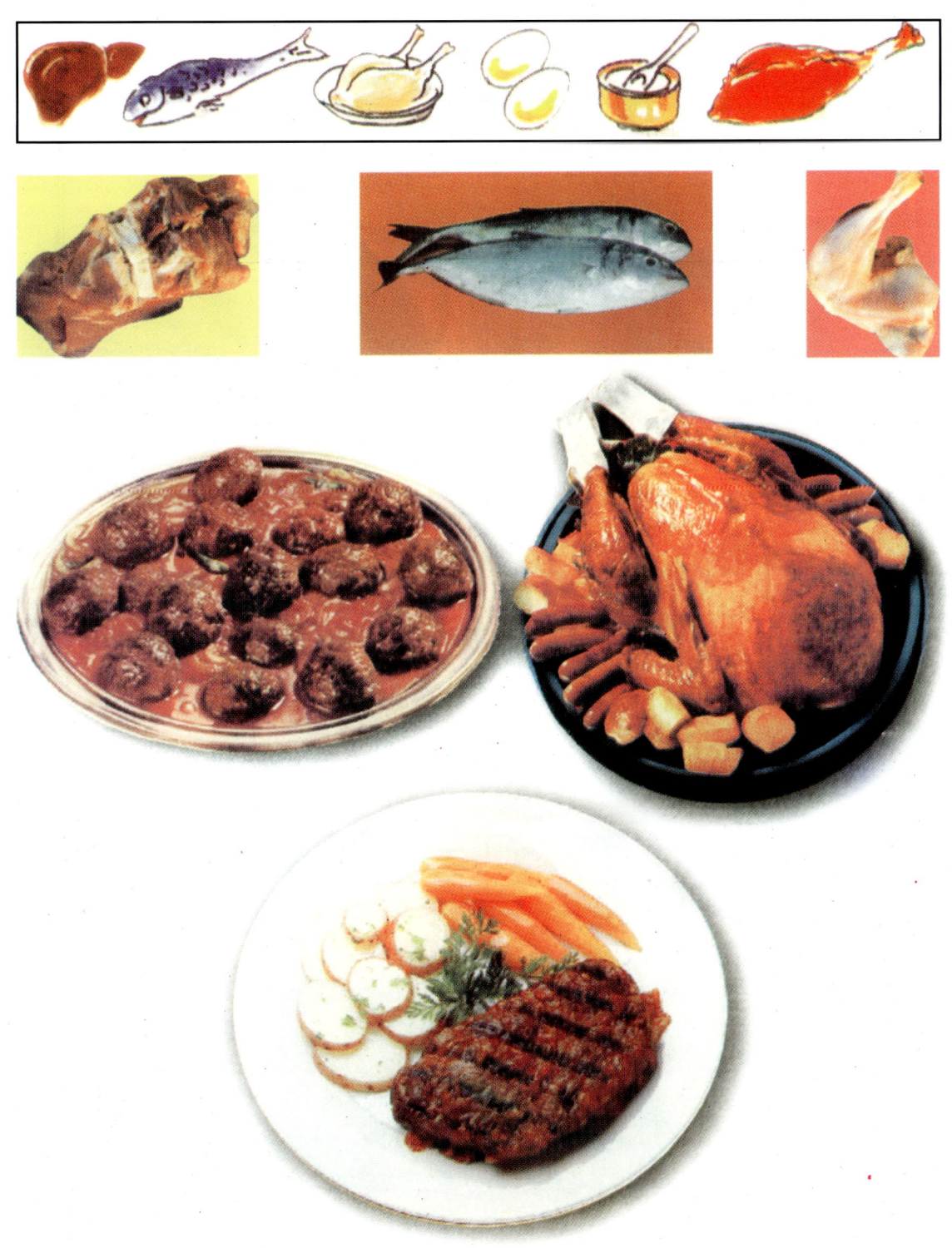

Plate X-E: Meat preparations

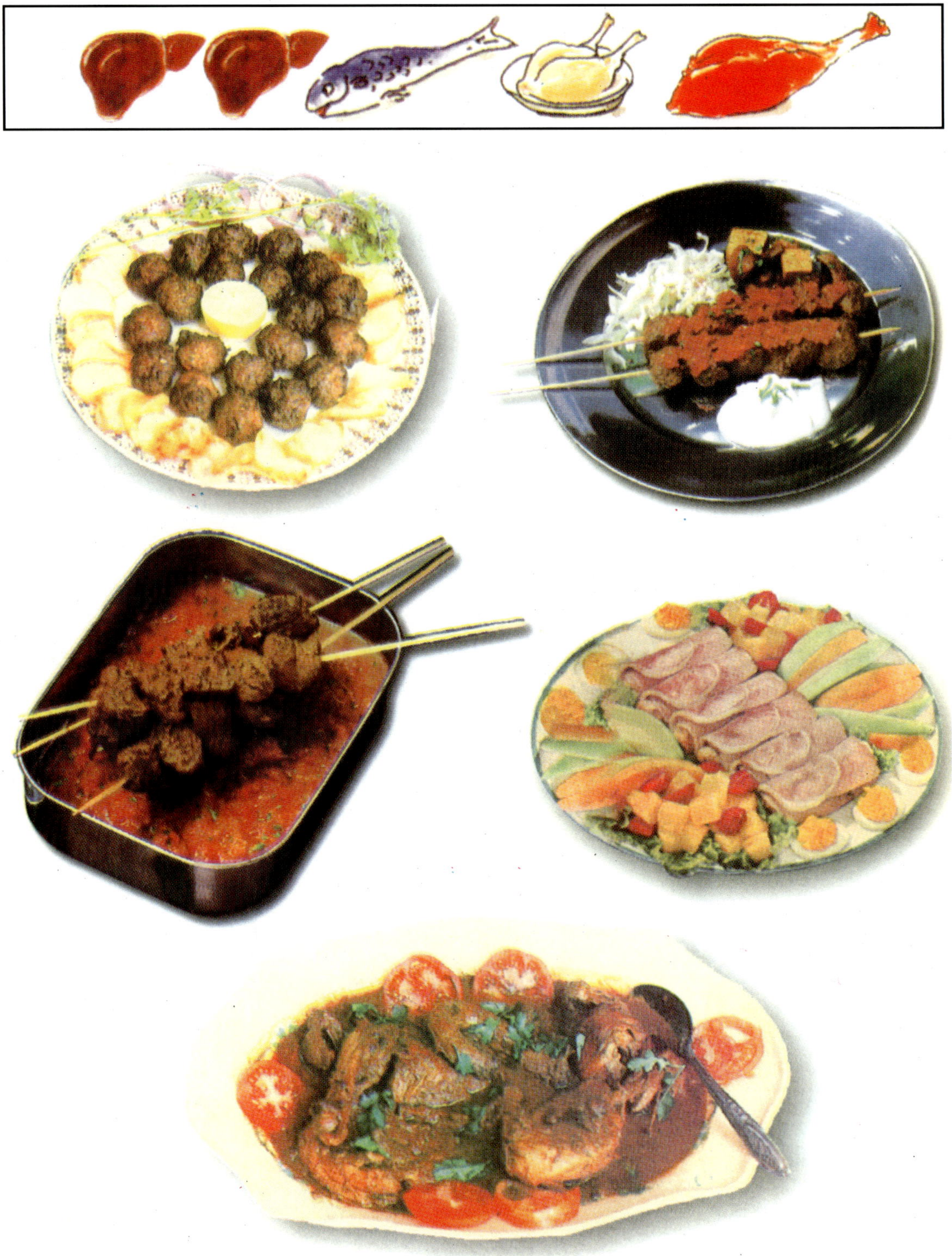

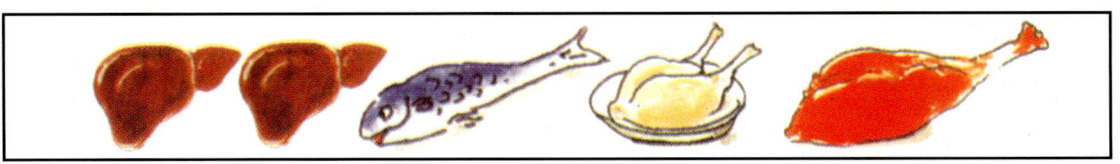

Plate X-F: Meat preparations

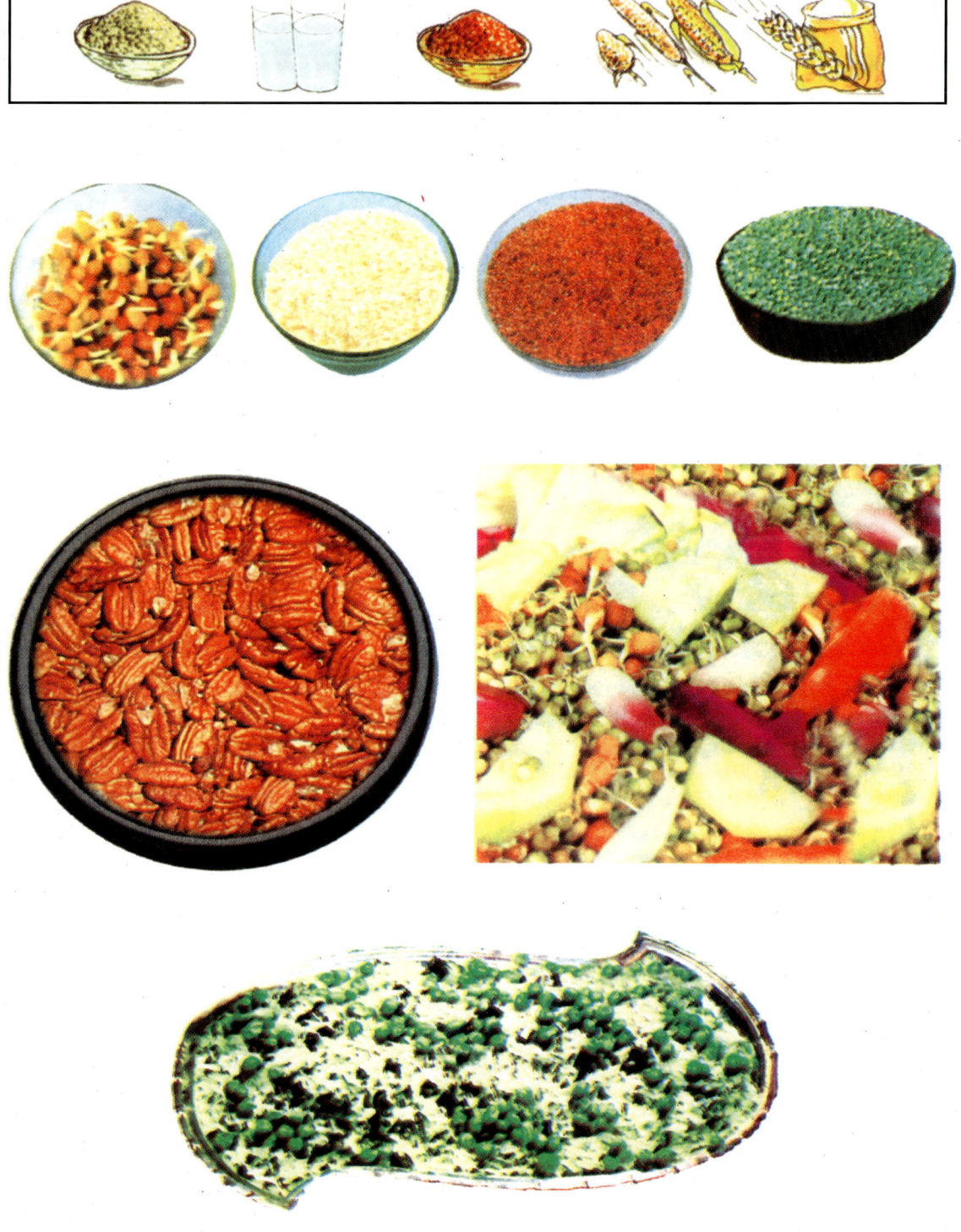

Plate X-G: Pulses, Legumes and Nuts

APPLICATIONS OF FATS AND OILS

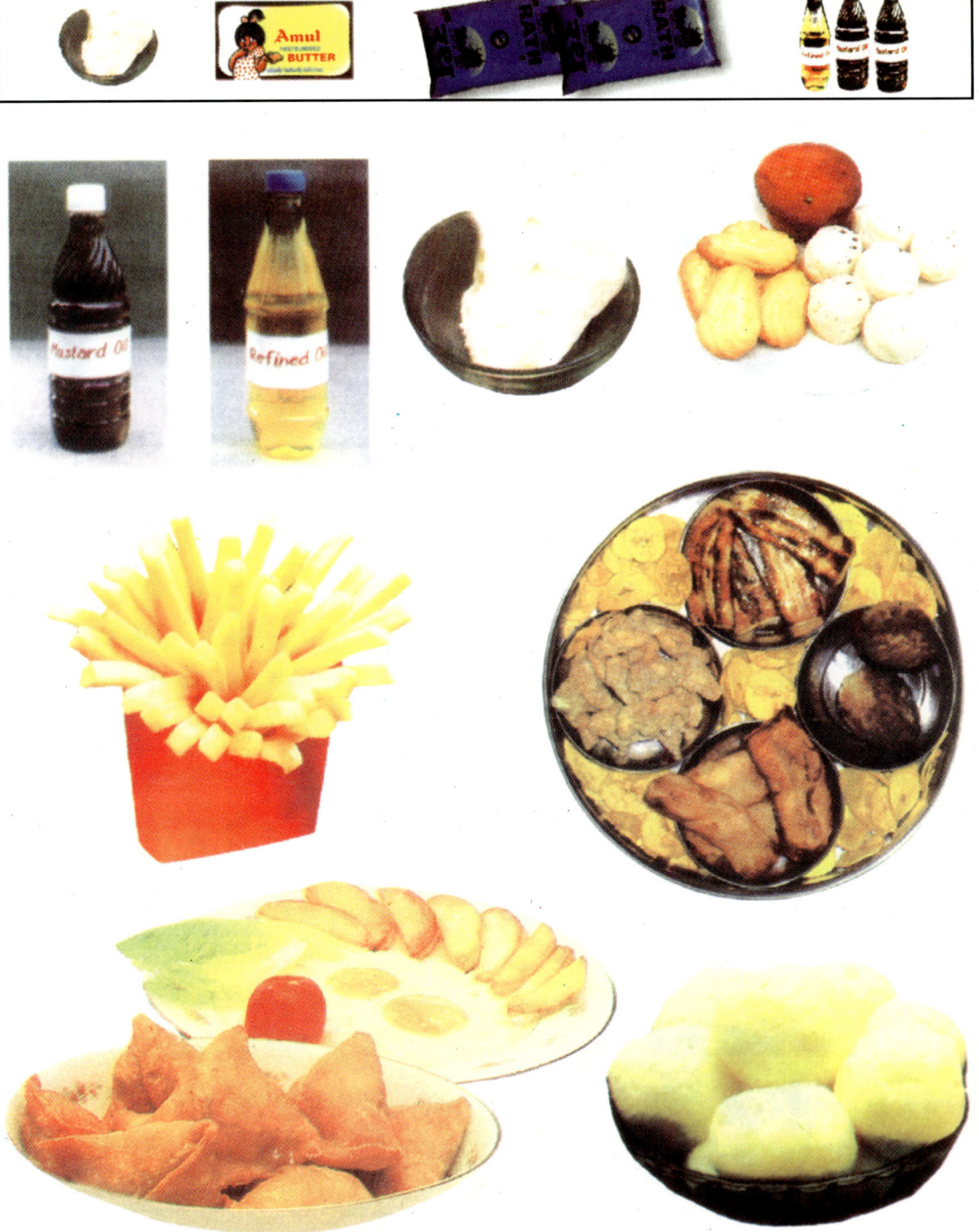

Plate XI: Food products containing fats

with moist heat methods. When a pulse or legume curry is cooled even at room temperature it thickens and at refrigeration temperatures tends to set. Refer to chapter 2 for other properties of starches using moist and dry heat cooking methods.

Denaturation

This property pertains to the effect of heat on the protein of grains, which also results in irreversible coagulation depending on the cooking methods employed. Other properties of proteins apply to these foods as well, and are discussed in the introduction to Unit 2.

Viscosity

Grains when prepared as gravies or stews tend to have smooth flow properties. This is mainly due to the binding of free water by the starchy constituents, as well as the formation of protein structures which keep the fat globules in emulsified form specially when the grains are cooked whole and include the germ portion as well. Some grains provide thicker consistencies in foods than others mainly due to the differences in the proportions of starch, proteins and fats. The de-husked varieties are less viscous than the whole grains.

Germination

All whole grains possess the property of germination, and the germinated foods are commonly called sprouts. This is an important property as it provides pulses and other grains in forms, endowed with the qualities of fresh greens in slack seasons. The content of vitamin C and B-group vitamins get enhanced and digestibility of proteins increases. The toxicity present in some grains also gets removed and the grains can be eaten raw or with only slight steaming.

Fermentation

Combination of cereals and pulses in ground form, given the conditions of temperature and humidity as present in most tropical countries, give rise to useful fermented batters and doughs that can then be suitably cooked or processed for consumption. In India, air fermentation is common for products like *idli, dosa* and the like. Cereal flours are also subjected to bacterial or yeast fermentation of which *bhatura* and *naan* are suitable examples.

Leavening

Flours are subjected to aeration when air or gas is incorporated in them by mechanical or chemical means as in the production of bakery goods. Leavening is brought about by beating, whisking, creaming, rubbing in fat into the flour or by the use of yeast as in breads raised by the carbon dioxide released during yeast fermentation. Chemically, products are leavened using baking powders, cooking soda and so on as done in the preparation of cakes, of different kinds.

Products are also prepared through partial leavening such as pie bases, muffins, pancakes where no agents are added for aeration but the steam released from the dough or batter acts as the leavening agent. To achieve the variety of products mentioned, flours are combined with liquid and other ingredients in the prescribed proportions to form batters and doughs which are then used for the preparations.

Grain Flours

Flours are largely composed of starches unless the cereal is ground whole in which case it contains its original properties and nutrients, with minor losses that take place during milling. Wheat flour contains 65-80% starch, 8-12% protein and 1-2% fat. The percentage of starch increases as the flour gets finer till only the starchy endosperm remains as in the case of *maida*. The proteins decrease in direct proportion to the decrease in aleurone layer during extraction, therefore coarser cereals contain more protein. In refining, the fat, vitamins and minerals get removed with the germ. Whole wheat flour contains thrice as much fibre as refined flours because of the presence of the bran.

Of all the flours wheat flour is the only one which has the natural property in its dough to entrap air or gases required for the preparation of raised breads like, *naan, kulcha, phulka, chapati* and many similar preparations used in the subcontinent, Turkey and the Middle East countries. Composite flours with part replacements have been tried, with binders such as gums and proteins to achieve gas retention, but found unsuitable.

Apart from cooking them as such, the most common use to which cereals and pulses have been put is by using their flours or mixtures for preparation of batters, doughs and pastes. These are therefore being discussed in detail to provide an understanding of how the properties of different grain foods can be utilized creatively.

Batters and Doughs

Batters and doughs are mixtures of various raw ingredients which form the basis of a number of baked, fried or steamed products in our diet. The difference between the two are mainly in their consistency or flow properties, batters flowing more easily than doughs which can be handled and manipulated into different shapes, sizes and forms.

Batters can usually be dropped or poured into cooking pans or heated oil or other media depending on the proportion of liquid present in the mixture which is usually 1:1. Doughs on the other hand are hard or soft according of the ratio of liquid to other ingredients used in their preparation and the end product desired. In bread dough however, the relation between gelation, coagulation and emulsification or foaming is not easily or clearly defined.

Most batters and doughs are foams, the size and shape of the air cell formed determining the texture of the final product prepared from them. Flour forms the base ingredient for batters and doughs in which other items such as eggs, sugar, salt, leavening agents, and even vegetables or fruits in dry or fresh forms may be added to provide different textural and organoleptic qualities to products prepared from them.

Structure. The structure of the batter or dough largely determines the structure of the final products. Factors which are responsible for the structure are:

(*a*) Ingredients and the proportion in which they are combined.
(*b*) Kind and amount of leavening agent used.
(*c*) Temperature of ingredients when mixed.
(*d*) Extent of mixing.
(*e*) Method of combining them.

The characteristic property of batters and doughs related to their structure is viscosity, which is affected by many factors such as concentration, temperature, degree of dispersion, solvation, electric charge, beating, presence of colloids, electrolytes and so on.

Role of Ingredients

Each ingredient plays a role in imparting characteristic qualities to the end product.

Flour

This gives elasticity to a dough enabling air to be entrapped in it. On cooking when the air is released the product acquires a spongy soft texture, as in the case of a bloated *Phulka*. The protein in flours provides the structure and rigidity as also seen in the case of well risen cakes, or steamed *idlis*.

Eggs

Beaten eggs act as leaveners in batters and doughs as the proteins impart elasticity and help to incorporate air making the end product spongy yet firm in texture. The final volume of a product is determined largely by the concentration of eggs in the batter or dough, which is directly proportional to the amount of air incorporated. In addition, the presence of emulsifying components in egg yolk helps to keep immiscible liquids like water and oil together in batters and doughs resulting in smooth textural qualities of products.

Liquid

Liquids act as the vehicles for dissolving or dispersing ingredients like sugar, salt, spices and for ionizing them to release gases as in baked products.

Fats

These act as shortening agents that cover particles of the structural ingredients thus preventing the development of protein strands in doughs. By this process elasticity is decreased and tenderness and *break* of the products increases as in the preparation of biscuits or *mathris*.

Sugar

Apart from the sweetness that sugar imparts to products it also makes them tender because of its hygroscopicity. Sugar takes up the moisture instead of the flour, and this interferes with gluten development in doughs, thereby reducing elasticity and increasing crispness and tenderness of products. Sugar is also the only ingredient that has the ability of incorporating air into fat as in making batters through creaming for preparation of cakes. Further it is responsible for imparting the brown colour to products, through the Maillard reaction occurring between the protein and sugar. If no sugar is present in the batter or dough the browning that occurs is less even on the surface of the product because it results from dextrinization of the starch present.

Acid

The presence of acids in batters or doughs reduces the rate of browning. It is for this reason that a little sugar or baking powder is added along with the acid to counter the slow browning effect on the product.

A variety of minor ingredients can be added to batters and doughs to enhance flavours, however, the main ones described can only be substituted by ingredients with similar properties. Liquid may be in the form of juices, or milk while eggs may be substituted by protein foods like curds, the sugar by jaggery or brown sugar, honey or other syrups, the flours of different cereals used as such or mixed in different proportions depending on the qualities desired in the finished product. Whatever the ingredients used the important factor is their *balance* in the dough or batter. The structural ingredients like flour and eggs should balance the tenderizing ingredients like fat and sugar. Similarly the liquid and the dry ingredients should be balanced to enable easy handling of doughs and batters for cooking as required, as well as for taste and other sensory qualities of the cooked product.

Combining Ingredients

The method of combining ingredients will depend on those given in standard recipes for different products according to the characteristics desired in the final product. What is worth remembering is that, while dealing with doughs and batters the amounts of various ingredients in a recipe cannot always be multiplied for preparing products in quantity, and the method of combining alone will not give desired results. This is specially true for cakes and similar products, such as pop-overs, fritters, muffins and so on. Methods used vary from the conventional creaming to pastry blending, sponge and quick-mix methods.

Effect of Heat

A stable shortened cake batter in contrast to a foamy meringue batter, can be kept covered in a baking pan for some time without much loss in quality. The gas is only lost if it is kept in a bowl and later transferred to a baking pan. However, a number of changes take place during baking.

(a) Air bubbles from a creamed batter are released to the aqueous phase even before the fat is completely melted or reaches 40°C.

(b) The carbon dioxide released from the baking powder collects in the air bubbles, and as heating is continued these are set in motion by convection currents established in the oven, as well as by the pressure of the expanding gases.

(c) The batter next to the sides and bottom of the pan get heated first and set up convection currents within the batter although the motion of these is not discernible because the movement is very slow.

(d) Heat enlarges the gas cells rapidly at 80°C. The colliding and coalescing of these cells brings about the visible rising of the cake.

(e) Steam formed adds to the leavening in the product. At this stage if the oven door is opened the temperature of the batter falls and the cake is likely to collapse. When a cake batter is rising its stability is critical for the formation of a quality crumb.

When cakes are baked at high temperatures the volume tends to be greater though the crumb is fine in contrast to those which are baked at lower temperatures. This is because in the latter heat penetration is slower and there is more time for the gas bubbles to expand and the batter to be overstretched before the proteins coagulate and set, forming the crumb and giving a larger, coarser grain to the product. Other factors too play a role in texture such as the metal and size of pan determining the type of heat energy that dominates the cooking. Fast baking pans tend to give a humped product with irregular browning. Tunnels too get formed in cakes if the pans are not the right size or when the mixture contains a low sugar to flour ratio.

Experiments 36-40 have been designed to impart an understanding of the effect of using different leavening agents, methods of mixing, temperatures and other factors on quality of whole cereal and flour based products.

EXPERIMENT 36

Aim

To study the time, temperature and water required for sprouting whole pulses and legumes.

Equipment

Weighing scale, pans, bowls, thermometer, measuring jar, muslin cloth, sprout maker.

Materials

Whole green and red gram (*moong* and *masoor*) and kidney beans (*rajma*).

Principle

Whole unwashed pulses and legumes are like any seed which when provided the right temperature and humidity will sprout. This process called germination, requires different periods of time to split depending on the hardness of the outer layers of the grain, legumes or beans usually requiring more time than smaller pulses.

Procedure

A. (*i*) Weigh 10g each of the whole green gram, red gram and kidney beans.
   (*ii*) Pick, clean and wash them.
   (*iii*) Soak in 50 ml water for few hours or preferably overnight in a covered pan, to allow them to swell completely. Weigh each sample, and not/the amount of water absorbed.
   (*iv*) Drain out any remaining liquid and tie each sample loosely in a wet muslin cloth and hang in air. Sprinkle water on the muslin if dry patches are seen.
   (*v*) Keep sprinkling over 1-3 days till sprouts begin to appear. Remove from muslin when the sprouts are 1/2-3/4 inch in length. Weigh the sprouts again and note the water absorption.
   (*vi*) Note the room temperature and the time taken for each grain to sprout.
   (*vii*) Place in covered bowls and refrigerate for evaluation.

B. (*i*) Repeat experiment A (i-vii) but instead of hanging the grains in muslin cloth use a sprout maker.
   (*ii*) Note the time and temperature when sprouts are equal in length to those in A.
   (*iii*) Examine samples of experiments A and B and make your observations. Note : This experiment can be done side by side with other experiments.

Observations

Tabulate the observations made with respect to amount of water absorbed, time taken, temperature of sprouting, and sensory characteristics of the sprouted grains. Draw your inferences regarding acceptability for use as such, or after steaming for 10 minutes.

Precautions

1. Drinking water should be used for soaking and sprouting.
2. Weights and time should be recorded accurately.

3. Sprouts should be of the same length before refrigeration.
4. Evaluation should be done as soon as the experiments are completed.

Practice Exercises

1. Steam 10 g samples of the prepared sprouts, and note the changes in colour, texture, flavour and applicability in food preparation. Compare with the unsteamed samples.
2. Prepare a salad with the sprouts using two different salad dressings.
3. What is the utility of sprouting in meal preparation. Explain.

EXPERIMENT 37

Aim

To study the effect of cooking on whole and washed or dehusked/decorticated pulses and legumes.

Equipment

Cooking pans, weighing scale, measuring cup, bowls.

Materials

Green gram whole and decorticated, beans (*lobia*), water, turmeric, ginger, cumin seed, salt to taste and fat.

Principle

Whole and decorticated (*dhuli*) pulses and legumes absorb different amounts of water at different temperatures of cooking. The time taken for achieving a certain consistency is also affected by the pulse components. The greater the amount of starch the more mushy the consistency of the end product.

Procedure

A. (*i*) Take 25 g each of whole and decorticated pulses and beans.

(*ii*) Pick, clean and wash the pulses and legumes, and soak them for 30 minutes in 200 ml of water. Strain the water into cooking pans and weigh the pulses and legume. Note the amount of water absorbed by each.

(*iii*) Put the pulses into the soaking water on the burner, add a pinch of turmeric, fresh chopped ginger and salt, and allow them to cook till the water is completely mixed with the pulses and does not separate out.

(*iv*) Remove from burner when done and note the time taken for cooking. Put the readv pulses in separate bowls, record the final weight and keep aside covered.

(*v*) Heat 1 T oil or fat in a pan, add 1/2 t cumin seed, and pour the hot fat on top of the boiled pulses.

(*vi*) Evaluate for colour texture, taste, consistency as well as total water absorption and cooking time.

B. Repeat A(i-vi) but this time do not soak the pulses, directly cook and evaluate.

C. Repeat A(i-vi) but keep cooking time constant, evaluate.

Observations

Tabulate your results as learnt in previous experiments, indicating the differences observed in sensory characteristics of each pulse under experiments A, B and C. Draw your inferences and show how you would apply the knowledge gained in the cooking of other pulses and legumes.

Precautions

1. When boiling pulses and legumes reduce the source of heat as soon as it begins to foam to prevent boiling-over.

2. Weigh and measure accurately.
3. Avoid overcooking and lump formation.
4. Record the time as soon as the pulse is ready and water does not separate out when mixed.

Practice Exercises

1. Prepare any pulse as learnt, but add tomatoes to it and then boil. Note the time taken to cook and the differences in sensory attributes. Compare results.

2. Sprout whole pulses and any type of dried beans. Comment on their sensory quality and acceptability on sprouting and after cooking.

3. Prepare a snack using a combination of cereal and pulse. Show how one complements the other in texture, taste and nutritional quality.

EXPERIMENT 38

Aim

To prepare batters using different flours and study the effect of deep frying them.

Equipment

Burner, bowl, wooden spoons, measuring spoons, standard cup, weighing scale, skillet, perforated ladle, sieve, brown paper.

Materials

Refined flour (*maida*), gram flour (*besan*), soya flour, water, salt, chilli powder, *garam masala,* oil for frying, baking powder, sugar, egg, fat and milk.

Principle

The affinity of flour for water is so great that when they are combined they interact to form films of protein which get separated into fibrils which can be seen emerging from the fractured surface of the endosperm cells. These fibrils carry with them grains of starch with which they unite to form a network.

When a high proportion of liquid is added to flour as in a batter, the gluten gets hydrated and a network does not form. It only helps in the formation of steam during cooking which gives a hollow structure to the,product when it escapes. Sometimes a large amount of fat added to batters also prevents glutenization, resulting in a tender and richer product.

Procedure

A. (*i*) Seive 30 *g maida* into a bowl.

  (*ii*) Make a well in the centre and add 15ml water.

 (*iii*) Mix together and beat well till a thick batter is obtained.

 (*iv*) Add the salt and spices to taste and mix. Rest the batter covered for 20 minutes.

  (*v*) Measure and heat oil in a *kadai,* testing readiness for frying by dropping a little batter in it. If it rises to the surface immediately the oil is ready for frying. Note the temperature of the oil.

 (*vi*) Drop teaspoons of the batter into the hot oil and deep fry till golden brown. Note the time taken.

 (*vii*) Drain the oil using the perforated ladle and place the ready product on a brown paper to completely drain the oil. Note the weight.

(*viii*) Place on a plate and keep aside.

B. (*i*) Repeat A (*i-viii*) using besan; soya flour/urd/moong flour.

  (*ii*) Compare the products for weight, time taken for the same amount of browning, and assess their sensory qualities.

 (*iii*) Strain the oil, cool and measure it, to determine the amount absorbed.

Observations

Tabulate your observations for colour, texture, flavour, taste, degree of aeration, time taken to cook the product and acceptability. Explain your observations in the light of the theory learnt and suggest ways of improving the product using different combinations.

Precautions

1. Add the liquid gradually and mix continuously till the batter is smooth, light and of coating consistency.
2. Ensure thorough mixing of the batter to avoid lump formation.
3. The batters should be rested for the same time period.
4. Test oil before frying and record the temperature before frying each batter.
5. Thermometer should be vertically fixed to dip into the oil for taking readings.
6. Oil should be thoroughly drained before weighing each product.

Practice Exercises

1. Prepare batters as learnt and cook in boiling water instead of oil.
2. Place batters in a bowl in the microwave oven without water or oil. And cook till done. Compare the results with those obtained in the experiment.
3. Slice potatoes 1/4 inch thick, dip in the batters and deep fry. Comment on the sensory characteristics of the product.
4. List 5 foods that are made from batters and indicate why their results are different.

EXPERIMENT 39

Aim

To demonstrate the effect of different methods of making dough on the quality of Indian breads like *chapati.*

Equipments

Weighing scale, bowl or flat plate (*paraat*), burner, iron griddle (*tawa*) and measuring cup

Materials

Whole wheat flour, refined wheat flour, soya flour water, salt and oil.

Principle

When cereal flours are mixed with water, they absorb a certain amount and the starch grains swell. It is therefore necessary to rest a flour mixture before manipulating it into a dough. In wheat dough. the proteins develop on kneading to form gluten, which imparts the property of holding air incorporated during kneading. This leavens or aerates the product giving it a light, spongy and-soft texture. Thus, many types of breads both flat and leavened can be prepared from flours of different types.

Procedure

A. (*i*) Weigh 50g of wheat flour into a bowl, make a well in the centre and pour 50 ml water into it.

  (*ii*) Gently mix the water and the flour together from the centre outward till you can make a ball. Place the ball in the bowl, cover with a damp muslin cloth and let it rest for 20 minutes at room temperature.

  (*iii*) Place the ball on a flat plate or surface and knead with knuckles of the hand repeatedly till the dough becomes elastic and can be pulled or stretched.

  (*iv*) Make small balls and roll them into flat rounds or *chapatis.*

  (*v*) Preheat griddle plate and cook the flat bread partially on both sides.

  (*vi*) Cook one *chapatti* fully on both sides, and convert the 2nd into a bloated *phulka* by placing it directly on the burner after both sides are partially cooked, or pressing the edges of the *chapati* on the griddle plate with a napkin and allow it to bloat. Keep aside covered.

B. (*i*) Repeat A (*i-vi*) using refined wheat flour.

C. (*i*) Repeat A (*i-vi*) using a mixture of wheat flour and soyaflour in the ratio of 5:1.

  (*ii*) Evaluate the products from A, B and C for colour, stretchability, texture, chewability, softness and acceptability for various applications.

Observations

Tabulate your results and comment on the reasons for the differences observed. What kind of browning takes place, why does one *chapati* bloat and not the other, when the dough is the same.

Precautions

  1. The dough must be allowed to rest before kneading.

2. Ingredients should be measured accurately.
3. The bloated *chapati* should be left on the hot griddle for some time to enable proteins to coagulate around the air and keep it enclosed even after it has bloated, otherwise it will collapse on removing from heat.
4. The *tawa* should be preheated till a sprinkling of flour on it turns brown. Brush this off before placing the *chapati* on it.

Practice Exercises

1. Prepare chapati and phulka using different cereal flours, and their mixtures. Comment on their quality characteristics comparing them to the products from whole wheat flour.
2. Prepare wheat flour dough using a little oil or fat in making it. Note the differences in sensory and other qualities.
3. Deep fry small *chapatis* making dough with and without oil using different cereal flour and flour-pulse combinations. Record your observations.
4. Prepare refined wheat flour dough as learnt but, replace some of the water with 1 T beaten curd. Measure the amount of water used. Rest the dough for 1 hour at room temperature. Then knead and make into equal sized balls and rest them for another one hour or until nearly double their size. Now roll out chapatti and cook one in a preheated oven, one on a hot griddle till done and deep fry the third. Comment on their sensory qualities, and explain the reasons for the differences in the products.

EXPERIMENT 40

Aim

To study the development of gluten in fermented doughs.

Equipment

Baking tin, oven, weighing scale, standard cups and spoons, muslin cloth, *thali* or deep plate cooking thermometer.

Materials

Refined flour or *maida,* yeast, sugar, salt, water and fat.

Principle

The functional protein of wheat flour is gluten which when hydrated and manipulated forms an elastic dough, due to the linkages which form between the protein molecules. The greater the kneading, the more linkages form and the stronger is the dough structure. The elasticity also increases and the dough can be stretched in opposite directions to form a sheet or film or in all directions under the pressure of expanding gas or air which then gets trapped to provide lightness to products. However, if excessively manipulated the gluten films become weak and break, and the product becomes dense. On exposure to heat the protein coagulates and forms a semi rigid structure. The lightness of a product therefore, depends on the degree of kneading and the amount of gas liberated during fermentation of dough prior to cooking.

Procedure

A. (*i*) Weigh and sieve 300g flour, place in a plate and make a well in the centre.

(*ii*) Heat 165ml water to 40°C or till luke warm.

(*iii*) Crumble 6g fresh yeast and 6g sugar into the well and pour 65 ml water preheated to 40°C over the yeast sugar mixture.

(*iv*) Leave, till it starts to froth and using the remaining water knead into dough by stretching and folding.

(*v*) Cream together 6g fat and 6g salt and incorpoate into the dough while stretching and folding for approximately 50 strokes.

(*vi*) Cover the dough with wet muslin and keep aside for 45 minutes away from light, allowing it to proof.

(*vii*) Punch and stretch the dough again and place in a bread tin. Cover and allow to proof 2 hours.

(*viii*) Preheat the oven to 425°C and bake for 1/2 hour after brushing the surface with water. Cool the bread in the tin, then turn out, and leave to cool in air till room temperature.

B. Repeat experiment A using a mixture of refined and whole wheat flour.

C. Repeat experiment A using wheat and soya flour in the ratio of 10 : 1.

Observations

Make observations with respect to the volume, crust, cut, evenness of baking, colour, taste and flavour. Draw your inferences with respect to effect of yeast fermentation on wheat flour and other flour mixtures. Tabulate your results.

Precautions

1. Hydration of yeast should be done at 40-60°C.
2. Avoid using shiny pans for baking as they affect the rate of heat transfer.
3. Bread dough should contain approximately 40% moisture.
4. Salt content should not exceed 2% of the weight of the flour as it inhibits gas production.
5. Sugar is essential for fermentation but should not exceed 10% of flour weight.

Practice Exercises

1. Prepare fermented products using air, lactic acid and yeast for the fermentation. Compare the results and comment on the extent of glutenization in each.
2. Prepare *idli, dosa* and *dhokla* combining cereal and pulse flours. Discuss the appropriate methods of fermentation and explain why the products are so different in their sensory qualities.

9

Nuts and Oilseeds

Nuts and oilseeds are the edible fruits or seeds of plants consisting of a kernel surrounded by a hard or brittle shell and usually grow on trees in areas where other crops cannot thrive. The only exception is the groundnut, which is similar to a pulse crop. Nuts are important food resources because they are not only a source of edible oil, but the deoiled meal is a good source of protein, vitamins and minerals. Those most commonly used in diets are coconut, groundnut, almond, cashewnut and walnut among others. Most nuts and oilseeds contain 3-8% moisture and 25-60% oil or fat, and are therefore more popularly eaten during winter months, or in cold climates, when high energy foods are required.

Composition

Nuts are very variable in their size and composition. The kernel is usually rich in oils and fats, proteins and minerals, the amounts varying with each type of nut or seed. Nuts are often grouped according to their composition, some being rich in fats others in proteins with chestnut containing about 50% carbohydrates mainly starches, although relatively poor in proteins and fats. On an average they contain 2% minerals being good sources of phosphorus and potassium. Table 9.1 indicates these differences.

Table 9.1 Composition of some commonly used nuts and oilseeds (per 100g)

Nuts/Seeds	CHO g	Protein g	Fat/Oil g	Ca mg	P mg	Fe mg	Energy kcal
Nuts							
Almond	10.5	20.8	58.9	230	490	4.5	655
Cashewnut	22.3	21.2	46.9	50	450	5.0	596
Chestnut*	54.24	10.9	1.84	–	–	–	54
Coconut (Dry)	18.4	6.8	62.3	40	210	2.7	662
Groundnut	26.1	25.3	40.1	90	350	2.8	570
Pistachio	16.2	19.8	53.5	140	430	7.7	626
Walnut	11.0	15.6	64.5	100	380	4.8	687

(Contd.)

Nuts/Seeds	CHO g	Protein g	Fat/Oil g	Ca mg	P mg	Fe mg	Energy kcal
Seeds							
Gingelly	25.0	18.3	43.3	1450	570	10.5	563
Linseed	28.9	20.3	37.1	170	370	2.7	530
Mustard	23.0	20.0	39.7	490	700	17.9	541
Safflower	17.9	13.5	25.6	236	823	–	356
Sunflower	17.9	19.8	52.1	280	670	5.0	620

Sources: NIN, Nutritive value of Indian Foods, ICMR, 1999.

*Manay and Shadakharaswamy, Foods. 1987.

Apart from the above values for macronutrients and some minerals indicated the Table 9.1, nuts and oil seeds contain B-vitamins as well, especially thiamine, riboflavin and niacin. But, since they are consumed only in small amounts in meals or snacks, they do not contribute appreciably to the diet. However, the deoiled cakes of nuts and seeds form an important protein source for fortification and enrichment of processed foods. They do however, form fair sources of calcium, sodium, magnesium and iron in the diet if used on a regular basis. In addition, they provide concentrated sources of energy supplying from 350-800 kcals per 100g depending on the variety used.

Properties

Nuts and oilseeds exhibit three important properties for consideration in food preparation and processing.

Perishability

Nuts are very perishable in nature and therefore it is important to process, package and store them in conditions which will not lead to deteriorative changes.

Rancidity

Nuts and oilseeds tend to turn rancid if stored over long periods and develop off flavours, because of their high fat content. It is therefore important to buy those marked with seals of quality, and once a pack is opened it needs to be stored in airtight containers. In hot tropical summers they should be refrigerated.

Toxicity

Many nuts and seeds tend to become toxic on long storage especially when piled up in large amounts as in national reserve storages or at processing plants. Sometimes agricultural contaminants such as insecticides, biocides, growth promoting sprays or substances can remain in the crop and cause toxicity.

Fungal, mold or bacterial growth may take place if humidity is not controlled, as often happens in tropical countries. Toxic effects of *Aspergillus flavus* in groundnuts is well documented, which imparts a bitter taste to nuts. Oxidative changes and enzyme activity can also cause changes in colour, flavour and texture of nuts and oilseeds.

Storage

Nuts are usually stored in cool, dry and dark conditions as light may lead to oxidation of lipids present leading to rancidity. Rodents may also contaminate grains, nuts and seeds in storage, their urine and droppings spreading diseases. They can also be attacked by insects, which eat away portions making them hollow.

Effect of Heat

Direct heat as in roasting or frying improves the taste of nuts, as it separates out the oil from the cells which then gives the nuts a crispiness and flavour. The B-vitamins are however lost to different extents depending on the time and temperature of cooking. The digestibility of nuts and oilseeds is increased on heating as in the case of cereals, pulses and legumes.

Uses

Nuts find a number of uses in meals and as ingredients for preparation of snacks.

1. They enhance the nutritional value of the dish.
2. Improve colour, flavour and other sensory qualities of the meal.
3. Eaten as such the provide excellent snacks with beverages.
4. Used as garnishes, for rice dishes, desserts and sweet snacks.
5. In deoiled form they can be used for low energy meals, while still adding to taste and flavour.

Experiments 41 and 42 is designed to provide an exposure to changes that take place in cooking nuts and oilseeds through the preparation of snacks in which they form the main ingredient.

EXPERIMENT 41

Aim

To demonstrate the effect of roasting on nuts and oilseeds.

Equipment

Iron kadai or wok, perforated ladle, strainer, oven and tray.

Materials

Groundnuts, cashewnuts, gingelly seeds, salt.

Principle

Nuts and oilseeds are generally not eaten raw and have to be processed in some manner before being consumed. The heat treatment improves colour, flavour and general acceptability as well as their digestibility. Nuts also provide a good source of energy, protein and other nutrients.

Procedure

A. (*i*) Weigh, clean and pick 10g each of groundnuts, cashewnuts and gingelly seeds.

  (*ii*) Heat the iron *kadai* without oil, and lower the flame of the burner.

  (*iii*) Add the groundnuts to the hot *kadai* and keep turning them over till the outer paper-like skin gets easily removed and a roasted flavour and aroma is noticeable. Remove one nut, coo 1 in air and test for readiness.

  (*iv*) Remove the nuts from the *kadai* into a plate, sprinkle salt to taste, cool and weigh. Note down the difference in weight.

  (*v*) Repeat (*i-iv*) for cashewnuts.
Repeat (*i-iv*) for gingelly seeds.

B. (*i*) Repeat A(*i-vi*) but this time use a preheated oven at 200°C for roasting, turning the nuts over occasionally to prevent scorching.

C. (*i*) Repeat A(*i-vi*) but roast the nuts in salt pre-heated along with the kadai.

  (*ii*) Place all the samples together and evaluate their sensory attributes. Comment on their applicability in food processing and cooking.

Observations

Tabulate your observations and determine the best method of roasting nuts and oilseeds.

Precautions

1. When roasting nuts and oilseeds the heating should be even.
2. Temperatures should be adjusted to the nut or seed to prevent scorching or incomplete cooking.
3. Constant turning over is important.
4. Weighing should be accurate, to determine the weight change during roasting.

Practice Exercises

1. Use a little thickened milk or khoa alongwith the nuts to make a burfee, and compare for differences in the various attributes of the product with those obtained in the experiment.
2. Prepare coconut burfee using fresh and dry coconut. Comment on the sensory characteristics.
3. Prepare carrot burfee and differentiate between one made with and without nuts.
4. Roast the nuts and seeds in a microwave oven and evaluate the quality of the product. Cover the dish when roasting seeds as spluttering will occur.
5. Prepare a salad and use suitable nuts in it. Explain why you selected particular nuts only.
6. Prepare a pulao and garnish with nuts. Comment on its advantages and acceptability.
7. Prepare laddus with the roasted gingelly seeds, using any basic recipe. Comment on the product.

EXPERIMENT 42

Aim

To prepare sweet a sweet snack (*burfee*) using nuts as a major ingredient.

Equipment

Weighing scale, grinder, kadai, ladle, rolling board and pin, knife, quarter plates and burner.

Materials

Cashew nuts, almonds soaked and peeled, sugar, water, kewra essence (optional).

Principle

Since nuts contain a high proportion of fat or oil, they can be cooked with sugar to make sweets which do not exhibit recrystallization The products are therefore soft in texture and have the characteristic flavour of the nut, If deoiled nuts are used there is little or no fat to interfere with the recrystallization process and therefore the texture becomes grainy. Such sweets can be stored at room temperature for weeks without developing off flavours. The sugar being hygroscopic in nature also acts as a preservative to extend shelf life of the product.

Procedure

A. (*i*) Grind 20g chashewnuts finely.

  (*ii*) Add 2T water to 20g sugar in a kadai and cook on medium heat till the syrup is of 2-thread consistency (p. 3).

 (*iii*) Add powdered cashewnut and a drop of kewra essence. Mix well with a ladle and remove from fire.

 (*iv*) Apply a little oil on hands and make ball of the mixture.

  (*v*) Roll while still warm on a greased rolling board to an even thickness of 3mm, making a square shape as you roll. Cut diagonally into triangles.

 (*vi*) Refrigerate half the portions and keep the other half aside, for observations after 1/2-1 hour.

B. (*i*) Repeat A (*i-vi*) using roasted groundnuts.

C. (*i*) Repeat A (*i-vi*) using unroasted pistachionuts.

Observations

Place all the samples refrigerated and other side by side in plates and evaluate for colour, texture, flavour, mouthfeel and general acceptability. Observe the state of crystallization through appearance and mouthfeel. Tabulate results and draw your inferences.

Precautions

1. Grind nuts finely.
2. Only enough water should be added to the sugar to bring out its water of crystallisation.
3. Cooking should be done on medium heat to prevent caramelisation of sugar.

4. Testing sugar for 2-thread consistency is important before adding the ground nuts.

Practice Exercises

1. Use a little thickened milk or khoa alongwith the nuts to make a burfee, and compare for differences in the various attributes of the product with those obtained in the experiment.

2. Prepare coconut burfee using fresh and dry coconut. Comment on the sensory characteristics.

3. Prepare carrot burfee and differentiate between one made with and without nuts.

4. Roast the nuts and seeds in a microwave oven and evaluate the quality of the product. Cover the dish when roasting seeds as spluttering will occur.

5. Prepare a salad and use suitable nuts in it. Explain why you selected particular nuts only.

6. Prepare a pulao and garnish with nuts. Comment on its advantages and acceptability.

7. Prepare laddus with the roasted gingelly seeds, using any basic recipe. Comment on the product.

UNIT III

DIETARY FATS

Fats and oils are present in virtually every food and are a concentrated source of energy in both plants and animals. When they occur as part of the structure of the food they are called invisible fats I and when isolated or extracted from foods for the purpose of using them as ingredients for cooking or processing they are termed as *visible fats.* Dietary fats and oils may be classified as indicated in Fig. 10.0.

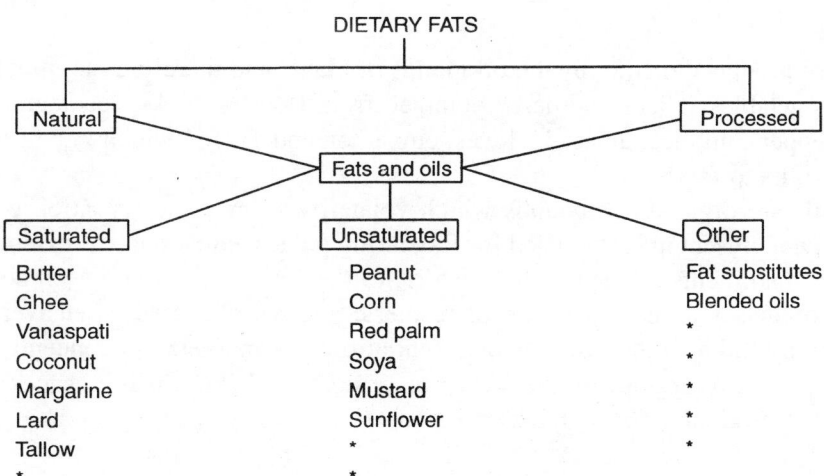

Fig. 10.0. Classification of Dietary Fats.

Figure 10.0 shows that fats and oils occur naturally in foods, but are also processed in forms that can impart desired properties to a food product. Processing involves not only extraction of fats from natural sources, but also the manufacture of products like blended oils, margarines, fat replacers and the like, which are being increasingly used as ingredients in cooking and food production. At present, there are 17 major fats and oils being processed including those from animal sources. Vegetable oils contribute 80% of the total global production followed by soya oil (21%), butter (20%), palm oil (17%), and rapeseed oil (10%). It has however, been estimated that 25% of the fats produced are consumed by the affluent because of their high cost.

Structure

Like carbhydrates, fats are composed of carbon, hydrogen and oxygen and are esters of fatty acids and glycerol, but are different from them in that, they are not polymers of repeating molecular units and do not form long chains. Natural fats are not made up of one type of molecule but are mixtures of many types. There are many different fatty acid molecules connected to glycerol which differ in length and in the number of atoms they contain. Longer fatty acids form harder fats, and chemical variations lead to a wide variety of different functional and other properties.

Types of fatty acids

There are basically two types of fatty acids, saturated and unsaturated, the latter being further subdivided according to the number of double bonds present in their structure. The saturated ones do not contain any double bonds and therefore provide stability to a fat or oil. Some fatty acids cannot be synthesized in the body and therefore need to be provided through dietary sources, these are therefore called *Essential fatty acids* (EFA). A totally fat free diet is therefore not recommended under any circumstances.

Fats and oils exist in invisible forms as lipids or mixtures of triglycerides, unless extracted from the foods. The terms *fat* is used for those mixtures which are solid at room temperature, whereas those which remain liquid are called *oils*. Besides fats however, some oils are found in plants which are not triglycerides and called *essential oils*.

Essential Oils

Essential oils are produced mainly by the oil glands of plants and therefore the important sources are fruits and vegetables, spices and herbs obtained from flowers, barks, seeds and roots. Some examples are peppers, nutmeg, aniseed, cloves, cinnamon and saffron which impart characteristic colours and flavours to foods.

Essential oils are organic compounds which volatalize to give the sensation of flavour. An example is *Eugenol* present in cloves used for flavouring pulaos, curries and as essences for baked products. Other condiments and spices are also rich in essential oils, some even contributing to characteristic colours as seen in the case of turmeric and paprika used extensively in tropical countries especially India. Today extracts of essential oils are marketed in concentrated forms to acts as flavouring or colouring agents, the former being commonly known as *essences* and resemble the flavours of the original herbs and spices.

Properties

Dietary fats and ails exhibit some common physical and chemical properties which are detailed in chapter 10.

Nutritional Importance

Fats are important sources of energy, fat soluble vitamins and phytochemicals. The nutritional value of the fats however, varies depending on their source and the processes used for their extraction, fortification, blending and packaging. For example, the oil bearing fruit of the palm produces two types of oils, one from the fruit and the other from its kernel, the latter being 85% saturated.

Being similar in structure and most properties, fats and oils have been discussed together through chapters 10 and 11. Wherever the term fat is used it applies to oils as well, unless otherwise stated.

10

Fats and Oils

Fats are organic compounds derived from reaction of trihydric glycerol with organic acids which are widely present in foods. The term *lipid* is often used to cover all types of food fats and fat-like substances. A lipid of significance in nutrition is cholesterol, which plays a structural role in biolgoical membranes and is a precursor of important hormones. Cholesterol is present in all animal foods, plant foods being devoid of this lipid.

Structure

The simplest structure of a fat contains one molecule of glycerol and three molecules of fatty acid, and is therefore termed as *a triglyceride*. The type and length of the fatty acid structure be it the

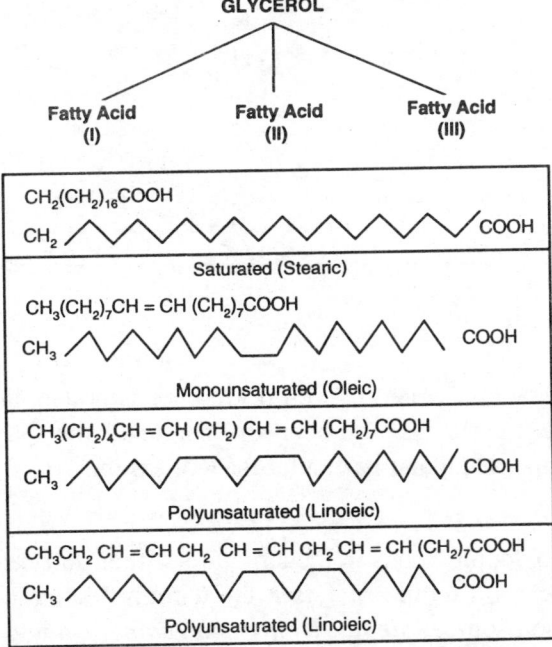

Fig. 10.1. Schematic structure of a fat molecule and some fatty acids.

185

same or different and their arrangement all determine the properties of the fat. The general formula being RCOOH where "R" stands for the feature which makes fatty acids different from each other. Glycerol has three reactive OH groups and each fatty acid has a reactive COOH group. The structure represents a hydrocarbon chain simply illustrated in Fig. 10.1 along with some fatty acids.

There are about 40 fatty acids identified as naturally occuring in food fats, some common ones are presented in Table 10.1.

Table 10.1 Dietary fatty acids

Food oil/fat	Fatty Acid (FA)	Carbons (C)	M.pt C	Saturated	Unsaturated Mono	Poly
Butter	Butyric	4	−8	+		
Coconut	Lauric	12	44	+		
Palm, butter Coconut	Myristic	14	54	+		
Meat fats, Palm, butter	Palmitic	16	63	+		
Cocoa butter, animal fat, butter	Stearic	18	69	+		
Soya, sunflower, safflower, corn cottonseed oils	Linoleic	18	−5			+
Olive, peanut, animal fat corn, palm, rapeseed	Oleic	18	14		+	
Soya, canola	Linoleic	18	−11			+
Fish oils	Gadoleic	20	−		+	
Animal fat	Arachidonic	20	−40			+
Animal fats	Behenic	22	80	+		
Fish oils	Erucic	33	33			+
Some fish					+	

Adapted from H. Lawson (1997) P.9.

Composition

There are two types of fatty acids present in a fat or oil one, saturated and the other unsaturated, in which double bonds are present. The number and nature of the fatty acids present in a fat molecule determine the properties that a particular fat will exhibit.

Saturated fats

Those fats which contain no double bonds in the structure of their fatty acids are called *saturated* and are responsible for the solid nature of fats even at room temperature. Examples of some saturated fatty acids with their sources are *lauric, myristic, palmitic and stearic* acids. Coconut oil is rich in lauric acid (49%) and a good source of myristic acid (18%). Palmitic acid constitutes 20-30% of all animal fats as against 4-48% in vegetable oils, being richest in palm oil, followed by cottonseed (24%), soybean (12%), coconut (8%) and canola (4%) oils respectively. Stearic acid forms 5-20% of the fatty acids present in all animal fats, as against 2-4% in vegetable oils. Examples of saturated fats include butter fat, palm oil, cocoa butter, palm kernel oil and all animal fats.

Saturates are different in their effects on cholesterol. *Palmitic acid* is the most common dietary fatty acid and does not increase cholesterol. Simopoules (1998) offers a classification of common fats which is adapted and placed in Table 10.2.

Table 10.2 Classification of Common fats and oils used in India

Saturated	*Mono unsaturated*	*Poly unsaturated*
Butter*	Olive	Corn
Lard*	Canda	Safflaower
Coconut oil	Safflower**	Sunflower
Palm oil	–	Flax seed
Cocoabutter	–	Groundnut nut
Palm kernel oil	–	Cotton seed
		Canola***
		Soyabean
		Fish
		Walnut
		Sesame
		–
		–
		–

Note:

*   Solid fats, rest are oils.

**   Only high oleic oil is safflower oil.

***   High in Poly + monounsaturated oils.

For composition of margarines the labels on packages give a good indication through the types of oils used in their manufacture.

Olive oil has only recently been adopted for cooking in homes and in well known hotels. It is however advantageous to know that if used for salads the virgin variey should be used, while the pomace variety is good enough for cooking. At present a few brands of pomace oil are imported packaged and marketed in India, under brand names of *Bertdi*, *Leonardo* and others, since olives do not grow in India. At present it is manufactured, packed and imported from Italy, but is soon expected to be packaged in India after bulk importation, till such times as olives are grown here.

Unsaturated fats

Unsaturated fats are classifed into two categories mono and polyunsaturated named according to the number of double bonds in the fatty acid structure, and are generally liquid at room temperature or when kept under refrigeration. The monounsaturated fatty acid (MUFA) most commonly present is *oleic* acid found abundantly in animal and vegetable fats. The monounsaturated oils include olive oil (80%), canola (70%), safflower, sunflower and avocado oils, while regular safflaower and sunflower oils are classified as polyunsaturated. The *high oleic* labelled varieties are newer oils in the MUFA category.

The polyunsaturated fatty acids (PUFA) contain more than one double bond in their structure as the name suggests. Of those present in fats and oils and fat-rich foods such as nuts, oilseeds and some legumes, there are only three which the body cannot synthesize and therefore they need to be provided through dietary sources. These are *linoleic, arachidonic* and *linolenic* acids and are termed as *Essential Fatty Acids* (EFA). Of these linoleic is the most important EFA as its presence is necessary for synthesizing arachidonic acid in the body. Dietary sources are animal fats and vegetable oils, the acid constituting 1-10% in the former and 55% in the latter, examples of which are corn, safflower, sunflower, peanut, cottonseed, soyabean, fish, flax seed, walnut, sesame and grape seed oils.

With such wide ranging melting points of fatty acids, their mixtures may thus produce fats and oils of different consistencies depending on the overall degree of saturation. These differences can be observed in *ghee,* butter, lard, hydrogenated fat, mustard, coconut and other oils at room temperature. The degree of unsaturation of a fat or oil can be measured through the determination of its *Iodine value,* because a molecule of iodine reacts with each double bond present in the fat or oil.

In the past little distinction was made between the various polyunsaturated oils because all were low in saturated fatty acids and cholesterol which were the most important characteristics attributed to them. This belief allowed free choice of oils on the basis of cost, habit, flavour and cooking qualities. However, recent research shows that the various different PUFA oils can have varied effects on health depending on their ratio of omega-6 to omega-3 fatty acids. The basic difference is that omega-3 fatty acids have an extra double bond in their structure, located three carbon atoms from the end of the molecule and this accounts for the difference between sickness and health. Soyabean oil is the only one which belongs to both omega-3 and omega-6 categories. Oils in the former category include fish oils, walnut, canola and flaxseed oils, whereas those in the latter category are corn, safflower, peanut, sesame, sunflower and cottonseed oils.

Properties of Oils and Fats

Fats and oils exhibit physical and chemical properties according to their fatty acid composition and their arrangement in the structure of the oil or fat. Monounsaturated oils are liquid at room temperature but may become cloudy or semisolid at referigeration temperatures.

Colour

The colour of fats and oils ranges from light yellow through amber and various shades of brown. Its viscosity varies with the source from which it is drawn, animal fats being solid at room tetrf rature compared to oils from plant sources. Processed fats however may vary widely in their consistencies depending on the end use for which they are manufactured.

Flavour

Fats usually act as vehicles for releasing and enhancing flavours of other ingredients with which they are combined in foods, since most flavouring compounds are fat soluble. Fats with lower viscosity and sharp melting points release flavours more readily than those with higher melting points. Butterfat, mustard and coconut oils are examples of fats which possess distinctive flavours and aroma. Unsaturated gamma-lactones have been identified as contributing to the flavour of deep fried foods.

Feel

Fats feel oily to the touch and exhibit lubricating properties. They form a greasy film around foods and prolong shelf life, prevent shrinkage in storage and impart a sheen on vegetables making for aesthetic quality. This lubricating function is important in grilling foods as it helps in moisture and flavour retention. Fats act as lubricants and help in swallowing foods making them slippery and soft which may otherwise irritate the mucous membranes of the mouth and throat.

Satiety

Compared with other energy giving foods, fats provide greater satiety value. This is because they are digested slowly and therefore remain in the stomach longer, warding off the feeling of hunger Besides, they also provide twice as much energy as carbohydrates or proteins and therefore help to relieve hunger for longer periods while at the same time increasing palatability of foods and meal satisfaction.

Solubility

Fats and oils are insoluble in water, but in the presence of an emulsifier can be made to mix and remain in dispersion (see emulsions, p. 106). However, they are soluble in organic solvents, a property used in their extraction from foods.

Aeration

Fats possess the property of aerating foods by forming a film around the fine grains of flour being used in batters and doughs, creating spaces for air or gas and thus helping to improve the volume of foods when heated, resulting in soft spongy textures.

Viscosity

Viscosity of oils decreases with increase in unsaturation of the fatty acids present. Fatty acids of relatively low molecular weight are less viscous than those of high weight, irrespective of the degree of unsaturation. Polymerization of fats also increases viscosity.

Heat Conduction

Liquid fat is a good conductor of heat with the advantage that the temperature attained is not self limiting due to the heating since fats do not evaporate as in the case of water. Thus foods cooked in fat get evenly browned, this being due to other factors as well such as Maillard browning and caramelization.

Melting

Most fats melt between 30-40° although a distinct melting point is not discernible especially in the case of oils. The melting point of oils is usually the temperature at which the viscosity or flow increases and the oil becomes more transparent and clear. The longer the carbon chain in the structure of the fat the higher is its melting point. For example, the melting point of cocoa butter ranges between 29-34°C, palm oil is also less than 37°C while vanaspati varies from 31-41°C.

Fats which melt above body temperature are tallowy. Fats like cocoa butter are solid at 31°C and have a melting point below 37°C or body temperature, a property that makes chocolates melt in the mouth. Coconut fat also has a sharp melt as experienced when eating coconut *burfee* or other preparations.

Emulsification

Fats exhibit the property of emulsification if beaten with water or any liquid and air (see P. 88 on emulsions). It is due to this property that it is possible to cream fat with sugar or other ingredients in food preparation.

Smoking

When a fat or oil is subjected to high temperature a smoke or haze starts appearing from its surface. The temperature at which this starts is known as the smoking point. This is accompanied the formation of *acrolein,* a breakdown product of glycerol which has a strong acrid odour and Often irritates the throat when frying is done under uncontrolled temperatures. This phenomenon indicates that the fat or oil has started to decompose, the process being irreversible. Smoking points of different oils and fats vary between 185-230°C, vegetable oils having higher points than animal fats.

Repeated heating of fat or the burning of food particles as occuring during frying, lowers the smoking point of the fat in addition to producing oxidative and hydrolytic changes that impart undesirable colours and flavours to foods. When the smoking point is lowered the fat becomes more viscous and begins to foam, leading to greater fat absorption by the foods fried in it.

Flashing

When fats are heated to a very high temperature the vapours given off ignite into a flame. The temperature at which this happens is called the *flash or fire point* which varies for different fats and oils usually occuring between 340-360°C. This is important in commercial frying operations and therefore temperatures are automatically monitored to prevent accidents. The PFA Rules do not permit use of any fat or oil whose flash point is less than 250°C.

Plasticity

Fats are plastic at certain temperatures and therefore provide spreadability which however, varies in degree with each fat depending on the melting points of the triglycerides present. At any one temperature therefore, some fats are liquid while others are in a crystalline solid state. Fats with smaller crystals as formed by rapid cooling and agitation during manufacture, and are more plastic than those cooled slowly.

A mix of triglycerides which show a wide range of melting points exhibit a large plastic range, and therefore spread and cream better than hard fats with a narrow range of plasticity. This property of fats is made use of in the manufacture of margarines so that they spread easily even if just removed from the refrigerator.

Hydrolysis

This is the process of breakdown of fats that takes place due to faulty storage of fats or foods containing them. Hydrolysis is primarily a reaction of lipases in which fats break up into glycerol and fatty acids in the ratio of 1:3 per molecule of fat or oil. However, as the water is reduced in the reaction medium the equilibrium shifts towards synthesis resulting in esterification and interesterification. When fats or products with a high fat content are stored in a warm place the enzyme activity gets accelerated (Khare et al., 2000).

Rancidity

Rancidity is associated with unacceptability in fats, oils or products in which they are present. There are two types of changes that take place in fats namely oxidative and hydrolytic which are responsible for rancidity.

Oxidative Rancidity

This refers to the reaction between unsaturated triglycerides and oxygen from the air, leading to the formation of aldehydes and ketones responsible for the unpleasant rancid taste and odour. The more the unsaturation of the fat, the greater is its susceptibility to oxidative rancidity.This reaction is increased in the presence of heat, light and metallic ions such as copper and iron, therefore fats should be stored in a cool dark place because of the prooxidant effect of light. Commercially processed butter and other fatty products therefore, contain added antioxidants to prevent oxidative changes and increase the shelf life of the products. Those aoproved for use in fats are butylated hydroxytoluene (BHT), butylated hydroxyanisole (BHA) and propyl gallate.

Hydrolytic Rancidity

In this kind of rancidity the fats are hydrolyzed by enzymes such as *lipases* and broken down into glycerol and fatty acids. The enzymes may be present naturally in the fats or through microorganisms in foods cooked in the fats. The unpleasant taste and smell in the products is due to the formation of short-chain fatty acids like butyric acid as found in rancid butter. It is therefore not advisable to fry repeatedly in the same oil, as the degradation of the fat or oil takes place both due to heat as well as the crumbs that remain in the oil, from foods.

Consistency of Fats

The melting point and plasticity of fats greatly affect their consistency, which has a bearing on the functional properties in foods, prepared or processed. The consistency of plastic fats depends on the ratio of crystals to oil. In fact cooling a liquid fat may cause crystallization in the fat, as seen in salad oils cooled under the chill tray of a refrigerator. Good quality salad oils are usually chilled and any crystals f6rmed removed before packing and marketing, so that the oils do not crystallize on normal refrigeration. This treatment given to fats is called *winterizing. In* salad oil manufacture the addition of crystal inhibitors in the form of heat oxidized saturated fats, such as *oxystearin* are now permitted.

Fats which exhibit a wide range of plasticity have some crystals even at high temperatures, while others may remain liquid at low temperatures. In production, processes where creaming is required such as for cakes, a wide plastic range and small crystals in the fat are desirable. In contrast, a narrow plastic range is required for products where spreadability is the desired feature as in butter, margarine, sandwich spreads and so on.

Visible and Invisible Fats

All fats used for cooking or added to products during processing are called visible fats. Those present as part of the structure of foods are called invisible because they are not all visible to the naked eye, or handled to be used as ingredients for cooking. However, invisible fats may be processed to visible forms by extraction from foods rich in them such as meats, fish, grounduts, soybean, safflower, gingelly seeds and many more. In most countries extracted animal fat called lard is used.

A new product combining the price advantage of vegetable oil, vanaspati and lower fatty acid quality of refined oils, has been prepared by the Vanaspati Manufacturing Association (VMA), called *Randhan*. This is a *ghee*-like product marketed under different brand names. This low cholesterol *ghee* has been approved by the Health Ministry, Government of India, and has the texture and taste of *desi-ghee*, or the pungency of mustard oil or flavour of groundnut oil depending on the additives used (Industry News, 1999).

The Oil Technologists' Association of India (OTAI) has urged the government to tap realisable potential of 3 m. tonnes of vegetable oil from ricebran, cotton seeds and oilseeds of tree & forest origin and oilcakes. Rice bran alone has the oil potential of 8 lakh tonnes.

Cooking with Fats

Fats and oils provide as very good cooking medium for the uniform transfer of heat to foods, and since they provide temperatures of 170-180°C, the heat penetration is uniform and cooking is quick. With high protein foods the surface proteins coagulate almost instantly at these temperatures and the surface gets sealed off, so the flavours and moisture remain in the foods. This makes the products crisp on the outside but tender and aromatic within.

Frying

Frying is the most common method of cooking used for food preparation. When the food is dipped in hot oil during the process it is known as deep frying, and if a small amount of fat is used the term employed is shallow frying. A method of cooking using very small quantities of hot oil in which food is tossed occasionally during cooking is called sauteeing.

Deep fat frying is an economical, fast and convenient method and retains food flavour and texture as well. The products acquire aesthetic and palatability characteristics because of even heat transfer and are also microbiologically safer than foods prepared by other methods. However only fats with high smoking points are suitable for frying, as the high frying temperatures result in less oil absorption by foods. Fats like butter which have low smoking points are therefore considered unsuitable.

The frying medium however undergoes degradative changes due to continued exposure to air or oxygen, high temperatures and contact with metals or moisture from the products being fried. In order to prevent breakdown of fats a process called *refreshing is* used in which a little fresh oil is mixed with the used oil for refrying. But this is not encouraged continuously. Fats must be discarded when they show signs of degradation like darkening or a waxy appearance with decrease in viscosity.

Shortening

Fats provide a crumbly texture to foods by forming a film around the starch and protein particles in flours, preventing the formation of long gluten strands in them. This is accomplished when fat is rubbed into a flour gently using the tips of the fingers only. Such treatment to flours before dough formation makes products soft and tender or short after cooking. This effect is called *shortening* and is used for making biscuits, cakes, pie bases, pastry products, *mathris and* so on, where a golden colour and crisp texture is required through baking or frying.

Leavening

When fats are creamed with sugars as in preparation of cake batters, they help to incorporate air into the batter making it light and foamy. On baking the protein films coagulate enclosing the air, and making the end products light in texture and soft in mouthfeel. In biscuits since foaming is not required the fat is rubbed into the flour gently to provide slight aeration to impart a light crisp texture.

Creaming

Fats are also used for creaming ingrediends into cake batters, sandwich spreads and dips. The method improves textural and mouthfeel qualities of products through aeration, leavening and emulsification properties of fats.

Changes in fats

A number of changes occur in fats during repeated frying, some more apparent than others. The changes in colour, flavour, viscosity, smoking, foaming are easily noticeable, but some structural changes occur as well. Some of these are:

Polymerization

When fat is heated above 200°C molecules may unite to form long chain polymers. If unsaturated fats form cyclic compounds, polymerization is visible as deposits of a gum-like material around the sides of a frying equipment, especially where fat, metal and air come in contact.

Foaming

When polymerization is allowed to continue by repeated frying it causes foaming of fat, which decreases surface tension and increases viscosity. When foaming occurs the fat should be discarded because polymerization increases the unsaturation in the fat. However, techniques have now been evolved whereby relatively high polyunsaturates can be made to resist foaming.

Hydrolytic breakdown

Hydrolytic and oxidation products form which tend to reduce interfacial tension between fat and the water from products being fried, and also change the viscosity of the oil. This favours penetration of fats into the foods making them greasy and unpalatable.

Experiments 43 and 44 have been designed to provide some insight into the choice of fats for household use considering their properties.

EXPERIMENT 43

Aim

To determine the smoking point of fats and oils.

Equipment

Measuring and weighing equipment, pyrex beakers, thermometer and stands, burner, tripod stand and gauze, stop watch.

Materials

Hydrogenated fat, mustard and refined vegetable oils, margarine.

Principle

When a fat or oil is heated to high temperatures the triglycerides gradually breakdown to free fatty acids and glycerol. The glycerol then gets dehydrated and deco os to form an unsaturated aldehyde called acrolein which results in a blue haze or smoke. The temperature at which this appears on the surface of the oil is known as the smoking point, and depends on the percentage of free glycerol present in a fat and the rate at which the molecules get dehydrated. Monoglycerides if present in the oil or fat get hydrolysed more easily than triglycerides. Acrolein has a strong odour and irritates the mucous membranes indicating that the fat is decomposing and has been heated under uncontrolled conditions.

Procedure

A. (*i*) Take 100g of hydrogenated fat in a pyrex beaker.

 (*ii*) Fix the thermometer on a stand so that the bulb will dip vertically in the melted fat when the beaker is placed over the flame.

 (*iii*) Place the beaker of fat over a steady flame and keep on moderate heat throughout the experiment. Note the temperature of the fat every 2 minutes.

 (*iv*) Continue to heat the fat till a blue haze is noticed rising from the surface of the fat. Switch off the burner and read the temperature immediately. Record the smoking point and the time taken for the oil to smoke.

B. (*i*) Repeat experiment A (*i–iv*) using 100 ml mustard oil instead of 100 g fat. (*ii*) Note the smoking point and the time taken.

C. (*i*) Repeat experiment A (*i–iv*) using 100 ml vegetable oil. (*ii*) Note the smoking point and the time taken.

D. (*i*) Repeat experiment A (*i–iv*) using 100 g butter.

 (*ii*) Note the smoking point and the time taken to reach it.

 Note the volume, colour, viscosity and flavour of the fats and oils before and after they are heated to smoking point and then cooled to room temperature. Record the differences in their smoking temperatures.

Observations

Record your observations according to the format presented in Table 10.2. From your observations determine the fat or oil with the highest smoking point and comment on the changes in volume, and other sensory qualities. Which is the best oil to use for frying. Give reasons for your choice. Draw inferences with respect to the changes observed in each oil and discuss the applicability of each medium in food preparation.

Table 10.3: Smoking point of fats and oils.

Fat/Oil	Smoking pt. °C	Time taken minutes	Volume I	II	Colour I	II	Viscosity I	II	Flavour I	II
Hydrogenated										
Mustard										
Vegetable										
Butter										

Plot a graph showing time on the X-axis recorded every 2 minutes for each fat and the corresponding temperatures on the Y-axis. Show the differences observed and how they can be employed in food preparation and processing with the least damage to the fat.

Precautions

1. Take equal amount for each experiment.
2. Heating should be carried out with a constant flame.
3. Note temperature every 2 minutes and stop the flame as soon as it starts to smoke.
4. Read off the smoking temperature immediately.
5. Use a stop watch for noting time accurately.

Practice Exercises

1. Repeat the experiment learnt using other fats and oils such as canola, sunflower, coconut and so on and compare the smoking temperatures and suitability of the oils for frying.
2. Preparepooris using fats and oils with low and high smoking points. Compare the products and comment on their palatability and acceptability. Give reasons for your comments.
3. List five foods in the preparation of which different oils or fats are used. How can you improve the quality of the foods with your knowledge of fats and oils.

EXPERIMENT 44

Aim

To determine the best frying temperature for different fats and learn a household test for oil readiness for frying.

Equipment

Pyrex beakers, thermometer, stand, stop watch, fork knife, chopping board.

Materials

Hydrogenated fat, vegetable and mustard oils, butter and 2 bread slices.

Principle

Fats and oils are good conductors of heat so foods cooked in them get evenly browned on the surface and moist and tender within. The browning is due to a number of changes that take place during heating depending on the composition of the foods being fried. These are dextrinization of starches, the Maillard reaction between breakdown products of starches and proteins and caramelization of the resultant sugars formed or those present in the product being cooked. The temperatures for cooking in oil or frying are usually 25-40°C below their smoking point and range from 114-220°C for different fats.

Procedure

The readiness of an oil or fat used for frying can be tested using household tests or a cooking thermometer.

A. (*i*) Place bread slices on the chopping board, remove the crusts and cut into even sized cubes.

   (*ii*) Heat l 00ml fat in a beaker with a thermometer suspended from a stand so that its bulb dips in the oil. Record the initial temperature of the melted fat and then after every two minutes during heating, using a stop watch for accuracy.

   (*iii*) When the temperature reaches 117°C drop a cube of bread in the hot oil, and if it rises to the top immediately the fat is ready for frying. Fry till the cube is golden brown.

   (*iv*) Lift the browned cube with the help of a fork so that the oil is drained back into the beaker Place the cube on a brown paper and leave for 15 minutes.

   (*v*) Note time taken for browning using a stop watch and record the end temperature of the oil.

   (*vi*) Repeat steps (*iii-v*) dropping one cube in the hot oil at each of the following temperatures: 117, 170, 180, 190, 200 and 210°C, removing each cube as it is browned.

   (*vii*) Keep samples labelled for evaluation.

B. (*i*) Repeat experiment A (*i–vii*) using mustard oil. (*ii*) Keep aside on brown paper.

C. (*i*) Repeat experiment A (*i–vii*) using vegetable oil.

D. (*i*) Repeat A (*i–vii*) using butter. Stop heating if the butter starts scorching, and note the temperature at which the last cube was fried.

(*ii*) Evaluate the results of frying in different fats and oils at the various temperatures, to determine the ideal frying temperature for each medium. Compare the time taken for frying and sensory qualities of the products.

Observations

Record your observations according to the format presented in Table 10.3. Cool the oil in each beaker to room temperature and measure after frying, to determine the amount of oil absorption during frying for each oil.

Table 10.4 Evaluation of suitability of fats for frying

Fat/Oil	Temp. °C	Time min/sec.	Product Quality			Fat/Oil absorption	Inference
			Appearance	Colour	Texture		
H. fat	117						
	170						
	180						
	190						
	200						
	210						
Mustard	117						
	170						
	*						
	*						
Vegetable	*						
	*						
Butter	*						
	*						

Determine the ideal temperature to use for frying with different fats and oils, by evaluating the temperature at which the fried product was best browned. Draw your inference on the oils best suited to frying, and those unsuitable, giving reasons. Also evaluate the oils after frying in terms of volume, appearance, clarity, viscosity, colour and odour.

Precautions

Same as for experiment 43.

Practice Exercises

1. Use coconut, groundnut, saffola, soya and palm oils for frying. Comment on their suitability by evaluating the products for their quality and acceptabiliy.
2. Use the different oils for shallow frying *tikkis,* and sauteeing vegetables. Evaluate the products and comment on the suitability of the fats for use in these methods of cooking.

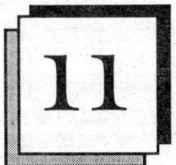

11

Fat Substitutes

Fat substitutes are fat-like foods specially processed to replace true fats in dietaries, in order to reduce the calorific value of the foods. Many new products have been manufactured and marketed to substitute for true or natural fats such as margarines for butter, or low calorie foods designed according to customer demand.

Fat substitutes can be categorized into two distinct classes one, those which are less energy dense than the natural fats and two, those that behave like a fat but are not readily absorbed by the body. These are therefore useful for formulating low energy diets and food products without compromising the textural and other sensory and functional properties of the fats normally used in food preparation. Some examples are, fats designed with high smoking points for better suitability for frying, or low melting points for better spreadability, changing textures of oils for longer shelf-life, storage and easier transportation.

Thus fat substitutes are macromolecules that physically and chemically resemble triglycerides which can replace conventional fats and oils. These are derived from conventional fats by enzymatic modification or chemical synthesis. Chemically synthesized lipids provide no calories as they are not metabolized and can be used in high temperature applications such as in frying operations. For example, *salatrim* which is a modified triglyceride containing one long chain and two short chain fatty acids. It is partially digested and provides 5 kcal per gram (Sharma et al., 1998).

Fat Modification

Fats are modified in a number of ways to serve intended goals in terms of their usage in food preparation and processing. This may be done through mechanical, chemical or enzymatic processes such as hydrogenation, esterification, superglycerination, rearrangement, acetylation, halogenation or isomerization.

Hydrogenation

The process by which unsaturated oils or their blends may be saturated by passing hydrogen through them during processing is known as hydrogenation. The double bonds decrease in the process while some may even migrate to other positions in the fat molecule. Temperature, pressure and the degree of agitation all influence these changes. After the hydrogenation process is complete the liquid fat is subjected to nitrogen gas under pressure. The fat is then rapidly cooled to 18°C and agitated to bring about crystallization. With the sudden release of pressure the gas gets dispersed through the fat, which is then warmed to change the crystals first formed to a more stable form. After this warming or *tempering* the consistency of the fat does not change during storage. The process makes the oils become solid at room temperature and acquire the properties of solid fats as seen in the manufacture of *vanaspati* processed from vegetable oils.

Hydrogenation increases the melting point, improves flavour, stability and plasticity. But, the process introduces a number of isomers which increases HDL cholesterol due to the formation of trans fatty acids.

Esterification

This is the reverse of hydrolysis and involves the combining or recombining of free fatty acids with glycerol to form mono-, di- and triglycerides. Mono- and diglyceride formation is called glycerolysis or super glycerination.

Superglycerination

This is a process of converting true fats into ones which contain monoglyceride in the form of 2-3% glyceryl mono stearate with smaller amounts of diglyceride.

Rearrangement

When fat is heated in the presence of nitrogen and a suitable catalyst, fatty acid radicals migrate and recombine randomly with glycerol to form new glycerides making it more heterogenous. The process which is also referred to as *interesterification*, brings about changes in consistency and plasticity that remains over a wide range of temperature.

Migration or interchange of fatty acid radicals from one fat to another or one point in the molecule to another, leads to ester interchange reactions. These may occur randomly or be directed, but do not change the degree of unsaturation of the fat, inspite of a change in its fatty acid positions.

Acetylation

This is a process in which the acetic acid radicals replace fatty acid radicals in a fat molecule. The resultant acetin fat may be liquid or plastic depending on the nature of the fatty acids present. The process lowers the melting point without affecting its stability. Acetin fats are transluscent and waxy rather than grainy on crystallisation. These fats form flexible films and are often used for coating dried fruits, meats, cheeses and nuts (Charley, 1982).

Halogenation

Halogens like chlorine, bromine and Iodine can readily attach themselves at the double bonds in the fat structure. This process is used in laboratories to determine the degree of unsaturation of a fat.

Isomerization

This takes place when two or more fats are composed of the same fatty acids although in different structural arrangements. Two important types of isomers have been identified, the *cis* and *trans* forms. The process is called geometric or positional isomerism (Lawson, 1997).

True fats may be partially or wholly replaced in natural or processed foods containing them. Schaefer et al. (1996) have described fat replacers as substitutes, mimetics and bulking agents, which may be carbohydrate, protein or lipid based. Efforts have been made to modify high energy properties of fats in four ways:

1. Combining water and surface active lipids or non-lipid additives of lower energy values. These include polysaccharides or proteins which have good gelling or emulsifying properties.
2. Adding compounds with low heat of combustion such as acetoglycerides.
3. Substitution with acaloric compounds such as silicones and paraffins, whose structure differs from triglycerides.
4. Replacing fat with substances exhibiting fat-like properties resembling those of ordinary lipids but with ester bonds modified, such as glycerol ethers, pseudo fats and carbohydrate fatty acid esters.

Fat Mimetics

Mimetics are substances that imitate the organoleptic and or physical properties of fats and oils, and cannot replace fat on a one-to-one basis. They are usually carbohydrate or protein based, such as starches and maltodextrins which may be chemically modified to mimic fat functionally (Akoh, 1998). They provide 4 kcal per gram and are totally digested. Protein based mimetics such as *simplesse* are minute and spherical in shape, and therefore provide smoothness to foods in which they are used as replacers.

Bulking Agents

These are substances which add body and texture to food products in which sugar has been replaced by high intensity sweeteners. They include food gums or hydrophillic colloids which easily swell up in aqueous systems to give thickening, gelling and creaming properties as required for a product.

A new source of conventional fat is derived from microalgae which have the ability to synthesize specific triglycerides that are more homogenous than those present in natural fats. Fats containing up to 50% of the omega-3 acids *eicosapentaenoic* (EPA) and *docosahexanoic* (DHA) have been obtained from this source. However, such fats cannot be produced in quantity as against fish oils which are also good sources (Lawson, 1997).

Carbohydrate based Fat Substitutes

Hydrocolloids not only resemble fats in physical and chemical properties but physiologically help to reduce blood cholesterol and moderate glucose responses in diabetics. These include gums, gels and other derivatives of starches and celluloses. Carbohydrate based substitutes give products which are stable to heat and safe for use in salad dressings, margarines, soups, desserts, dairy products and baked products.

Gums

Gums are not fat substitutes but their hydrophillic properties allows them to replace fat partially because of their water holding capacity, which helps foods to remain moist and soft. Carrageenan is extensively used in the processing of meat for low fat hamburgers in which it is responsible for reducing the fat calories from 30 to 9 per cent (Lawson, 1997).

Gums are used at 0.1-0.5% levels to dramatically increase viscosity and thereby provide stability particularly in food emulsions (Glicksmann, 1991). In food preparation and processing they find wide applications in bakery foods, breakfast cereals, sauces, dips and spreads, dairy and meat products, low calorie beverages, sweeteners and snack foods.

Cellulose gel

The microcrystalline form of cellulose obtained by partial depolymerization of cellulose, is marketed as *Avicel,* which when dispersed in water or other liquid, forms a colloidal dispersion of insoluble cellulose particles. The soft creamy gel formed is rheologically similar to an oil-in-water emulsion and used for processing of frozen desserts, salad dressings, sour cream and spreads (Pszczola, 1991; Penichter and McGinley, 1991).

Starch derivatives

Starch derivatives are maltodextrins, obtained by partial enzymatic hydrolysis of saccharides followed by spray drying. In the process, amylose and amylopectins of the starch form cleavages, the degree of polymerization determining the functions of the maltodextrins formed.

Starch degraded to lower molecular weight compounds with lowered dextrose equivalence (DE) has fat mimicking properties. DE is a measure of reducing sugar content calculated as percent dextrose on dry weight basis. The DE of starch is zero as against that of dextrose which is 100 (Glicksmann, 1991). The lower the DE value of the maltodextrins the better is its fat substitution ability. For example, potato starch maltodextrin has a calorific value of 16 kJ/g as against 28 kJ in fats used for icecream manufacture, bringing about a calorie reduction of about 30% in comparison to traditional icecream.

Other polymers are cornstarch maltodextrin which is non-sweet and produces a bland flavour, smooth mouthfeel and texture similar to that of hydrogenated oils, used in margarines and other table spreads. Tapioca starch derivatives form reversible gels with fat-like qualities. *Leanmaker* an oat bran based fat replacer has been reported to provide the texture, flavour and juiciness to lean meat products which closely resemble full fat meat (Inglett and Grisamore, 1991). LEANesse, a meat fat substitute is used up to 96% in various meat products (Lawson, 1997).

Polydextrose

A low calorie polydextrose derivative prepared from glucose, sorbitol and polycarboxylic acid catalyst is used as a substitute for replacing one or two of the fatty acids in the fat molecule. The polydextrose is a water soluble amorphous solid having bulking properties and providing only 1 kcal per gram. It is used for reducing the energy value of food products in the candy, confectionery, bakery and dairy industries through partial fat substitution.

Other carbohydrate fat replacers such as inulin from chicory roots, pectins and hemicelluloses from a variety of plant sources are also modified and used.

Protein-based Replacers

Protein based substitutes are manufactured from proteins of eggs especially white, and milk casein and whey proteins. *Simplesse* a low calorie substitute is produced from milk and egg white proteins and sugar by a process of heating and blending called *microparticulation,* in which the protein size is reduced to very minute particles. This enables the products to maintain their textural properties of smoothness, viscosity, mouthfeel and so on. *Simplesse* however, is not stable to heat and therefore not suitable for cooking. It is used only for processing foods like frozen desserts, icings, dips and sauces. Other replacers tested are *Lita, Trail blazer, Yoghurtesse* and some cereal protein products.

Lipid based Fat Substitutes

The properties of fats depend largely on their fatty acid composition and their attachment to the glycerol. The changes brought about in lipid based substitutes are either with respect to the substitution of glycerol or the fatty acids. The changes therefore result in two types of products.

Esterified Propoxylated Glycerol (EPG)

The structure of EPG is similar to that of natural fat but they are propylene oxide derivatives. EPG is a low calorie, heat stable fat substitute made by combining propylene oxide with a naturally occurring fat. The substitute is resistant to enzymatic digestion and therefore finds use in zero or low calorie products like spreads, frozen desserts, salad dressings and bakery products.

Polyglycerol Esters

These are obtained by the esterification of polyglycerol with fatty acids. The glycerol is first polymerized and then esterified with fatty acids. The resulting ester is more surface active than mono or diglycerides providing greater emulsification stability in products.

Polysiloxane

This is an organic derivative of silica and has a linear polymeric structure, the type depending on the organic radicals present such as methyl or phenyl groups or their mixtures. These compounds are chemically inert, not absorbed by the body and nontoxic. Their viscosity is maintained over a large range of temperature and are resistant to oxidation, hydrolysis and degradation.

Structured Lipids

Structured lipids in the form of medium chain triglycerides (MCT) as a fat alternative has been considered for broad usage. Coconut oil is a good source of C8 and C10 acids, which comprise 98% of the MCTs, and have unique properties of low viscosity, oxidative stability, are colourless, bland and provide only 8.3 kcal per gram. They act as important flavour carriers and therefore important for manufacture of any food. *Caprenin* has been developed as a reduced calorie replacer for cocoa butter, and contains the fatty acids caprylic, capric and behenic obtained from peanut oil and butter fat.

Synthetic Fats

Fats which completely substitute the natural fat or oil in a product are called synthetic fats and contribute zero calories. Such fats are structured to increase oxidative stability and provide a wide range of plasticity required for food processing operations. They are made by a process of introducing acetic acid into the triglyceride molecule by interesterification and are therefore called *acetin fats*. They are prepared from sucrose and 6-8 long chain fatty acids. Like sucrose polyesters, acetin fats are heat stable and not absorbed by the body. An example is *Olestra* which is used in shortenings and oils for the preparation of snack foods.

Fats are modified to produce special melting characteristics required in products like chocolates and ice creams. While genuine chocolates are based on cocoa butter, ice creams get their smoothners and eating quality from milk fat.

The cocoa butter substitutes (CBS) derived from vegetable fats are now permitted in chocolate manufature from 5-25% levels. Fats are extracted from unconventional sources such as kokum, sal, mango kernel etc. all forming an excellent base for creating CBS fats. (only IFI, 2005).

Blended Oils

The term suggests that a number of oils from different sources may be mixed together, refined and packaged. This is done to give the qualities of fats desired for specific processing needs. Further, it helps to get the best combination of fatty acids essential to health, prolong life of the oil in storage and remain in usable condition at high temperatures of use as in frying and so on. Besides it helps to reduce prices because cheaper edible oils can be blended for good acceptability.

Experiments 45 and 46 are based on the use of a fat substitute as used in food preparation since most fat placers are used in processing industries the experiment will give an idea about household uses for commonly marketed products like margarine.

EXPERIMENT 45

Aim

To demonstrate the method of preparing peanut butter.

Equipment

Weighing scale, grinder, electrical or hand beater, *kadai,* burner, mixing bowl and glass jar.

Materials

Groundnuts, ghee or clarified butter, salt, sugar.

Principle

Butter is a liquid in oil emulsion, and nuts have over 50% fat or oil and some moisture in which the proteins and other elements are dispersed. They therefore form a good vehicle for butter making. Whether the emulsion remains stable or not depends on the quantity of oil or fat and moisture in the product. When roasted nuts are used the moisture present in further reduced and therefore the oil may rise to the surface on keeping, as all of it is not used up for emulsification. The butter prepared is stabler if the nuts are not subjected to heat treatment as there is enough water and solids to be dispersed in the oil. However, aroma, flavour and palatability are enhanced on roasting. Besides all nuts cannot be used for making butter without prior heat treatment, as this is necessary for better acceptability and keeping quality. Temperature too is a determinant of stability.

Procedure

A. (*i*) Weigh 100g groundnuts, roast them in a kadai, cool and weigh again. Note the difference in weight.

(*ii*) Grind-the nuts fine, and place in a mixing bowl.

(*iii*) Add 2T melted ghee, 1/8T powdered sugar and a pinch of salt and mix well.

(*iv*) Use a beater and continue beating the mixture till creamy in texture. The oil present in the nuts will be released and get emulsified.

(*v*) Transfer the butter to a preweighed jar and record the net weight of the product, Keep aside.

B. (*i*) Repeat A (*i-v*) with cashwnuts and keep aside for evaluation.

(*ii*) Place half the samples from A and B in the refrigerator and the other half at room temperature.

C. (*i*) Repeat A (*i-v*) with coconut but do not roast the nut.

(*ii*) As in B (*ii*).

Observations

Note the differences in the net weights obtained and compare the results of A, B, and C with respect to colour, texture, flavour, stability and spreadability. Keep all the samples and observe for shelf life every week, recording any sensory or other changes as they occur, both under refrigeration and at room temperature.

Tabulate the results obtained and draw inferences as to applicability of the products for home or industry use.

Precautions

1. Clean the bowl thoroughly before making each of the products.
2. Mix for the same amount of time so that comparisons can be made.
3. Keep the products in the refrigerator for use as required if room temperature is above 22°C.

Practice Exercises

1. Prepare butter as learnt using other nuts and study their shelf life and applicability.
2. Use shelled and deoiled almonds and prepare butter from both separately. Compare products for colour, texture, taste, spread, stability, acceptability and shelf life.
3. Prepare the butter as learnt using coarsely ground peanuts and compare the texture, mouthfeel and stability of the emulsion with that prepared from finely ground nuts.

EXPERIMENT 46

Aim
To use a fat substitute in the preparation of plain biscuits.

Equipment
Bowl, baking sheet, oven board, rolling pin, biscuit cutter and wire rack.

Materials
Refined wheat flour, butter, margarine, castor sugar, baking powder, egg and milk.

Principle
Biscuits are prepared from dough which has been shortened with fat, but can easily be rolled out and cut into desired shapes and sizes. The usual fat used is butter or hydrogenated fat, but fat substitutes are also in processing. The type of fat largely influences the textural properties of biscuits besides other sensory attributes for acceptability.

Procedure

A. Biscuit preparation using butter.
  (*i*) Sieve 50 g flour and baking powder together.
  (*ii*) Cream 25g butter with 25g sugar till light and fluffy and beat in 1/4 egg.
  (*iii*) Add flour to the above mixture and make a dough with milk as required.
  (*iv*) Roll the dough to 1/4 in thickness on a floured board, and cut into desired shape. Prick each biscuit with a fork.
  (*v*) Place on lightly greased baking sheet and bake at 180°C for about 10-15 minutes or till golden in colour.
  (*vi*) Remove and keep to cool on a wire rack.

B. Biscuit using margarine.
  (*i*) Repeat A (*i-vi*) but use margarine instead of butter.
  (*ii*) Place both the prepared products and test for colour, break, texture and mouthfeel. Comment on the similarity or difference between using the natural fat and the substitute on the quality and acceptability of the products.

C. (*i*) Prepare biscuit as learnt and use the rubbing method for fat incorporation.
  (*ii*) Compare the product with those from A and B.

Observations
Tabulate your observations as learnt.

Precautions
  1. Weigh the ingredients accurately.
  2. Cream butter and sugar till fluffy to enclose maximum air.

3. Preheat the oven before baking.
4. Let biscuits cool before evaluation.

Practice Exercises

1. Make toasts and apply butter on one and margarine on another. Evaluate the products for acceptability.
2. Prepare home made butter and bake a cake with it using a standard recipe. Repeat using any fat substitute in the market. Evaluate for sensory and acceptability characteristics.

FOOD PRESERVATION

Food preservation literally means preserving or preventing foods from any kind of spoilage. Early attempts to preserve foods were based on readily available foods and processes. Food preservation was thus limited to methods used by households to condition fresh seasonal foods in different innovative ways, not only to preserve them for consumption when not in season but, also to add variety to meals at all times. This necessarily required, methods that could enable treated foods to remain wholsome, using the limited resources available at hand, to be stored for longer periods and used as and when desired or required.

A number of methods were thus developed by experience and the practice of sundrying or cooking to dryness, pickling, curing, syruping and fermentation were the conventional methods of preservation used in households for thousands of years. Even today, these are followed in every household and form part of daily meals. Examples are fermentation of milk to form curds and cheese, using dried pulses, grains and spices or their mixtures, and curing for pickling of vegetables, fruits, meats and preparation of jams and preserves.

Traditional methods and meal composition has thus led to further innovations using modern methods and equipment, used to prolong shelf life of produts and add convenience to meal preparation. Research and development efforts have resulted in new food products on market shelves for increasing variety in meals and eased transportation of the products throughout the country and globally as well, to satisfy the varying needs of consumers, considering the adoption of a variety of meal patterns from different regions.

Today, household food processes and preservation methods have shifted largely to the factory where processes have been streamlined through automated machinery and products produced in large scale. Newer equipment has also helped to standardize sensory and other qualities of products. Foods are now being manufactured, packed, labeled, branded and shelved for convenience and use, keeping in line with changing living, cooking and eating lifestyles.

Food Preservation

All foods when harvested contain different amounts of moisture and vary in their degree of acidity, thereby making them perishable to different extents. On the above basis, foods are classified as perishable, semi-perishable and nonperishable considering the average period for which they may be stored in wholesome condition prior to use. What is important however is, that foods especially plants, continue to respire even after harvesting, and therefore are vulnerable to contamination and spoilage by dust, dirt, microorganisms, chemicals, radiations and oxidation. Meats too are highly perishable and prone to spoilage, and therefore require special care in storage and use.

In order to extend the freshness, wholesomeness or fitness of foods for use, they have been treated traditionally in many ways in every country. This collective wisdom, which was aimed at getting the most out of food in terms of health, availability, variety and value for money provided the basis for the development of modern methods *of Food* Pr*eser*v*ation.* The term therefore implies, prevention of spoilage in foods by any means be it physical, chemical or microbial, that may take place even unknowingly, although the food in question may appear perfectly sound.

Principles of Food Preservation

The principles of food preservation are based on creating in or around the food, such conditions that will inhibit the growth or survival of harmful microorganisms, remove harmful chemicals or toxins from food, inactivate food enzymes and form barriers to entry of insects, rodents etc. that can spoil the food by mechanical or excretory action. The principles of food preservation are therefore based on:

- Maintenance of aseptic conditions in the food environment
- Inactivation or destruction of microbial or enzymatic activity
- Prevention or delay of self decomposition of food
- Prevention of damage to food due to insects, rodents, animals and mechanical causes

Different foods require preservation treatments according to their specific structure and composition but the principles remain the same.

Methods of Food Preservation

All methods of food preservation are aimed at keeping food wholesome and fit for human consumption, whether practiced at household or manufacturing level. The method chosen for each food depends largely on the time for which the food is required to be stored in wholesome condition for future consumption. The time may vary from one day to one year depending on the purpose for which the food is being preserved such as extending its shelf life for:

- Making foods available for off-seasons
- Reducing meal preparation time
- Taking the price advantage when foods are in season
- Adding variety to the diet
- Stabilizing market prices of foods
- Making foods easy to transport for better nutrition or trade
- Making food available in emergency, difficult or disaster situations

The methods of preservation are basically categorized as *bacteriostatic* and *bactericidal,* the former providing conditions for inhibiting the growth of microorganisms and the latter bringing about their destruction.

Bacteriostatic methods

These basically prevent microbial or enzymatic growth in foods and prevent their spoilage by keeping the number of bacteria present static or by inactivation of enzymes present in foods. They work through adjustments made in the food and its environment in a manner that growth or activity is inhibited and food preserved for longer periods. This is done by:

- Reducing the moisture content of foods and controlling the humidity in its environment
- Maintaining temperatures at which microbes cannot thrive
- Lowering pH and increasing the acidity in and around foods
- Removing oxygen partially or totally from the food environment
- Inactivating enzymes
- Addition of hygroscopic agents like sugar, salt and spices

These goals have been achieved through traditional and modern methods developed from time to time through research and development efforts in food science, technology and food engineering.

Bactericidal methods

These methods involve the destruction of microbes in foods by subjecting them to suitable heat and cold treatments depending on the optimum temperatures for the growth of specific microorganisms present in different foods. These methods were traditionally carried out in home kitchens and supplemented by using the heat of the sun to preserve foods for longer use. The preservation methods commonly used are outlined in Fig.12.1.

All methods are thus based on the above mentioned principles, which attempt to ensure aseptic conditions throughout the procedures followed for handling foods through all the processes from harvesting till they reach the consumer. Hygiene and sanitation practices at every stage are important and suitable treatments are therefore necessary for increasing shelf life of foods and their continuous availability.

Today, food processing technologies have made it possible to control temperatures, humidity, volume, water activity, acidity, oxygen supply and even change the atmospheres within storages and packages to strictly control the quality and enhance storage life of foods.

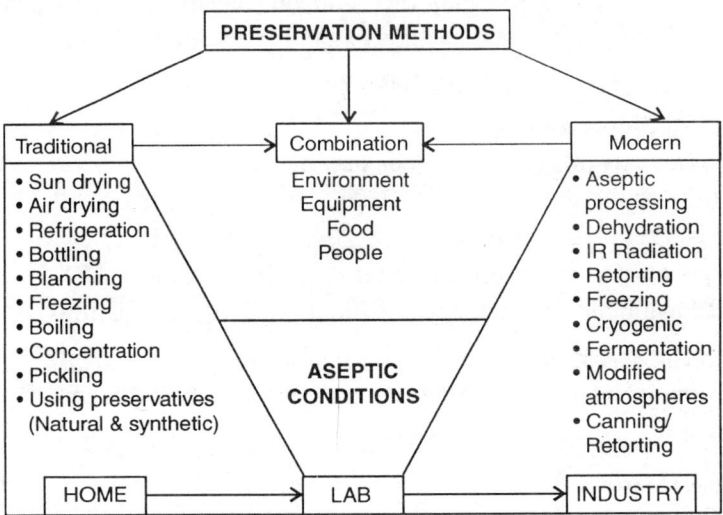

Notes: 1. All processes need to be followed under aseptic conditions.

2. Any of the methods may be combined to develop a process.

3. Home freezing is possible only if a deep freezer is available.

Fig. 12.1. Methods of food preservation.

Discussing the details of each method is not within the purview of this text, but some methods of preservation are discussed briefly for clarity, namely *physical methods, asepsis, chemical methods, controlling microorganisms* and *combination methods.*

Physical methods

These involve the physical handling of foods right from farm to table, the aim being to retain their freshness and safety along the way, whether they are prepared at home or manufactured in the form of ingredients, ready to use or ready-to-eat foods. These handling methods involve cutting and trimming inedible parts of plants from which foods are then packed according to their textures, sizes etc. as required, and subsequently transported to markets for the consumer.

The handling of foods in bulk can lead to physical damage in the form of bruises and cuts that can cause spoilage through entry of pathogenic microorganisms from dust and soil adhering to foods. Tropical climates with high temperatures and humidity can accelerate spoilage, to prevent which the damaged pieces need to be sorted out manually and discarded immediately before the spoilage spreads.

Physical changes do not form any new compounds in foods, but include the impact of gravity that manifests them. These changes are usually seen in the form of heavier particles settling down, molecules going out of solution, free water getting released and moving through evaporation, osmosis, diffusion or leaching. Some of these changes are reversible as in the re-mixing of separated salad dressings while others are not, as when milk separates out into cheese and whey.

The nature of physical changes that are commonly observed in the process of food preservation are of three kinds, namely, a change of state, separation and or dissolving out of certain soluble components of foods.

Change of state

This is seen in foods when:

- The water present changes to solid as in a frozen food. This causes damage to its structure due to ice formation. The result is hardening of the food inhibiting activity required for preservation.
- Water evaporates to different extents depending on the exposure to air and temperature differentials, resulting in a shriveled surface and reduced weight and volume. This is seen on the surface of a refrigerated uncovered food or in dehydrated fruits like raisins, dates and figs.
- Foods take up moisture and the vapour turns to liquid increasing the moisture content of the foods and hence their perishability.
- Sugars present in syrups like corn, honey and so on, crystallize and affect their texture, taste and flavour. Jellies, jams and candies are also prone to this change of state if not prepared and preserved under controlled conditions.

Separation

These are general physical changes in which chemical interactions may sometimes be involved. The food shows two distinct layers of ingredients that were used to prepare it. This phenomena can be seen in:

- Unstable emulsions as two distinct layers of water and oil.
- Milk when left out in tropical summers and separates into the solid fraction and water.
- Cheese manufacture when the protein coagulum is separated intentionally from the liquid whey.
- Salad dressings when the solids settle and the lighter water soluble ingredients rise to the top.
- Batters kept aside for a while before use. This is of course reversible by mixing them again and using immediately.
- Gels that show a watery layer and a compact solid portion especially on refrigeration.

Dissolving

Water-soluble compounds such as sugars, some nutrients, salts, pigments and flavors may leach out during food preservation processes. It is for this reason that colors and flavors are added to processed foods to make them as attractive as the fresh foods.

Asepsis

Asepsis describes an environmental situation in and around foods that keeps them protected from agents of spoilage. This involves safe handling of foods to inhibit the activity of enzymes in foods, and prevent them from respiring normally by reducing the oxygen available to them. The immediate environment around the foods are subjected to a level of cleanliness that can ensure the elimination and thereby absence of harmful microbes, insects, rodents etc. Nature has provided most foods with aseptic covering in the form of peels, shells, skins and so on.

Antiseptic chemical formulations are however sometimes used for cleaning the food and its environment to provide spoilage free conditions. Some formulations commonly used are classified as chlorine based, iodine based, ammonium compounds, acid ionic surfactants and phenolic sanitizers.

Chlorine based

These are inexpensive bactericides such as hypochlorites, chloramines, and others used for rinsing equipment and are active against all microorganisms and spores. They are used at a concentration of 25mg per litre, at pH 10 or less and at a temperature of 50°C.

Iodine based

These are stable and do not deteriorate easily and have a long shelf life. They destroy most bacterial cells but not spores, are effective in hard water and non-corrosive. They do not leave residues or irritate the skin. The formulations work slowly at pH 5.0 or above and may stain some surfaces. Ideally used in concentrations of 12-25mg per litre at 24-49°C.

Ammonium compounds

These are also known as quarternary ammonium compounds (QUATS) and were developed to destroy organisms in food industries. They are water soluble, lower surface tension of solutions and can therefore contact and kill organisms that are not accessible to non wetting germicides. In addition, they are highly stable, non-corrosive and possess low odour, high germicidal activity and low toxicity, when used in specified concentrations.

Ammonium compounds are however sensitive to pH and work best at pH 9-10 destroying all coliform bacteria. In acid environments however, they are active against some pseudomonas organisms. Although these compounds are non-corrosive and non irritating they are not effective in hard water, and are not recommended for use in food handling environments as their residual effect is not fully known.

Acid non-ionic surfactants

These are stable compounds, active against microorganisms, are odourless, nonstaining and effective in hard water. If they do leave a residual film it is antibacterial and of low toxicity. Most effective at pH 1.9-3.0, but they corrode metals except stainless steel and aluminium. Spores survive their action even in concentrations of 100-200mg per litre and at temperatures of 24-43°C.

Phenolic compounds

These compounds are more stable used with synthetic anionics. They act as deodourizers but are not so effective in sanitizing food handling equipment.

Chemical methods

As the name suggests these methods make use of chemical compounds that are destructive to surface microbes and or toxins, although care has to be exercised in removing the chemicals before preparation or processing the raw foods. Chemical changes that take place during handling and processing are however generally non-reversible and therefore the safety of the food for consumers is a prime consideration in their use. Sometimes chemical reactions take place between compounds already present in foods and produce irreversible changes that may or may not be considered favorable to the quality of the food. Some of these are briefly described.

Maillard Browning

This is a reaction named after its French scientist, in which a chemical reaction takes place between proteins and reducing sugars present in foods or their mixtures during during roasting, baking, cooking or processing. Due to this reaction browning takes place and may also be accompanied by changes in colour, flavor and texture of foods. Since no enzyme activity is involved in the reaction it is called a non-enzymatic reaction.

The Maillard reaction is responsible for the desirable browning of most foods upon heating such as on the crust on breads and cakes, roasted meats coffee beans, soya sauce and roasted nuts. The browning occurs slowly at room temperatures, but is accelerated by low moisture and heat and retarded by refrigeration temperatures.

The browning reactions that occur during long term storage of foods are a major cause of quality concern in preserved foods, as very small amounts of both carbohydrates and proteins present in food enzymes and cell walls are enough for the reaction to take place. The effects of the reaction are more pronounced in foods which are light in colour, the browning increasing with time of storage. This is undesirable and is called non-enzymatic browning.

The chemicals used in food preservation are termed as *preservatives* and their use is determined according to the nature of the foods and the methods of processing used for each category or type. Preservatives are chemical salts or compounds used according to the Food Laws prescribed in every country. Some follow international standards in terms of minimum and or maximum levels present or added during processing, for safety of consumers. In India, the PFA Act, 1954 lays down the rules to be followed by food processing industries. The Act is amended from time to time and newer rules formulated as required. Some commonly used preservatives permissible in any product are presented in Annexure.

The choice of chemicals used should normally have no effect on the structure and composition of the foods, nor react with the packaging material or disagree in any way with the consumer of the food.

Controlling microbial spoilage

Spoilage in foods can be caused by several types of micro-plants and organisms including molds, yeasts and bacteria. Controlling the growth of microorganisms on or in foods requires an understanding of what each one of these require for their growth. In general, their inactivation or destruction can be brought about by decreasing the available moisture required for their activity, reducing the pH of the foods to levels at which they cannot grow and removing oxygen from the environment in which the foods are kept, handled or stored.

Molds

Molds grow on foods particularly in warm, damp and dark places as they grow well between 25-30°C and some types even at refrigeration temperatures. Their presence can be noticed by a fuzzy or cottony appearance on food surfaces appearing as gray, white or even green and red-orange patches, comprising of a mass of branching multi-cellular filaments. A small number of species however, produce toxic materials in the form of *mycotoxins*.

If grains are not properly dried after harvesting *aflatoxin* is produced in peanuts, wheat, millets and other grains. Bulk storage of grains and nuts as done in FCI godowns, in cramped spaces in wholesale markets or in food industry bulk storages, can produce toxicity in the foods as they are piled one over the other. The temperatures and humidity in such storages become conducive to mold growth, especially at contact surfaces between the layers of grain. Special care therefore needs to be taken to provide well ventilated, lighted and temperature controlled storages. Bulk transportation of grains too, requires attention.

Yeasts

Yeasts reproduce by a process of cell budding usually in the presence of oxygen and sugar. They grow rapidly between 28-30°C and during spoilage, hydrolyse the sugar in foods to acid and carbon dioxide. Yeasts therefore grow in sweet or sweetened foods such as fruits, doughs and batters in which they cause fermentation.

Bacteria

These are unicellular microorganisms smaller in size than molds and yeasts, but differing in their shapes and sizes, on the basis of which they are generally classified. Bacteria with round shaped cells are called *cocci*, cylindrical are *bacilli* and spiral are *spirilla*. Each type have different requirements of food, moisture and pH for their growth which is usually rapid between 20-53°C. Bacteria may also be classified according to the temperatures at which their growth is optimum for example, those that grow best at or above 45°C are called *thermophils*, between 20-25°C are called *mesophils* and those growing below 20°C are termed as *psychrophils*. The optimum pH ranges also vary for each category of bacteria.

However, all microorganisms are not harmful and do not necessarily cause spoilage in foods. Some strains have been successfully used for a long time to bring about desirable changes in foods in an effort to provide variety in flavours, textures and colours in diets, in addition to some even enhancing the nutritive value of the foods so treated.

Food science research has created foods and food combinations suited to all types of needs, by not only using microplants and organisms but also using the specific enzymes they produce in the foods or as isolates.

Enzymes

Enzymes are organic catalysts produced by living cells working to activate many reactions that take place in foods, both favourable and unfavourable which can be used in various ways by the food industry. Enzymes act within a wide range of temperatures varying from 0-60°C with optimum activity at 37°C. Some enzymes such as papain and bromelin from raw papaya and pineapples, help to tenderize tough cuts of meat, yeast enzymes ferment sugars for production of alcoholic beverages and vinegar, or help in leavening breads and are considered useful. Even those organisms that degrade or spoil foods are now being favourably used in the reduction of huge volumes of organic wastes by the food industries for waste management.

Combination methods

Some combination methods have been used traditionally for centuries such as blanching and sun-drying, pickling, preserving with sugar, salt and spices, all of which require the food to pass through various methods of handling, part cooking to destroy microorganisms or inactivate enzymes naturally present in foods. Some of the processes used are briefly described as examples.

Drying

Traditionally drying was carried out through the use of air drying with or without solar rays, as foods treated in different ways were left in the sun to dry, for many days till the products lost most of their moisture. Many vegetables and fruits were cut, washed and blanched to inactivate enzymes, then left covered with a muslin cloth and placed in the sun to remove moisture. Vegetables and fruits like cauliflower, turnips, figs etc were strung into a garland and hung in the sun to provide enough air circulation around every piece to prevent humid spots. This was done for several days till the fruit or vegetable dried up enough to become rigid in texture. It was then stored in airtight jars to use for variety in cooking during off seasons.

The disadvantages of traditional methods were however, that foods dried unevenly and the final products were shrunken and often darkened to different extents, since the time, temperature and exposure to sunlight could not be strictly controlled. Most products also had to be rehydrated before use in order to soften the texture.

Today, advancement in processing technologies have made it possible to bring foods to us around the globe, in forms wholesomeness and sensory qualities that were not imagined a few decades ago. This has been made possible only through research in food science and food engineering which has helped a great deal to enable us to understand how spoilage takes place and how it can be prevented without jeopardizing the quality of the food that comes to the table.

Methods of preservation thus, have become assembly line processes as foods have been taken fresh from farm to manufacturing units. This is evident from the large variety of food products seen on supermarket shelves and consumed in the form of cereal products, preserved fruits, meat, fish, poultry, seafoods, sauces, dressings, soups, mixes and so on.

This has been made possible by newer technology and methods that have helped to increase the shelf-life of foods which would otherwise have perished. In addition lifestyle changes of consumers demanding more and more convenience has prompted food industries to provide convenience foods, ready to mix, cook and serve or ready to eat from the package as desired.

Experiments 47-49 that follow, have been designed to familiarize the student with both traditional methods of preservation as well as those using newer equipment through which conditions of preservation can be controlled in the laboratory to help maintain product quality.

EXPERIMENT 47

Aim

To Prepare a fruit squash.

Equipment

Juice extractor, stainless steel (s.s.) cooking utensils, s.s.strainer or sieve, jug, washed and sterilized squash bottles, corks, screw caps, corking machine, s.s. knife, funnel, Clean kitchen cloths, chopping board, pH paper.

Materials

Lemon 1 kg, orange 1 dozen, guava 1 kg, grapes 1 kg, or other seasonal fruit, sugar and water as calculated using squash composition, potassium metabi- sulphite (KMS), sodium benzoate, citric acid, colour, essence as required.

Principle

Fruit beverages such as squashes, cordial, ready-to-serve beverage etc. are prepared from fruit juices or pulp and preserved by chemical preservatives or by application of heat. They need to be diluted with water or soda before converting to a beverage. The degree of dilution depends on individual tastes. Basically they are a combination of fruit juice and sugar syrup to which preservatives may or may not be added depending on the duration for which the squash needs to be stored. A squash generally contains 25% fruit juice or pulp, 50% total soluble solids (TSS), 1.5-1.6% acid and approximately 25% water.

Squashes remain in good condition for months if preservatives are added. This is important when fruits and vegetables are available seasonally and need to be stored for use till the next season. Once a bottle is opened for use it needs to be stored in the refrigerator especially in tropical summers. The main preservatives added to squashes are sugar, acid and KMS. Where squashes are made from dark coloured fruits like black grapes, *phalsa* or *jamun* sodium benzoate is used instead of KMS, because the latter will bleach the colour of the squash. Colour and flavour are added just before bottling if the product is to be stored for use as natural colours fade and flavours decrease on storage.

Procedure

The experiment is divided into sections A, B, and C to enable students to compare the products for sensory quality using different fruits.

    A. Method of preparing lemon squash.
   (*i*) Choose good quality smooth skin lemons.
  (*ii*) Wash well and wipe clean and dry.
 (*iii*) Cut lemons horizontally at right angles to the proximal end, using a stainless steel knife.
 (*iv*) Extract juice with the help of a conical juice extractor or a lime press.
  (*v*) Strain the juice through a s.s. sieve, and weigh it.
 (*vi*) Determine the pH using pH strips and the T.S.S. of the juice using a refractometer. From the refractometer reading calculate the amount of sugar and water required as follows:

Wt. of juice = 500g

Wt. of prepared squash (Juice being 25%)   = $500 \times 4 = 2000$g or 2 kg.

Refractometer reading of T.S.S.   = 7 %

Then T.S.S. from juice $= \dfrac{7}{100} \times 500 = 35$g

T.S.S. of squash is 50% $= \dfrac{2000}{2} = 1000$g

Amount of KMS required   = 1-2g

Therefore sugar required $= 1000 - (35 + 2.0g) = 963$g

Water required for the squash $= 2000 - (963 + 2.0 + 500) = 535$g

---

Note: No extra acid is necessary for lemon squash as the natural acidity of the juice is about 6%, and this will give the right pH in the final product. For other fruit juices if pH measurement requires addition of acid, it should be done in A(*vi*) when the syrup starts boiling.

(*vii*) Heat sugar and water and boil for 1-2 minutes, adding a few drops of the juice to clear the syrup. Keep aside to cool to room temperature.

(*viii*) Mix lemon juice to the cool syrup, measure the volume of the squash prepared, and its T.S.S.

(*ix*) Dissolve KMS in 1 t of water and mix to the squash.

(*x*) Pour into clean dry bottles using a dry funnel, then seal and label.

B. Repeat the steps in A using oranges for juice extraction instead of lemons.

C. Repeat the procedure using dark coloured fruit for the juice. Use sodium benzoate instead of KMS in step A(*ix*).

D. Keep aside 50 ml of juice from each of A,B,C and D, and mix them together to make mixed fruit juice. Use this to prepare the squash using the procedure in A.

E. Prepare squashes from each sample by dilution with same amount of water and make your observations. Using a refractometer determine the T.S.S. of the juices, bottled squashes and the beverages.

Observations

Record your observations for each squash in terms of number of bottles prepared or volume of squash bottled. Dilute to prepare the beverage and observe the sensory characteristics of the juice, squash and ready beverage. Make three separate tables as learnt and score the sensory qualities at each stage for colour, flavour, taste, likes or dislikes. Record your comments for general acceptability.

Precautions

1. Follow the calculations for the amounts of sugar and water required according to the weight of the juice extracted. Accuracy will give desired product each time.
2. Measurement of pH of juice is important to decide if acid needs to be added and how much.
3. Sugar must dissolve completely and the syrup allowed to boil for 1-2 minutes only.
4. Clarify the syrup with acid or lemon and cool it before mixing with the juice.
5. Tasting of the beverage should be done before adding the preservatives.

Practice Exercises

1. Prepare a squash using fresh guava juice and preserve according to the procedure learnt. Record your observations with respect to colour, taste, viscosity and pH. Keep one opened bottle each in the fridge and one outside screwed tightly. Use when required. Record any changes in taste, flavour etc every week and observe how long it takes for the product to remain in original condition.
2. Take a vegetable and fruit of your choice extract the juice and make squash from it. Record your observations.

EXPERIMENT 48

Aim

To prepare apple jam.

Equipment

Weighing balance, stove, refractometer, thermometer, wooden spoon, cooking pans, steel knife and jam jars.

Materials

Cooking applcs 2 kg, salt solution 2%, sugar 75%, citric acid 1½ t, essence and water.

Principle

Jam is a product made by boiling fruit pulp with sufficient sugar to a reasonably thick consistency, firm enough to hold the fruit tissues in position. Jam contains 0.5-0.6% acid and invest sugar should not be more than 40%. Jams set well if the proportion of sugar, pectin and acid are present in the right proportions. Since just ripe cooking apples have a good proportion of pectin in them, they make well set jams. Jams have pieces of fruit characteristic of the product and therefore the fruit should not be mushy when cooked. Jams need to be poured into jars when still hot so it is important to establish the right setting point before cooking is stopped.

Procedure

A (i) Weigh the apples accurately after washing and drying them.

(ii) Peel and cut into four segments, and remove the core and any blemishes.

(iii) Keep the fruit in 2% salt solution to prevent browning.

(iv) Cut each segment into small pieces and weigh them before placing them in the cooking pan.

(v) Add water equal to half the weight of fruit in the pan and cook till the fruit is tender but not pulpy.

(vi) Add sugar equal to 75% of the weight of the fruit to the pan and continue cooking with stirring.

(vii) Test the T.S.S. of the mixture using a Brix refractometer. At 66 degree Brix add the citric acid. Readiness can also be determined by noting the temperature of readiness with a sugar thermometer, or using the sheet or plate test as learnt on page 46.

(viii) Continue cooking till the T.S.S. reads 68°B. Stop cooking and remove from stove.

(ix) Add the apple essence, mix and fill sterilized dry jars with hot jam to the brim.

(x) On cooling seal jars with melted wax and screw caps.

(xi) Count the number of jars prepared. Determine the cost.

Observations

Assess the quality of the jam prepared and tabulate your observations with respect to colour, flavour, spreadability, texture and overall acceptability.

Precautions

1. During cooking the jam must be stirred constantly after addition of sugar to prevent burning at the bottom of the pan.
2. Only enough water to soften the fruit should be added to retain fruit pieces in the final product and prevent overcooking.
3. If the flavour of the fruit is strong enough , essence need not be added.

Practice Exercises

1. Test the pectin content of some fruits as learnt on p. 45 and list the high and low pectin ones separately.
2. Choose any high pectin fruit and prepare a jam as learnt. Make your observations and assess the product for sensory qualities. Comment on the acceptability of the product.
3. List the ways in which jams can be used in food preparation and processing.

EXPERIMENT 49

Aim

To prepare papaya chutney from raw papaya.

Equipment

Grinder, grater, peeler, refractometer, s.s. knife, spoons, stove, glass jars, stop watch and pH paper.

Materials

Raw papaya 1kg, sugar 1kg, garlic 5g, ginger 15g, onion 15g, dry dates 2, raisins 5-6, salt 25g, red chilli 5g, cinnamon 1g, cloves (headless) 2g, cumin seed 10g, black cardamom 1g, coriander 5g, black pepper 5g, glacial acetic acid 15ml. Red tomato colour and sodium benzoate 1/2t (optional).

Principle

Condiments, sugar, salt and acetic acid are the main preservatives in any chutney. No artificial preservatives are required unless the sugar content is lower than 65%, or the product is made in large quantity for storage, in which case sodium benzoate is added.

Procedure

A (*i*) Peel the green raw papaya, wash, wipe dry, cut and remove seed portion and grate.

   (*ii*) Weigh the grated fruit and place in a cooking pan with salt and water to cover. Salt should be added in the proportion of 250g per kg of fruit or 25% by wt of fruit.

  (*iii*) Place pan on stove and cook till fruit is tender.

  (*iv*) Add sugar equal to the weight of the grated papaya.

   (*v*) Cook the mixture till the refractometer shows a concentration of 65°B. Note the time taken.

  (*vi*) Add spices and condiments and continue cooking till the mixture reaches 68-70°B. Note the time taken to prepare the chutney.

 (*vii*) Remove from stove and add a pinch or drop of colour, 15ml glacial acetic acid and mix well.

(*viii*) Fill the hot chutney into sterilized and dry glass jars and leave to cool.

  (*ix*) Seal and store for use.

B. (*i*) Repeat A (*i-ix*) using 70% sugar in the preparation of the chutney.
Cooking for the same amount of time.

C. (*i*) Repeat B (*i-ix*) and add 50% sugar only. Keep all samples aside for comparison and evaluation.

Note: Measure the pH at each stage and comment on the differences in each sample.

Observations

Observe the differences in the products prepared in A,B and C with respect to colour, flavour, taste, texture and viscosity. Which is the best sample keeping overall acceptability in mind. Tabulate your observations recording the time, temperature, pH and concentration of the products as well. Indicate the applications of each product in food processing and cooking.

Precautions

The same precautions as in experiment 48 for jam preparation.

Practice Exercises

1. Prepare a chutney using tomatoes by procedure A. as learnt. Keep one jar aside and determine its shelf life.
2. Prepare chutney using any vegetable like brinjal, beetroot or carrot. How would you adjust the condiments and spices to get the maximum flavour from the product. Explain why this is necessary.
3. Compare the products of 1 and 2 and comment on their sensory qualities. Suggest modifications in ingredients for improving the products.

FOOD ADULTERATION

Food Adulteration is commonly thought of as the intentional or unintentional addition or subtraction of any substance to or from food, which alters its natural or original composition and quality. This alteration may or may not be detected by the consumer at the time of the purchase or consumption.

The Prevention of Food Adulteration Act, 1954 (PFA) with its numerous amendments and rules, goes a little further to include sanitary quality as being essential for any food at the point of its manufacture, sale and consumption so that it is not injurious to health.

Intentional Adulteration

Intentional adulteration is the act of knowingly adding substances to food, removal and or substitution of some of its ingredients changing its properties with the explicit purpose of making extra profits through deceitful means. Government of India records indicate that on an average 25-30% of edibles sold in the market are adulterated, the rate being more alarming in some states than in others.

Some examples of intentional adulteration are addition of water to liquid milk, extraneous matter to ground spices, or the removal and or substitution of milk solids from the natural product. The latter in its extreme is seen in the case of synthetic milk which is widespread today. Besides these, some colours, flavours, metallic residues from cooking vessels or processing equipment, water or soil can lead to symptoms of which the cause may not be easily detected.

Unintentional Adulteration

Foods can incidentally or unknowingly get contaminated during growth, harvesting, storage, processing, transportation and handling, as well as after it has been sold to the consumer. Incidental adulteration is usually attributed to ignorance, carelessness of lack of facilities for maintaining food quality. This kind of adulteration results from pesticide and insect residues or microorganisms entering the food right from the farm through other stages leading to the consumer.

In some cases toxins get produced in the food during storage even in the home if humidity and temperatures of storage are not maintained according to the perishability of the food. Since the appearance or other sensory qualities of toxic foods do not always show the changes, their consumption can produce illnesses varying from simple diarrhoea to fevers, gastrointestinal disturbances, organ failures and even death depending on the type or nature of the infestation or contamination.

Natural Adulteration

This occurs due to the presence of certain chemicals, organic compounds or radicals naturally occurring in foods which are injurious to health and are not added to the foods intentionally or unintentionally, such as toxic varieties of pulses, mushrooms, green and other vegetables, fish and sea-foods. About 5000 species of marine fish are known to be poisonous and many of these are among edible varieties.

In addition there are a number of chemicals synthesized by plants or present in animals that act as toxins when the foods are consumed. Some get destroyed during cooking and processing while others remain latent in their action till they reach body temperature, when they begin to show symptoms of disease.

Today, with almost every food we eat having a chance of being adulterated it is apt to quote Dr. T Venkatesh of St. John's Medical College, Bangalore (Outlook, 1998):

There are no natural deaths now. I am convinced that every death is caused by the adulteration of food.

Of course not all types of adulteration causes death, thanks to the immunity developed by people living and eating adulterated food as they have no choice, but surely there are health hazards from the clinical point of view, some treatable others not.

The common adulterants present in different types of foods are discussed in chapter 13 along with what we as consumers can do about the problem and how to ensure we are eating healthy food.

13

Adulterants in Foods

All foods are subject to some kind of adulteration or other depending on the ethical values and goals of the adulterators. In fact, the range of adulterants added to our foods by profiteers simply for immediate monetary gains is mind boggling. Adulterators often forget that their own actions might trigger off a chain reaction and give ideas to somebody else who would probably be poisoning their food and that of their families, injuring health of the people at large. The common adulterants which have been identified in different foods are discussed briefly.

Water

Water is the most important vehicle for carrying adulterants in plant, animals and humans, and is therefore the focus of attention for food scientists. If water is contaminated it can make all other foods a source of disease, through carrying, pesticides, fertilizers, insect residues, microorganisms, metallic residues or others. Water may also be unintentionally adulterated if taken from an unhygienic environment such as a contaminated well or other water source. Water borne diseases are well documented. So if food is prepared with utmost care and the water used is contaminated dire consequences can result.

Even so-called mineral water may be bottled and found contaminated with mineral acids, heavy metals like arsenic, copper, lead, fluorides, chlorine, microorganisms and much more. Soft drinks too are not all safe, sometimes containing colours, flavours, sweeteners that are non- permitted and may be injurious to health if consumed regularly over long periods of time.

Soft drinks prepared from pure water may also get contaminated if processed in unhygienic environments, or seals broken filled with substitutes and coloured, then resealed by unscrupulous traders. These are prone to microbial, heavy metal and harmful dye contamination.

Milk and milk products

The simplest form of adulteration in liquid milk is the addition of water, which in many cases may be infected. Contaminated water can be a source of pathogenic bacteria and unless pasteurized and packed by a standard dairy can become hazardous to health. Today, it has become common practice to replace milk solids by adding caustic soda, urea and soap solution. Commonly referred to as *synthetic milk* it may also contain pesticide and antibiotic residues.

Cases have been reported in which the hormone oxytocin is injected into buffaloes to increase milk yield, and if even a small quantity of the hormone is secreted in the milk, it acts as a slow poison. On regular consumption it can lead to loss of uterine contractability and diseases of the liver and kidney.

In addition, reports of unhygienic animal fat from buffalo, goat or pig being used to make milk more creamy have appeared in the literature (Industry News, 1997), in addition to detergents, urea, starch and soda ash. Sugar is often added to satisfy the specific gravity and relative density requirements.

Strong evidence suggests that the use of DDT for control of malaria, increases the levels of the insecticide in bovine milk, fatty foods and even in the milk of mothers residing in the area. Of 30 samples tested in Bangalore, 88.3% were found contaminated with organochlorine insecticide residues also, which are nerve poisons. To make things worse tests on baby milk and baby foods too performed by scientists of Gujarat Agriculture University showed contamination levels above the maximum residue levels (MRL) prescribed.

Such malpractices and others using animal fats in milk, not only deprive children of nutrition but lead them to nervous disorders, blurred vision, nausea and other gastrointestinal problems which in the long term may cause cancer.

Meat, fish and poultry

This group of foods is most vulerable to adulteration by microorganisms like E. coli, and other pathogens, mycotoxins, hormone residues, antibiotics, pesticides, and heavy metals. Even in countries where there are very strict Food and Drug laws, poisoning from meat products has been detected. Hamburger poisoning due to E. coli was detected in the U.S. and attributed to weak safety standards and risky practices in the processing plant. This led to the closure of the food company (Industry News, 1997). If left unchecked contaminants can lead to liver or other organ damage and cancers.

The toxins in poultry may come from the feeds or be ingested through air, infected water and unsanitary surroundings.

The toxicity from fish is known as *ichthyotoxism* and the toxins usually come from blue-green algae present in marine environments. Shell fish have concentrated toxins which they derive from *plankton* on which they thrive. The toxins however, are also heat stable and not completely destroyed by normal cooking temperatures.

Cereals pulses and legumes

These foods are available in many processed forms but are extensively used whole or as flours. It is much easier to clean and wash them before cooking if whole but when ground into flour may be mixed with items of poorer quality, drought resistant varieties which are hard to digest, not so nutritious and cheap.

Rana et al. (1999) tested market samples of different pulses and found that black gram *dal* exceeded the permissible limits of PFA in moisture, foreign matter, other edible grains and damaged grains. Also 40% of the pulse samples were polished with charcoal dye, while 60% used metanil yellow both of which are strictly prohibited as they have carcinogenic effects. Some grains were also weevil infested.

There are a variety of pulses and legumes which contain natural toxins that are released in the body when consumed, depending on the methods of preparation used. Those of concern are two thermolabile factors in the form of enzyme inhibitors and haemagglutinins. These factors inhibit the action of the enzymes trypsin, chymotrypsin and alpha-amylase affecting the digestion and thereby absorption of carbohydrates and proteins. Besides these, legumes also contain toxic substances known as *saponins* and some cyanogenic glycosides and alkaloids.

Trypsin inhibitors

These are proteins found widely in pulses and inhibit the release of amino acids which then cannot be absorbed thus affecting normal growth in children. Because of the fixation of the amino acids the pancreas may get stimulated to produce more trypsin leading to damage of the organ and its malfunction.

Haemagglutinins

These are also proteins and combine with the products of digestion preventing their proper absorption and thereby utilization by the body.

Saponins

Saponins are substances which when shaken foam and leave a lather like residue on the sides of the pan, commonly seen when boiling pulses and legumes. These substances are structurally glycosides of high molecular weight and are found in beans of various varieties. Toxic saponins cause symptoms such as nausea, vomiting or diarrhoea. The toxic effects can however, be removed on soaking of the legumes prior to cooking as they are water soluble. In addition to legumes potatoes sometimes contain green areas which contain toxic saponins and should be discarded before cooking.

Alkaloids

These are found in the seeds of some pulses and legumes but are not significant in their effects on health. Some compounds in seeds however, may lead to iodine deficiency as they bind the iodine preventing it from being taken up by the body.

Of all toxic substances identified in foods those of particular concern are two factors that cause serious disease conditions. These are present in *kesari* dal, the over consumption of which leads to the disease lathyrism, and the other factor usually in broad beans known as the haemolytic factor causing *favism* characterized by severe haemolytic anemia.

Grains like *bajra, jowar* and *rye* easily get infected with a fungus, *Claviceps purpurea* commonly known as *ergot,* responsible for the toxic symptoms of *Ergotism.* Eating fungal grains also causes symptoms of the alimentary tract referred to as *Alimentary Toxic Aleukia* (ATA).

Lathyrism

In *lathyrism,* the toxic factor interferes with the normal formation of collagen fibres and results in weakness and or paralysis of the lower limbs. The condition is not curable and affects people especially in drought areas who thrive on *kesari dal* as this is drought resistant and grows when other crops fail.

This crop being cheaply available is used by adulterators and mixed with *tuar dal* which it resembles. Fortunately, the toxicity can be removed by soaking, and discarding the water although some nutrients of the *tuar* may get lost. Besides, only high doses of the toxin taken through about 250-233 g of kesari dal alone per day over a period of more than 6 months can produce severe disease symptoms.

Favism

This is a condition of severe anemia which can be brought about through excessive consumption of broad beans or even through pollen of its flower. The toxic factor affects the metabolism of glutathione in the red blood cells because of a deficiency in the activity of the enzyme glucose-6-phosphate dehydrogenase. In haemolytic anemia the red blood cells get destroyed faster than they can be produced leading to other pathological complications.

It is heartening however, that pulses and legumes are eaten only after cooking, and this removes most of the toxic effects. Fermentation before cooking in some varieties is further helpful as in the preparation, of *idli, dhokla* and the like. Cooking also improves digestibility of cereals, pulses and legumes, although the method of heat application is important.

Fruits and Vegetables

The sources of adulteration in fruits and vegetables are those passed on from soil and water, infested seeds and pollutants in the environment, for example pesticides, heavy metals and carbon monoxide.

Saponins are present in spinach, asparagus, potato and other vegetables, while goitrogens in the form of glucosides appear in cabbage, rapeseed and mustard. Spinach and beet are also high in oxalic acid and may cause oxalic acid poisoning. All protein rich foods like cereals, pulses, nuts and edible seeds may act as allergens in sensitive people,

Nuts and oilseeds

Nuts and oilseeds can get contaminated the same way in storage godowns as cereals, pulses and legumes. The fungus *Aspergillus flavus* specially develops in groundnut cotton seed, their flours and cakes producing aflatoxins which are injurious to health. There are 14 chemically related toxins of which one, *Aflatoxin B* is most frequently found in food and is a known carcinogen that can cause liver cancer (Manay and Shadaksharaswamy,1987).

Nuts being generally expensive items are easily adulterated, for example almonds are mixed with apricot kernels which resemble certain varieties, and sold at the price of almonds. The kernels of apricot have a bitter compound that when consumed regularly can lead to slow cyanide poisoning.

Fat and oils

Incidents have been reported of contamination of mustard oil with argemone oil, both seeds growing together in the same field and getting mixed during harvesting. Since they resemble each other so closely it is difficult to seggregate them easily and the oil extraction process mixes the two together. If on testing the level of argemone oil is higher than permitted levels disease symptoms appear, finally leading to dropsy. Other contaminants in this group of foods are addition of cheap rancid oil, castor oil, mineral oils, non-permitted colours and so on, consumption of which may cause stomach upsets, damage to eyes, bones or other organs.

Almond oil too, which is expensive and commonly used for medicinal purposes or for flavouring foods is adulterated with apricot kernel oil which contains poisonous hydrogen cyanide.

Sugar and confectionery

This group includes sugar and syrups of all description and products manufactured from them. The contaminants are basically in the form of non-permitted colours such as lead chromate, textile dyes like metanil yellow, artificial sweeteners, aluminium foil all hazardous to health. Also beware of sherbets with fluorescent colours added to make them attractive.

All Indian sweets are traditionally topped with fine silver foil called *warq*, especially on festive occasions, which because of the high costs is often replaced by aluminium foil that is hazardous with long term use.

Spices and condiments

This group of ingredients used most commonly in cooking is sold mostly in ground or powdered form. There is virtually no spice used in India which is free from adulteration, some not harmful other hazardous especially when sold in loose attractive heaps at cheaper rates. This however does not exclude some packaged brands that are not quality branded. Some examples are red chilli powder which may have mixed with it, rice flake powder, corn flour, rice husks or old spent chillies. All these are not injurious to health but the bright *Sudan Red* colours added certainly are. Similarly the oil soluble colours added to turmeric, the gum and resins in asafoetida or *heeng* are injurious.

Even whole spices are not spared such as black pepper seeds often mixed with dry papaya seeds that resemble them, the practice being profitable and not harmful. Similarly saffron is mixed with stigma of other flowers, coriander with husk and cumin with grass seeds. The list is virtually endless.

Packaged foods

Even packaged foods are suspect and adulterants do act as slow poisons. Canned foods especially those which are non acidic are particularly prone to bacterial toxins of which the fatal effects of *Clostridium botulinum* are well documented. Other bacteria involved are *Staphylococcus aureus* and *Bacillus cereus,* which produce sufficient toxins to cause food poisoning. Some act almost immediately on ingestion of food, others have different incubation periods and therefore symptoms surface after some time. Fortunately the toxins especially those causing *botulism* are thermolabile and destroyed on heating at 80°C for 30 minutes.

Detection of Adulterants

Both sensory and objective methods have been used for detection of adulteration in foods. House holders used their senses and vast experience with buying, handling and cooking foods of various types, rejecting those items which did not appear fresh, or smelt foul, or had any signs of deterioration or insect infestation. But, this was possible when foods went straight from farms to markets for sale and they were handled by the users for inspection.

Today, with technological advancements in processing, preservation, packaging and storage it has become possible to make available foods of all descriptions around the year which were unheard of, except seasonally. In addition, global influences in eating and living patterns have changed the variety of foods which were limited in households. The media too have played its role in influencing people to purchase packed foods, the contents of which the majority cannot inspect for acceptance or rejection when buying. But habits die hard and the majority of illiterates and poor in India, still purchase loose items from cheaper neighbourhood stores or vendors, who try to compete for sales through unfair and unscrupulous means. It is the ignorant who are most affected and educationists, media, NGO's all need to join hands to educate the people against exploitation by whatever means possible especially when it affects health and well being.

Food scientists are doing their bit by developing some simple tests which can be conducted for the detection of adulteration in commonly consumed items. Some of these are presented in Table 13.1.

Table 13.1 Adulterants in Foods

S.No.	Name of Food Article	Adulterant	Simple Method for detection of Common Adulterants	Caution
1	2	3	4	5
1.	Whole spices	Dirt, dust, straw, insect, damaged seeds, other seeds, rodent hair and excreta.	These can be examined visually.	
a.	Black pepper	Papaya seeds	Papaya seeds can be separated out from pepper as they are shrunk, oval in shape and greenish brown or brownish black in colour.	
		Light black pepper	Float the sample of black pepper in alcohol (rectified spirit). The mature black pepper berries sink while the papaya seeds and light black pepper float.	
		Coated with mineral oil	Black pepper coated with mineral oil gives kerosene like smell.	
b.	Cloves	Volatile oil extracted (exhausted cloves)	Exhausted cloves can be identified by its small size and shrunken appearance. The characteristic pungent tests of genuine cloves is less pronounced compared to exhausted cloves.	
c.	Mustard seed	Argemone seed	Mustard seeds have a smooth surface. the argemone seed have grainy and rough surface and are black and hence can be separated out by close examination. When Mustard seed is pressed inside it is yellow while for argemone seed it is white.	Use magnifying glass for identification.
2.	Powdered spices	Added starch	Add few drops of tincture of Iodine or Iodine solution. Indication of blue color shows the presence of starch.	Iodine test for added starch is not applicable for turmeric powder.
		Common Salt	Taste for addition of common salt.	

(Contd.)

1	2	3	4	5
3.	Turmeric powder	Colored saw dust, yellow earth, sand or talc, prohibited colour	Take a teaspoonful of turmeric powder in a test tube. Add a few drops of concentrated hydro-chloricacid. Instant appearance of pink colour which disappears on dilution with water shows the presence of turmeric. If the colour persists, metanil yellow (an artificial colour) a non-permitted coal tar colour is present.	This test is only for Metanil yellow.
		Lead chromate used for polishing.	Take 2 g of whole turmeric and add 10 ml of (1:7) sulphuric acid. Boil for 5 minutes and filter. Take 5 ml of filtrate and add 0.5 ml of diphenyl carbazide solution.	Dark pink colour shows presence of lead chromate.
		Chalk powder or yellow soap stone powder	Take a small quantity of turmeric powder in a test tube containing small quantity of water. Add a few drops of concentrated Hydrochloric acid, effervescence (giving off bubbles) will indicate the presence of chalk or yellow soap stone powder.	
4.	Chilly powder	Brick Powder, salt powder or talc powder, powdered bran, mineral oil, prohibited colour.	Take a teaspoonful of chilli powder in a glass of water. Colored water extract will show the presence of artificial color. Any grittiness that may be felt on rubbing the sediment at the bottom of glass confirms the presence of brick powder/sand, soapy and smooth touch of the white residue at the bottom indicates the presence of soapstone. Take chilli powder on a wet filter paper. Add a few drops of ether or alcohol. A red colour shows presence of Rhodamine B. When heated a large quantity of ash is left behind if talc or brick powder is added.	This test is only for earthy material.
		Water soluble coal tar color	Water soluble artificial colour can be detected by sprinkling small quantity of chillies or turmeric powder on the surface of water contained in a glass tumbler. The water soluble colour will immediately start descending in colour streaks.	
		Oil soluble coal tar color	Grind 5 g of chilli powder with 25 ml of 2% ammonium hydroxide and 70% alcohol, keep for 2 hrs, filter and	Presence of coal tar dye gives a colored solution.

(Contd.)

1	2	3	4	5
			evaporate to dryness. Dissolve the residue in 15 ml water containing 4 ml acetic acid, add 20 cm piece of neutral wool, boil for 15 min and wash with tap water. Transfer to 100 ml beaker and add 20 ml dilute ammonia solution.	
5.	Cardamom	Horse dung powder	Soak the sample in water. Horse dung which floats can be visually detected.	
6.	Heeng	Soap stone or other earthy matter, sand, chalk, foreign resins and gums.	Shake little portion of the sample with water and allow to settle. Soap stone or other earthy matter will settle down at the bottom. When ignited pure sample burns with a bright flame.	In compounded heeng due to presence of starch, a slight turbid solution, may be produced. However, this will settle down after keeping.
7.	Saffron	Dried tendrils of maize cob	Genuine saffron will not break easily like the artificial one. Artificial saffron is prepared by soaking maize cob in sugar and coloring it with coal tar colour. The color dissolves in water if artificial. A bit of pure saffron when allowed to dissolve in water will continue to give its saffron color as long as it lasts. Dry the water extract and streak sulphuric acid across the sample.	Blue color turning purple to reddish brown indicates a pure sample.
8.	Ghee or butter	Vanaspati	Take about one teaspoonful of melted ghee or butter with equal quantity of concentrated Hydrochloric Acid in a test tube and add to it a pinch of cane-sugar. Shake well for one minute and let it stand for 5 minutes. Appearance of crimson colour in lower (acidic) layer shows the presence of 'Vanaspati'. In case no colour appears, dilute with water. Shake again and observe colour. Some coaltar colour also gives the test in dilute Hydrochloric Acid.	This test is specific for sesame oil which is conpulsorily added to Vanaspati. Some coaltar dyes also give a positive test. If the test is positive i.e. red colour develops only by adding strong Hydrochloric Acid (without adding crystals of cane-sugar) then the sample is adulterated with

(Contd.)

1	2	3	4	5
				coaltar dye. If the crimson of red colour develops after adding and shaking with cane-sugar, then alone vanaspati or sesame oil is present.
9.	Milk	Water	(*i*) The lactometer reading should not ordinarily be less than 1.026.	
			(*ii*) The presence of water can be detected by putting a drop of milk on a polished verticle surface. The drop of pure milk either stops or flows slowly leaving a white trail behind it whereas milk adulterated with water will flow immediately without leaving a mark.	The test is not valid if skimmed milk or other thickening material is added.
			(*iii*) Add tincture of iodine. Indication of blue colour shows the presence of starch.	
10.	Khoya	Starch	Boil the sample with some water, cool and add tincture of iodine. Indication of blue colour shows presence of starch.	
11.	Edible oils	Argemone oil	Add concentrated Nitric acid to the sample and shake carefully. Red to reddish brown colour in acid layer would indicate the presence of argemone oil.	Colourless (not yellowish) Nitric acid may be used. Artificial colour, if present with usually be a bright shade of colour, generally red or pink. The test may some time give misleading results.
12.	Sweetmeat, Sherbat Icecream etc.	Metanil yellow (a non-permitted coaltar dye)	Extract colour with luke warm water from food article. Add a few drops of concentrated hydrochloric acid. If magenta red colour develops the presence of metanil yelllow is indicated.	
13.	Dals	Kesari Dal	Add 50 ml. of dilute hydrochloric acid to dal and	The test is only for kesari dal. (Metanil

(*Contd.*)

1	2	3	4	5
			keep on simmering water for about 15 minutes. The pink colour, if developed indicates the presence of kesari dal.	yellow, if present will give a similar colour immediately without simmering.
		Clay, stone gravels etc. (lead chromate yellow)	Visual examination will detect these adulterants Shake 5 grams of dal with 5 ml. of water and add a few drops of hydrochloric acid. A pink colour shows the presence of colour.	
14.	Sela rice	Metanil yellow	Rub a few grains in the palms of two hands, yellow colour would get reduced or disappear. Add a few drops of dilute hydrocholoric acid to some rice grains mixed with a little water; presence of a violet colour shows presence of Metanil yellow.	
15.	Silver leaves (warq)	Aluminium leaves	(*i*) On ignition, genuine silver leaves burn away completely, leaving glistening white spherical ball of the same mass whereas aluminium leaves are reduced to ashes of dark grey blackish colour. (*ii*) take silver leaves in test tube, add dilute hydrochloric acid. Appearance of turbidity to white precipitate indicates the presence of silver leaves. Aluminium leaves do not give any turbidity or precepitate.	

Prevention of Adulteration

Prevention of adulteration is a marathon task which neither the government nor the consumer can tackle alone unless those involved in the act of profiteering through adulterating realise the gravity of the problem they have created. The country has to fight the malady on a war footing if the future citizens are to regain their confidence in the health and security provisions through the basics of safe water and food for everyone.

The legal system too must take the responsibility of not letting adulterators go scot free. All professionals need to pool in their resources to help tackle this problem to prevent crippling the nation in the future. Already things have gone too far. The government and the consumer both play a key role and therefore this is briefly discussed.

Role of Government

The government lays down the law and there are many laws to prevent adulteration and protect the consumers from exploitative, unfair practices especially those injurious to health. There have been strict rules and penalties laid down but they need to be implemented strictly, and that too immediately as an offence is committed.

The laws need to be amended according to new facts that come to light as a result of research or loopholes in the law. If one refers to the PFA, 1954, permissible limits are shocking especially with respect to rodent and insect residues in cereals and their products.

Simply making laws, rules and amendments cannot bring results, constant vigil and a sense of urgency, punishing adulterators in public through coordination of work of all departments concerned is required.

At the same time government cannot work alone, consumers, voluntary organization, media, manufacturers all have to assist the government, by making use of the law and influencing the changes required in it for the total good of the nation.

Consumer's Role

Consumers have a crucial role to play because the market gives them what they demand or accept without reservation. Each citizen has the responsibility of safeguarding their own health and that of the family. When they know what can affect children adversely people will be driven to gain more knowledge and act to ensure their family health. Some guidelines are presented in Table 14.1 by following which at least everyone can start to tackle the problem.

Table 14.1 Some guidelines for consumers

- Buy organically grown fruits and vegetables, avoiding purchase of polished vegetables.
- Use fresh produce where possible limiting use of packaged ones to those which do not contain preservatives.
- Avoid long storage.
- When eating out enquire about the oil being used.
- Avoid brightly coloured products especially sweets, desserts and snack foods. Reject pulses that leave colour when soaked in water.
- Recognize the shape and size of kesari dal and argemone seeds.
- Buy packaged products with government authorized standard marks of quality, or branded products known for their quality standards.
- Recognize quality marks like *Agmark, ISI, FPO, Ecomark* for agricultural products, other packaged products and fruit products respectively.
- Avoid processed meats and all foods available loose in the market, buy packaged ones from reliable sources.
- Avoid reheating cooked meat.
- Do not depend on mineral water and avoid colas. Use latest technology filters for drinking water to ensure that heavy metals are removed.
- Always boil milk before use unless bought from a reliable source. Don't consume street foods if exposed, especially those eaten raw.
- In case of complaints revert to the seller, manufacturer or go to the media, government department or consumer organisation but do not accept substandard foods. Take some action and tell others too.

Apart from following the above guidelines for food buying, consumers have a responsibility to pick up suspected foods and send them for analysis and testing to some of the laboratories closest to them.

When users are unhappy about a product, complain and return for replacement, write to the manufacturer with a copy to the health or PFA department or file a PIL through consumer organisations or resident associations. Most of all tell others not to buy the product. If one billion people boycott a product proved injurious to health a manufacturer will have no choice but to discontinue its production and improve it to meet demanded needs.

It is time every buyer and user of food wakes up and helps others too from their slumber. Remember we are important to the market but more important to the country, and must regain our driving seat, not allowing profiteers to take the upper hand. We must become choosers instead of accepting what is handed out to us. Quoting Swami Vivekananda: *Arise, awake and stop not till the goal is reached.*

EXPERIMENT 50

Aim

To detect *metanil yellow* in spices.

Equipment

Funnel, filter paper, test tubes and stand, dropper and filter paper.

Materials

Turmeric whole and powder, water, concentrated Hydrochloric acid (HCL).

Principle

Colours are often added to foods especially spices to enhance their brightness, but coal tar dyes like metanil yellow may sometimes be used which are injurious to health. Detection can therefore assist in educating the public about the hazard. Jacob (1976) has attributed the colour to testicular degeneration in males.

Procedure

A. (*i*) Mix ¼ t of turmeric powder in water, shake vigorously and then filter the solution.

  (*ii*) Dilute a part of the filtrate till it is almost colourless.

 (*iii*) Take some of the diluted sample in another test tube and add a few drops of concentrated HCl and observe the colour. A magenta red colour indicates the presence of metanil yellow.

B.   Repeat A (*i-iii*) with whole turmeric.

      Label the samples, and place on the stand for observation.

Observation

Record your observations with respect to the intensity of the change in colour that takes place in A and B. Draw inferences and state whether the sample is adulterated with metanil yellow or not.

Precautions

1. Use a dropper for adding concentrated acid, or it may result in bums.
2. The number of drops of acid added should be same for all samples.
3. Store acid in a cool dark place away from a flame.

Practice Exercises

1. Perform the test on other spices and pulses of yellow to orange colour and see if they are adulterated. Repeat the test 3 times to confirm your results. Keep a sample of the spice and the positive test results for record and necessary action.
2. What action would you take if they are found to be adulterated with metanil yellow.

EXPERIMENT 51

Aim

To test whole red chilli for the presence of *Rhodamine B* (red colour).

Equipment

Petridish, Cotton swab.

Materials

Whole red chilli, chilli powder, paraffin or mineral oil.

Principle

There are certain red colours such as amaranth, carmoisine, erythrosine, Fast red E and Ponceau 4R which are permitted under the PFA rules for addition to synthetic syrups and other foods. However, the addition of inorganic matter and pigments with lead salts, red or yellow earth are prohibited. Addition of artificial colours to pulses, spices, tea and coffee are strictly prohibited by the PFA Act. Impure colour preparations can contaminate food with lead, arsenic, copper, chromium and other dye intermediates. Depending on the contaminants symptoms ranging from anemia to brain damage can occur. Chillies and their powders are prone to addition of red colour.

Procedure

A. (*i*) Pour a little liquid paraffin or oil in a petridish.
  (*ii*) Soak the cotton Swab in it and rub the surface of a red chilli.
  (*iii*) Observe the cotton for colour. If the cotton becomes red then the sample contains added colour.
  (*iv*) Repeat (*i-iii*) twice to confirm your results.

B. (*i*) Test a teaspoon of chilli powder by shaking it in a test tube with paraffin oil.
  (*ii*) Let it stand for 15 minutes, shaking it intermitantly.
  (*iii*) Observe and check the degree of adulteration if present.

Observations

Record your observations and comment on the intensity of the colour in each sample.

Precautions

1. Take care to see that the sample is clean and dry.
2. Wash your hands thoroughly before and after the experiment.
3. Dispose off the paraffin oil carefully, so that it does not contaminate food or food surfaces.

Practice Exercises

1. Perform this test with other orange to red whole and powdered spices, pulses and legumes. Comment on the results.

EXPERIMENT 52

Aim

To test for adulterants in coffee powder.

Equipment

Beaker, coffee filter, test tubes and stand, holder, bunsen burner, funnel, filter paper, **measuring cylinder**, dropper.

Materials and reagents

Coffee powder, water, $KMnO_4$, Iodine solution, 2% NaOH solution, lead acetate, Selivanoff's reagent'

Principle

The common adulterants in coffee powder are starch, date and tamarind seeds and chicory, The starch responds to iodine solution, the seeds to 2% NAOH and chicory to Selvinoff's reagent and can therefore be easily tested.

Procedure

A. Testing for starch

   (*i*) Make a decoction of coffee.

   (*ii*) Take 10 ml in a test tube (tt).

   (*iii*) Decolourize it with acidified $KMnO_4$

   (*iv*) Observe the change in colour. Blue colour indicates the presence of starch.

B. Testing for roasted dates and tamarind seeds.

   (*i*) Take ¼ t coffee powder in a test tube.

   (*ii*) Add 10 ml of 2% NaOH solution and shake well. Keep on a tt stand for 3-4 minutes.

   (*iii*) Observe the colour. If reddish it indicates presence of date seeds, and if pink it shows adulteration with tamarind seeds.

C. Testing for chicory.

   (*i*) Prepare a 2% water extract of coffee and filter.

   (*ii*) To 5 ml of the clear filtrate in a tt, add 5 ml of Selvionff's reagent followed by 1 ml of concentrated HCl.

   (*iii*) Boil for 1 minute over a bunsen burner. Keep aside on tt stand.

   (*iv*) Observe any change in colour. If a red colour is obtained it indicates the presence of chicory.

Observations

Tabulate your observations as learnt and record your comments.

Precautions

  1. When handling acids care should be taken to pour them down the sides of the tt.

  2. Boil solutions on low to medium heat to prevent boiling-over.

3. Use a tt holder for heating.
4. Store reagents in a cool place.

Practice Exercises

1. Test for starch, and other adulterants in powdered tea as learnt. Comment on the colours obtained.
2. Take a blotting paper, moisten with water and sprinkle with dust tea. If yellow, red or orange spots appear the tea is adulterated.
3. Take a magnet and test tea leaves for presence of iron filings. Compare different brands of tea. Comment on your results.
4. What would you do if you found your beverages adulterated. Stop drinking them or take action against manufacturers.

EXPERIMENT 53

Aim

To test for presence of sugar in honey.

Equipment

Beaker, measuring cylinder, mortar and pestle, evaporating dish.

Materials and reagents

Honey, ether, resorcinol and concentrated HCl.

Principle

The presence of adulterants always brings about changes in reactions to various reagents depending on the composition of the food and the substances added.

Procedure

(*i*) Mix 2g honey with 5ml ether in a mortar and pestle.
(*ii*) Decant off the ether extract into an evaporating dish.
(*iii*) Repeat the process by treating the extract with ether and collect the residue.
(*iv*) Allow the ether to evaporate off at room temperature.
(*v*) To the remaining residue add resorcinol and 1 drop of conc. HCl.
(*vi*) The appearance of a cherry red colour indicates the presence of sugar.

Observations

Record your observations and comment on the honey sample as observed.

Precautions

1. As in experiments 51 and 52.

Practice Exercises

1. Take honey of different brands in the market and test for the presence of sugar. Comment on the best brand to buy.
2. Take any syrups sold in the market and test as learnt.
3. Add concentrated HCl to jaggery solution. A magenta red colour indicates adulteration.
4. To a little powdered sugar, add a few drops of conc. HCl. If effervescence occurs it indicates adulteration with washing soda.

EXPERIMENT 54

Aim

To Test for adulteration in fats and oils.

Equipment

Glass stoppered test tube, 5 ml graduated pippete, test tubes and stand, water bath, burner and gauze, measuring cylinder.

Materials and reagents

Ghee, butter, vegetable oil, conc. HCl, 7 N alcoholic KOH.

Principle

Fats and oils are easily adulterated with coal-tar dyes, mineral oil, argemone oil, vanaspati and animal fats. Adding vanaspati to ghee for instance may not be injurious, but when done with a purely profit motive, because the latter in expensive, is an act of adulteration to be reported against, if not indicated as an ingredient on the label of a package.

Procedure

A. Vanaspati in ghee.

(*i*) Dissolve a pinch of sugar in 10 ml of conc. HCI taken in a glass stoppered test tube (tt).

(*ii*) Add 10 ml of melted ghee and replace stopper.

(*iii*) Shake vigrously for 2 minutes.

(*iv*) Allow the tt to stand till the acid layer separates out.

(*v*) Observe the acid layer, if pink the sample contains vanaspati.

Such adulteration can also be detected by shaking 5ml ghee with 5ml dilute HCI and adding 0.2% furfural solution.

B. Coaltar dye in butter.

(*i*) Melt I t butter in a tt kept in a hot water bath.

(*ii*) Continue heating until the fat and water layers separate completely.

(*iii*) Decant off the fat layer from the top into a clean dry tt.

(*iv*) Dissolve 2 ml of the decanted fat in ether, and add to it 1.2ml of 50% HC1.

(*v*) Shake the tt vigorously and let stand.

(*vi*) Observe the acid layer. A wine red colour indicates the presence of coal-tar dye.

C. Mineral oil in vegetable oi!.

(*i*) Take 5 ml vegetable oil in a tt, and add 25 ml of 7N alcoholic KOH.

(*ii*) Saponify the mixture in a hot water bath.

(*iii*) When completed dilute with distilleď water.

(*iv*) Observe. If turbidity is present, the sample contains mineral oil.

Observations

Tabulate your observations as learnt.

Precaution

As in experiment 52.

Practice Exercises

1. Perform tests as learnt using different oils and blends. Record your observation. Which oil available in the market would you recommend for use in cooking.

2. Take samples of different brands of butter and margarine and test for adulteration using sensory evaluation and laboratory tests.

3. To 5 ml melted fat add 5 ml conc HCl, shake well and add 0.2% fluoroglucinal solution in ether. Pink colour shows rancidity in fat. Check other fats and oils for rancidity and comment on the results.

EXPERIMENT 55

Aim

Detection of $NaHCO_3$ (chalk) in flour.

Equipment

Beaker, test tubes and stand, burner, thermometer.

Materials and reagents

Whole wheat flour, maize flour, pulse flour, rice flour, dilute HCl, distilled water.

Principle

When any flour is adulterated with chalk or $NaHCO_3$, it gives off CO_2 when treated with hot HCl. An effervescence is noticed in the form of gas bubbles.

Procedure

A. Wheat flour

    (*i*) Take 1t of flour in a tt and shake it with 10 ml distilled water.

    (*ii*) Warm 20ml dilute HCl to 50-60°C in a beaker, over a burner.

    (*iii*) Add the warm acid along the sides of the tt containing the flour.

    (*iv*) Observe. If effervescence takes place the sample contains chalk.

B. Maize flour

Repeat A (*i-iv*) using maize flour instead of wheat.

C. Pulse flour

Repeat A (*i-iv*) using pulse flour.

D. Rice flour

Repeat A (*i-iv*) using rice flour.

Observations

Record your observations and comment on the degree of adulteration observed.

Precautions

Same as experiment 52.

Practice Exercises

1. Prepare chapati using wheat flour that is adulterated with chalk and one that is not. Evaluate for sensory characteristics. Record your observations as learnt.
2. Use soya and groundnut flours and test for adulteration.

FOOD EVALUATION

Food evaluation is the process of judging the quality and thereby the degree of acceptability of a food product or meal. This process may be done on a routine basis through the instant reactions of the consumer or carried out in a formalized planned manner to ascertain whether the food is of a predetermined or expected quality. There are as many criteria for evaluating food as the number of people consuming or judging it. Different foods too, are evaluated according to their characteristic structures, composition, properties and expected outcomes related to functions which the food performs in terms of its end-use. Cooking methods used also bring about structural changes which affect the palatability of foods.

There are basically two approaches to food evaluation, one based on the reactions of the senses and the other in which accurate measurements using calibrated instrumentation is carried out. The former is termed as sensory evaluation and is a subjective method of evaluation, while the latter is more objective, and being quantitative in nature is considered for its greater accuracy. Fig. 15.0 depicts clearly these two distinct approaches.

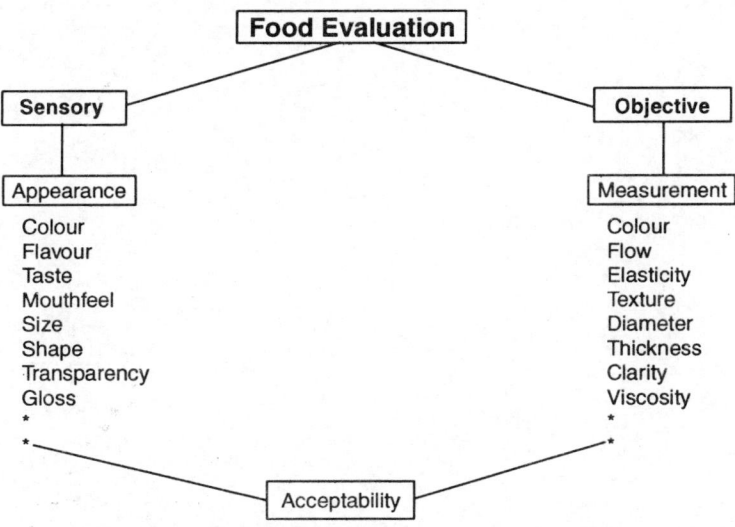

Fig. 15.0. Criteria and Methods for Food Evaluation.

Each food exhibits typical characteristics, and a basic knowledge of the important attributes is therefore essential for evaluation. Thus, the criteria for evaluation may be set up according to the characteristics of the food product being assessed. For example, the typical characteristics of meat products are appearance, flavour, texture, juiciness, and tenderness or doneness. These can be assessed using both subjective and objective methods.

Food is generally subjected to sensory methods of evaluation because it is the acceptability of the consumer that is the final determinant of whether it will sell or not, but at the manufacturing end, food products need to be accurately assessed to meet quality standards which will be consistent for production as well as adhere to the food laws of the country.

15

Subjective Evaluation

Subjective methods are methods of evaluating food quality. which have been developed scientifically through an understanding of the manner in which our sensory organs function to detect
colour, taste, flavour and so on, all affecting food acceptability. These methods are also called
sensory methods as they make use of the human senses. The evaluation techniques are based on
human sensitivity and acuity to perceive subtle differences in odour, taste and other attributes at
levels lower than the lowest instrumental sensitivity (Jellinek, 1985).

Thus subjective evaluation is highly dependent on the sensitivities of people be they trained
taste panelists or untrained consumers. However, other factors such as pH, temperature and so on,
also have their effects on the outcome of the evaluation and therefore, objective means may also be
used to control these variables during the preparation of the food samples.

Sensory organs and Sensations

The sensory organs consisting of eyes, nose, ears, mucous membranes of the mouth, tongue and
skin or the organs of touch respond to the sensations of sight, smell, taste, feel and sound of food.
But one can notice responses even at the thought of food, as in the case of favourites like icecream,
gulabjamun, biryani and so on. It is this thought response, that advertisers cash upon when they
produce mouth watering pictures of food products in a competitive market to lure customers.

Sight

It is well recognized that the appearance of what we see on a plate is an important factor in deciding
whether the food will be tasted or not. Appearance covers not only colour but also the shape, size
of portion, greasiness, transparency, brightness and so on, all of which must match a person's
expectations of that food or product. Imagine your response when a green coloured icecream is
presented to you as a strawberry icecream, or a yellow coloured thick paste as a cream of tomato
soup. Again a well prepared tasty cutlet shaped like a brinjal or a hot green chilli may be rejected
straight away even if it is delightful to taste. The foods therefore have to pass the sight test first
before they can be screened by other sensory organs. Eye appeal and therefore food presentation
is of utmost importance in evaluation.

Flavour

Once the food has appealed to the eyes, the sense organs of the nose and mouth take over in evaluating what is termed as *flavour*. This consists of three distinct components smell or odour, taste and the feel of food in the mouth known as *mouthfeel*.

Flavour is a complex sensation obtained from volatile food components such as hydrocarbons, alcohols, aldehydes, ketones, esters, amines, furans and pyrazines. Fats and fat-soluble substances have also been shown to be involved in flavour differences especially in meats from different species (Sharma and Wani, 1995). Thus, flavour has a significant effect on overall food acceptability.

Certain ingredients added during cooking affect flavour sensations in different ways. For example, salt subdues excessive sweetness, bitterness and tartness in food, and brings out delicate flavours and flavour differences. Similarly, a small amount added to vegetables or meat smoothens out and blends flavours together for better appeal.

Odour

This plays an important role in food acceptability as it stimulates appetite even before the appearance of the food. When one enters the home, the smell of good food or otherwise brings a reaction on the face because the elements responsible for odour are volatile and reach the sensors in the nose even from a distant source. The nose also picks up sensations of pain and therefore the smell of burning oil or hot chilli is detected immediately.

Odours from foods are important indices of freshness and even wholesomeness of the food, as stale food will not present pleasant odours because the substances responsible have been volatilized with time.

The odour constituents of foods are strongly perceived by tasting rather than by smell alone. This is because the samples become warm once in the mouth making the odour constituents more volatile.

Taste

Taste is the deciding index for food likes and dislikes, as it is a natural response of people to taste foods that are pleasing to the eyes and smell good. The organs responsible for taste are the *taste buds* situated in the epithelium and at various points on the tongue which the food touches most during mastication and swallowing. The front loose portion of the tongue is sensitive to touch but does not contain any sensitivity to taste. Most of the taste sensations are felt along the sides and back of the tongue where it is connected to the food pipe.

There are four recognized tastes that the taste buds can pick up-such as sweet, salt, sour and bitter, but depending on the acuity of the tongue many mixed, or fine differences in tastes can be detected by the nearly 10,000 taste buds present. Taste buds near the tip of the tongue detect sweet and salt sensations, while those on the sides are sensitive to sourness and the rear ones pick up the bitter tastes in foods. The sour sensations are associated with the low pH of foods like tamarind, fruits and vegetables, vinegar and acid salts.

The salt taste is associated with sodium chloride or other salts used in food preparation. The sweet sensation is due basically to the presence of sugars which being soluble in water impart the sweet sensation. The degree of sweetness may vary depending on solubility but mild sweet sensations are also due to the presence of organic compounds in foods such as alcohols (glycerol), amino acids and aldehydes such as cinnamic aldehyde in cinnamon.

Attention is now increasingly being focussed on non-calorie sweeteners possessing sweet taste-modifying characteristics, drawn from plant materials. Some examples are the use of dipeptides and other compounds used as salts of sodium, potassium or calcium which are 300-700 times sweeter than sucrose and used to manufacture non-nutritive sweeteners like *aspartame* and other non or low calorie substitutes.

The bitter taste in some foods is attributed to the presence of alkaloids such as caffeine, nicotine, quinine, theobromine, some salts of magnesium, ammonium, calcium, and glycosides of compounds.

Mouth feel

As the term suggests it is related to the feel of food in the mouth which strongly influences acceptability. Nerve fibres from the trigeminal nerve are responsible for this sensation which includes sensitivity to temperature, pain and touch, the latter helping to assess the shape, form and consistency of the food, often referred to as texture. Mouthfeel enhances taste sensations positively or negatively as seen when children spit out a food as soon as they take it in the mouth or become excited over flavour and taste.

Texture

Texture has been defined as *the attribute of a substance resulting from a combination of physical properties and perceived by the senses of touch, sight and hearing. The physical properties include size, shape, number, nature and conformation of structural elements* (British Standard Institution, 1975). Thus texture encompasses those properties of food, which are perceived by the kinesthetic and tactile senses in the mouth.

Apart from the touch sensation which gives an idea of food texture, it is the structure of foods which is responsible for their textural properties described as coarseness or fineness, brittle, chewy, crisp, hard and so on. Sometimes analogy is used to describe textures for want of precise expressions, such as a creamy sauce, or rubbery candy and the like, Consistency is described through viscosity, elasticity, plasticity, solidity etc. Instruments are now available to precisely measure and quantify certain aspects of texture.

Brennan (1984) categorized textural composition of animal foods into three distinct groups namely those with:

(a) *Mechanical characteristics,* which relate to the reaction of food to stress such as hardness, brittleness, gumminess, chewiness, elasticity and cohesion.
(b) *Geometric characteristics,* which relate to size, shape, particle orientation like grain, grit, fibrous and so on.
(c) *Moisture characteristics,* These relate to moisture and fat perceptions such as juiciness, greasiness and oiliness, resulting from moisture and fat released during mastication.

Teeth play and important role in the perception of texture as evidenced when biting, chewing and swallowing. Tenderness is assessed by the number of chews required to masticate a sample. They are counted till the food is generally ready for swallowing. Visual appearance and touch through food manipulation, provide some idea of firmness, fibrousness, crispness, mouldability through cut and knife penetration. The act of stirring, shaking, pouring or spreading also reflect viscosity and thereby texture.

Sound

The sound accompanying breaking of a food either by hand or while eating is perceived as crisp, short, heavy or light depending on the characteristics of the product being judged. Sound is an important indicator of quality for short crust products, biscuits, cookies, crackers, *mathris* and the like and reflects texture as well. Besides, the crackling sound of a sizzling steak indicated the temperature of the food as well.

Overall Palatability

Although this is not strictly a sensory attribute it is important for determining food acceptability, Palatability represents the cumulative perception or impression left on the evaluator of the food. It does not signify the sum total of all the attributes of the product being evaluated, although some attributes such as colour, flavour, size may strongly influence an overall palatability score. However, these characteristics may be different for different foods.

Sensory Assessment

Judging food quality is a matter of a panelist's reaction to the sensory qualities of foods and is not a property of the food itself. The assessment is affected by a number of psychological and social factors which play an important role in acceptance and thereby preferences. The selection of key characteristics for each food therefore, is important to the outcome of an evaluation.

Scientific methods of sensory assessment of food quality are becoming increasingly important as the variety of food products in the market are increasing and less and less products are available in loose forms to be handled and selected or rejected by the consumer at the point of purchase. The practical requirements for conducting any sensory assessment involve the following:

(*i*) Food Science laboratory

(*ii*) Experimental design

(*iii*) Taste panels

(*iv*) Sample preparation

(*v*) Assessment techniques

(*vi*) Product analysis.

For any exercise in sensory evaluation it is important to set the objective clearly, standardize the food product and earmark the characteristics of that food which need to be assessed.

Sensory Evaluation Laboratory

A reception area or room for sensory evaluation is an essential requisite to an evaluation laborartory. This should be adjacent to the sample preparation and testing booths, where each panel member can sit, take their own time and assess the product presented to them. Each booth should be so situated that interaction of any kind between the taste panelists is not possible.

The booths should be arranged with the products neatly placed with a plate and spoon or fork as required, and the evaluation form and pen for recording. No flowers or other table appointments should be present to distract the assessor. A clear glass of water should be placed covered, to enable the evaluator to rinse the mouth between tasting.

Experimental Design

Experimental design involves the systematic thinking through of the steps to be involved in the exercise of evaluation. The steps may be outlined as follows:

(a) Objective of evaluation.

(b) Standardization of food product and selection of food attributes to be assessed.

(c) Selection, agreement and communication with panelists.

(d) Fixing date of evaluation, preparing score cards with instruction for their completion.

(e) Preparation of samples and pretesting, to make modification in score sheets.

(f) Setting up the taste booths.

(g) Preparing and laying out samples properly coded, ensuring neatness and silence in the environment. Ensure that the number is limited to not more than 5 if possible, for each evaluation, so that the samples remain fresh throughout. This however, depends on the tests selected and the food tested.

(h) Receiving panelists, briefing them verbally and in writing regarding procedures, timing and so on.

(i) Supervising the evaluation.

(j) Deciding on the statistical tests to be used, colating data and final analysis.

If a clear randomized design is thus formulated scientifically, the results would be representative and enable the achievement of objectives fairly accurately inspite of minor differences in the scores due to some uncontrollable factors. Listing of the samples in the evaluation proforma should follow a coded statistical design.

Taste Panel

A taste panel consists of people who are requested to assess food quality of samples presented for evaluation and may vary in number from 3-5-10 depending on the testing technique used. In the case of preference testing with consumers the tasters may number in hundreds. For consistent results panel members should be endowed with certain qualities which are briefly listed.

(a) Possess good food standards and experience with foods.

(b) Be exposed to a large variety of foods

(c) Should not have strong likes or dislikes for any foods

(d) Be highly sensitive to small changes in odour, taste, flavour and other characteristics of foods.

(e) Have knowledge of quality characteristics and cooking methods for foods being evaluated.

(f) Be non-smokers and non-drinkers

(g) Be in good health

(h) Be literate and have a good memory for flavours etc. to make comparisons

Besides the above criteria certain rules need to be followed if sensory evaluation is to give reliable results. These are:

(a) Panelists should not be suffering from cold, cough or other infection at the time of the evaluation.

(b) They should not be very hungry and preferably eat at least two hours before tasting samples. The time when taste acuity is at its highest is between 11.30 a.m. - 4.30 p.m.

(c) Evaluators should have enough time to feel relaxed during evaluation.

All evaluation should be carried out in a quiet and comfortable environment preferably in natural light or under lighting in which the food is expected to be consumed. If cold foods are being evaluated the seasoning should be enhanced as flavours are not prominent at low temperatures.

Sample Preparation

Samples should be prepared as close to the evaluation time as possible to prevent any changes in their quality due to storage, temperature changes, reheating and so on. There should be uniformity in their preparation, care being taken to see that the food presented to the evaluators is prepared in the same lot under standardized laboratory conditions.

Accurate weights and measures of ingredients and temperature and time controls in the procedures followed are essential for reproduceability of the samples when necessary. The portion sizes for evaluation should be consistent for all samples.

The equipment used for the presentation of the samples should be clean and standardized in shape size, colour and filled with the product to the same level if liquid, or, same shape if solid. The shape and size however, should not detract the assessor away from the qualities of the product, and simplicity should be maintained.

Samples should be blind labelled with random 3-digit codes to avoid any bias and then presented in the order in which they are to be evaluated. A master sheet carrying the allotted codes and details of the attributes and number of samples for each panelist should be prepared before hand. This will help in decoding the results of the evaluations for a systematic statistical analysis of the results.

Assessment Techniques

A number of techniques and tests have been developed, standardized and used universally for assessing food quality. These are:

(i) Preference test

(ii) Difference test

(iii) Rating technique

(iv) Numeric scoring

(v) Hedonic scale technique

(vi) Composite scoring

(vii) Descriptive analysis

Preference test

This test involves a fairy large number of individuals who usually represent potential users of a product to be launched depending on the outcome of the assessment. It is usually conducted in the market place by a group of company representatives. A product specific evaluation proforma is designed and while customers randomly arrive to taste the product free of cost, their responses are closely recorded by one or two members of the company while others offer courtesies and ask each customer a few simple questions predesigned for the assessment. This is often seen when a new brand of beverage, pizza topping, salad cream or a sandwich spread is evaluated. The process is continued for 7-10 days in different markets and the results statistically analyzed. For customer preference scores, depending on the designed criteria.

Such testing enables adjustments to be made in the manufacture of the products according to customer acceptability criteria.

Difference test

This testing technique is also called discrimination testing, because the tests are designed to assess the differences in the various aspects of food quality of products such as differences, intensity or preference. The method requires a relatively small number of trained taste panelists (3-7), for the evaluation. Basically four methods are used for the performance of difference tests.

(*i*) Paired test
(*ii*) Rating test
(*iii*) Triangle test
(*iv*) Duo-Trio test
(*v*) Sorting test

(*i*) *Paired test* – There are two types of paired comparison tests, one indicates the direction of the difference and is called 2-Alternative Forced Choice test (2-AFC) and two, the simple difference paired comparison test, (DPCT). If it is known that a sample differs in a certain attribute then the 2-AFC method is used to find out the direction of the difference in terms of less or more sweet, coloured, crisp and so on. On the other hand if the attribute(s) in which the samples differ are not known the DPCT is applied even though it is less accurate (Lawless and Heymann, 1998).

This test requires two samples of the product being assessed, one control and the other experimental. The panelists involved may vary from 5-12 if trained and 70-80 if untrained. The evaluators are required to assess which of the samples has more or less of the attribute being judged. The samples are coded and presented to each panelist as designed in Table 15.1 using A as the control sample.

Table 15.1 Design for sample presentation in paired test

| Sample | Panelists | | | |
Number	*1*	*2*	*3*	*4*
1.	AB	AA	BB	BA
2.	BB	BA	AB	AA
3.	AA	BB	BA	AB
4.	BA	AB	AA	BB

The results may then be marked according to the number of correct judgements made each being given I point.

(*ii*) *Rating Test:* These are qualitative tests used for evaluating 2-3 samples at a time only.

There are four versions of this test the selection being made according to the attributes required to be tested and the accuracy desired.

(a) *Rank test:* Judges are asked to rank the samples on a simple 5-point scale for particular characteristics df the product under evaluation.

(b) *Single sample test:* This is particularly used for products which have a lingering after-taste. A single sample is required to determine the intensity of a particular flavour which is rated against certain criteria such as the time for which the taste remains in the mouth. A second sample cannot be used for such foods, as the taste lingers on.

(c) *Two sample difference test:* In this 4 pairs of the product duly coded are presented to the panelists. Two pairs contain one control and one test sample, while two other pairs contain two control samples only. The panelists are asked to record the degree of difference between the pairs.

(d) *Multiple sample test:* In this test 5-6 duly coded samples are presented of which one is the control. The panelists are asked to record the difference between each sample and the control.

(iii) *Triangle test:* This is also called the triad test and requires the preparation of three samples among which two are exactly the same and the evaluator is asked to indicate the odd sample. The format for evaluation is indicated in Table 15.2.

Table 15.2 Triangle test evaluation card

Panelist .... Food Product .... Date .... Time ....

Address .... Contact No ....

....

....

1. Three samples are presented of which two are identical, indicate the odd sample.

Sample	Odd one	Did you guess, say Yes or No
123	....	....
121	....	....
211	....	....

2. What was the difference in the odd sample:

None .... Very little .... Moderate .... Too much ....

3. Which sample did you prefer?

Odd one   Other

4. Any other comments you would like to make.

(iv) *Duo-Trio test:* The duo-trio test is basically a paired discrimination method although three samples are used of which one is a reference or control. The judges may be given an evaluation card as formatted in Table 15.3.

Table 15.3 Format for Duo-Trio test

Panelist .... Item code .... Date ....

The sample marked 'C' is the control for reference, taste it carefully then judge which of the two coded samples is the same as 'C'.

Set No.	Code	Numbers	Same as 'C'
1.	....	....	....
2.	....	....	....
3.			
4.			

The scoring for differences observed are compared as illustrated in Table 15.4.

Table 15.4 Format for testing differences in food samples by Duo-Trio test

Panel member	Day I matching	Day II matching
1.	–	+
2.	+	+
3.	+	+
4.		
•		
•		
•		
12		
	....	....
Total Points	....	....

The number of correct answers are allotted a point each and then totalled for each day. For 10 correct judgements among 12 panelists the level of significance is 5% for a 2-sample one tailed test.

(v) Sorting test: In this the panelists receive 5 samples and are required to sort them out into two groups, one with 2 samples that are different from the remaining three in the second group. This technique works well when only visual or tactile comparisons are required.

Rating Technique

When more than 3 samples need to be evaluated and accuracy is desired, then a score card developed with all the attributes of the samples is developed and marked with the relevant score against the attribute as indicated in Table 15.5. A number of samples of each food are presented to the evaluator and scored. The one which receives the highest average score from the panelists is taken as the most acceptable.

Multiple samples of the same product can be prepared by varying any one ingredient or its quantity in a recipe and getting it assessed for acceptability.

Table 15.5 Evaluating multiple food samples

Panelist	Food Item code............	Date ....
Contact No.	Address........................	

Sample. No.	Very poor 1	Poor 2	Fair 3	Fairly good 4	Good 5	Very good 6	Excellent 7
Colour							
Odour							
Flavour							
Texture							
Appearance							
Palatability							

Comments ....

....

Numeric Score Test

This test requires a card to be designed for scoring purposed on which a maximum score for a quality product is 100. The various general attributes are then allotted a maximum score and the sample judged against descriptive characteristics which apply to the product under assessment. A sample score sheet for evaluation is presented in Table 15.6.

Table 15.6 Sample score sheet for numeric scoring

Panelist	Food Item code............	Date	Contact
Contact No.	Address........................		Telephone
No.			

	Max. Score	Sample Score
1. Appearance (External)	20	
2. Appearance (Internal)	30	
3. Palatability	45	
4. Portion size and presentation	5	
Total Score	100	

Note: Detailed descriptions may be given for attributes desired in an excellent product that would get the maximum score.

This is not a suitable test for acceptability as it does not evaluate certain important food characteristics such as juiciness, texture, flavour and so on.

Hedonic Test: This is a test that focuses on general acceptability, in which the panelists record their likes and dislikes on a 5-10 point descriptive scale as indicated in table 14.7.

Table 15.7 Hedonic Scale for food evaluation

Characteristic	Like	Dislike
Colour	extremely	extremely
Texture	very much	very much
Flavour	moderately	moderately
Shape	slightly	slightly
Potion size	no comment	no comment

For children observations may be recorded on an illustrated scale as indicated in Fig. 15.1, the illustrations may be used as part of the Hedonic scale table in case children are involved in the evaluation.

Fig. 15.1. Illustrated Hedonic evaluation scale.

Composite Score Test

This is useful for grading batches of the same product and for detecting the defect in the production of a particular batch. A sample score card is presented in Table 15.8.

Descriptive Analysis

This is usually used on a single sample for the purpose of a detailed analysis of perceived sensory attributes. The terms are selected keeping in mind the desirable characteristics of the product. For example, the intensity of a flavour can be judged on a scale of 1-9 representing descriptions from weak to strong. For judging sweetness a 1-14 scale may describe minute changes in degree of sweetness. This is a very sophisticated tool used for sensory evaluation of each attribute.

Product Analysis

The coded sample scores should be statistically analysed through tests selected in the experimental design of the study. Depending on the tests used for the evaluation variance analysis, measures of significance through t-tests and so on may be used. For details Ranganna (1986) and Lawless and Heymann (1998) may be sourced.

Table 15.8 Score card for composite evaluation of a product

Mean Scores

Key: 5 : Excellent 4 : Very Good 3: Good

2 : Satisfactory 1 : Unsatisfactory

Panel Members	Evaluation the product and grade it								Overall rating Scores	Is there any thing you disliked about the product		If yes, what	Would you buy it
	Appearance	Colour	Shape	Taste	Texture	Odour	Flavour	Mouthfeel		Yes	No		
1.	4	4	4	5	5	5	5	4	5				Regularly
2.	4	3	4	4	5	4	4	4	4			Texture could be better and colour even	Regularly
3.	4	4	4	3	4	3	3	3	4				
4.	1	2	4	2	2	1	1	1	2			Flavour mouthfeel	Regularly Occasionally
5.	4	4	4	3	4	3	4	3	4				Occasionally
6.	3	4	3	4	4	4	4	4	4				Occasionally
7.	3	3	3	2	3	3	3	3.	3				Occasionally
8.	3	3	4	4	3	3	5	4	4				Occasionally
9.	3	3	2	2	3	2	2	2	3			Mouthfeel	Occasionally
10.	3	3	3	3	3	3	3	3	3				Regularly
11.	3	3	4	4	4	4	3	3	3			Mouthfeel	Occasionally
12.	4	3	4	4	3	3	3	4	4				Occasionally
13.	3	3	3	4	5	3	3	4	4				Occasionally
14.	4	4	3	4	4	3	3	3	4				Occasionally
15.	4	3	3	3	4	3	3	3	3				Regularly

Thus, sensory evaluation of food products requires skill, patience and practice to provide reliable information about products their development and acceptability.

Practice Exercises

1. What sensory characteristics would you look for while rating the acceptability of
   (*i*) Chapatti (*ii*) Cake (*iii*) Custard?
2. What tools would you use to carry out the evaluation of a midday meal or snack in a nursery school? State briefly.
3. Prepare a score card for the composite evaluation of any food product of your choice. Discuss its overall acceptability.

16

Objective Evaluation

Objective methods of food evaluation are non-sensory and depend heavily on instruments to measure the characteristics of different foods be it colour, shape, texture, elasticity and so on. They are usually used in testing or quality control laboratories attached to food processing units where accuracy is important for reproducing quality characteristics in particular foods. Besides this, instruments are used in academic institutions for teaching and research. There are three basic approaches to objective assessment:

- (*a*) Measurement using calibrated instruments.
- (*b*) Microscopic examination of structures.
- (*c*) Determination of the chemical composition of foods.

MEASURING INSTRUMENTS

The methods for measuring different attributes of foods vary widely, therefore a large variety of instruments from the very simple to complex have been designed for accuracy of measuring each attribute. Only the principle behind the measurement and some simple devices which can be used in an introductory food science laboratory are being discussed.

Weighing Balances

Balances of different types, sizes and accuracies are available, which can be used in a laboratory for standardizing a recipe or developing new products. These equipment are useful for establishing the right portion sizes for various food products.

Volumetric Equipment

Different types of glassware are used to measure volumes of liquids, reagents and fluids, varying from standard cups to volumetric cylinders of all sizes. The standard cups usually used in recipe development carry equivalents in fluid ounces or pints to suit the measurements for various recipes. This enables the experimenter to measure its equivalent in metric or any other measurement system. Standard cups are now available in polystyrene to avoid breakage and in enamel for very hot fluids. Flours, sugar, semolina etc. may also be measured in standard cups and spoons which are manufactured for accuracy using international standards for weights and measures.

A knowledge of the weights or volumes of substances dissolved in a liquid or solvent helps to establish its concentration in the final product. Determination of the specific gravity from volume measurements is an important index of food quality and involves simple arithmetic.

Thermometers

Thermometers are equipment used for measuring the temperature of foods during cooking and processing, because the texture and doneness of a product is largely dependent on the temperature. Temperature is the relative hotness or coldness of a food as compared with melting ice or boiling water. Many kinds of thermometers are manufactured each designed and calibrated to suit the range of temperatures required for various foods such as sugars, oils, doughs, meats and so on.

Temperature scales may be calibrated in °C (Celcius) or as °F (Fahrenheit) the scales used bearing 100 divisions on the former and 180 divisions on the latter scales. The temperature of melting ice and boiling water correspond to the temperature scales as calibrated being 0-100° on the Celcius and 32-212° degrees on the Fahrenheit scales.

Types of thermometers

Many models of thermometers are designed for measuring temperature varying from room temperature to the temperature of various foods as required in laboratories.

(a) *Room thermometer:* This is calibrated in °C or °F as mentioned above because the comfort temperature range varies from 18-22°C and the normal thermometer which contains either mercury or coloured ethanol for ease of reading is used. It is usually mounted on a wooden base and connected to a thermostat which maintains the required temperature.

(b) *Two-metal thermometer:* As the name suggests this is constructed using two types of metals and connected with a pointer which lies over a scale. With rise and fall of temperatures the two metals expand or contract moving the pointer on the scale and indicating the temperature that can then be recorded.

(c) *Maximum and Minimum thermometer:* This is usually used for recording the lowest and highest temperature as done in food storages to control food deterioration.

(d) *Cold storage or refrigeration thermometers:* Because they need to record low temperatures as in icecream parlours or cold rooms they are constructed with red coloured ethanol for easy reading in the presence of a cold mist that may settle on and around the device. The range of temperatures calibrated on these thermometers vary from −30 to −100°C.

(e) *Sugar thermometer:* These are like normal mercury (Hg) in glass instruments with a range of 10-230°C.

(f) *Oven thermometers:* These are same as sugar thermometers but their temperature range is 10-370°C marked on a brass scale, and suitable for baking, grilling and roasting foods.

(g) *Dough testing thermometer:* These have a temperature range of 10-43°C but are Hg in glass instruments.

(h) *Meat thermometer:* These are normal devices but protected in a metallic case to which a pointed probe is attached. The device is usually used for recording the internal temperature of large pieces of meat to know if they are cooked through, as in roast lamb. The internal temperature indicates the end of cooking depending on the degree of tenderness desired.

Hydrometers

These are simple instruments which help to measure the relative density (R.D.) of liquid foods. It has a weighted bulb and a graduated scale on the stem with a relative density calibrated on it. The instruments are allowed to float in the liquid and the depth to which it sinks is read off on the stem. Many versions are available being named according to the food for which they are calibrated, such as *lactometer* for measuring the density of milk, *saccharometer for sugar* syrups and so on.

Colour Measurement

Colour perception is subject to certain inaccuracies as far as sensory methods are concerned as it is difficult to memorize colours, therefore objective methods make use of instruments which are based on the principle of colour matching.

Photoelectric instruments: These devices are fitted with photoelectric cells which takeover the function of the human retina. A wide range of such instruments are available. For example, a wedge photometer is useful for measuring colour intensity in cereal flours which is mainly due to the presence of chlorophylls, xanthophylls and flavones rather than carotenes (Winton and Winton, 1999).

Spectrophotometers: In these instruments a curve relating to wavelength and colour intensity makes it possible to calculate a complete physical specification of colour. The Beckman spectrophotometer uses a prism while other models use a grating for isolating the spectral bands.

Ranganna (1986) has described the Hunter colour and colour difference meter, photovolt reflectance meter and some tranmittance methods for measuring colour accurately. Different instruments are adapted for the measurement of hues, brightness or lightness of colour.

Texture

Instruments have been devised to measure the rheological characteristics of foods, which are then accurately measured using mathematical or other means. Every texture measuring device has some basic parts such as a driving mechanism; probe element which comes in contact with the food; force directing element which controls the type and rate of force applied; sensing and recording system. Generally called *texturometers* they measure particular attributes of texture such as viscosity, ability to shear, tenderness, crispness and so on.

Texturometers

These provide an index of texture of foods by determining the resistance offered by the sample before being deformed. It is so designed as to simulate the movement of the teeth in chewing. The force gets recorded graphically along with the distance of each bite. From the graph formed the texture profile of the food can be determined for the required characteristics, whether they include hardness, cohesiveness, elasticity, brittleness, softness, adhesiveness and others.

A number of instruments have been designed to measure each attribute of texture to the accuracy desired. The devices are based on empirical methods measuring the force required for penetration, cutting, shearing and compression. Some of them are briefly dealt with below:

Shortometer: This measures the force needed to break a pastry crust, biscuit, cookie or *mathri*.

Penetrometers: These are instruments generally used for determining the internal tenderness of large cuts of meat. The important feature is a needle or a cone shaped probe which is inserted in the cut of meat. The instrument is calibrated and can be read off.

Mechanical models are also available attached with a thermometer on which the internal temperature of the food can be known, and this acts as the guide for judging the readiness of meat.

Viscometers or consistometers: These are instruments for measuring concentration of syrups, viscosity and consistencies of pulps, purees and sauces as well as flow properties such as elasticity and plasticity of doughs, batters, fats etc. The crumb of sponge cake however, while being elastic is reversible, and hence a cake is allowed to cool in an inverted pan before its texture is determined. A hydraulic press is sometimes used to measure liquids expressed from meats and other foods.

Jelmeter: This measures the flow time of a pectin extract used for making fruit jellies, the quality of products being dependent on the concentration of the extract.

Brix Refractometer: This is used to measure the concentration of sugar in the preparation of sauces and similar products, as these determine not only the readiness of the product but also its possible shelf life during storage. Used generally for products which are to be packed and sealed hot, when their concentration cannot be determined easily by sensory means. Sometimes sugar thermometers are fixed to equipment used for making, ketchups, sauces and jellies so that the temperature can be used to monitor the readiness of the products.

Line Spread test: This is sometimes used to measure the differences in consistency of batters, custards, sauces etc. The fluids are poured out on a tray and the degree of spread measured to determine differences in consistency.

Compressimeter: An instrument for measuring the firmness or staleness of bread.

Alveograph: This measures the strength of the dough by determining the pressure required to blow a sheet of dough into a bubble.

Farinograph: This instrument simulates dough mixing conditions and determines absorption, dough development, mixing time and dough stability. The device is computer attached and a graphic representation of the desired attributes appears. The farinograph indicates the type of cereal from which the flour for dough is made and tests the dough, with the gluten strands still in the development or excited state.

Extensograph: This tests the dough while it is at rest and with gluten strands relaxed as during fermentation, effect of different ingredients on fermentation characteristics, the fermentation tolerance of different flours in addition to product volume potential. The dough extensometer thus, measures the stretchability of a dough more accurately, recording the behaviour of the stretch graphically on a chart.

pH meter: This is used for measuring the acidity or alkalinity through measurement of hydrogen ion concentration of foods being tested. Since pH affects food attributes to a large extent the accuracy of measurements become important especially for standardization of products for large scale production where quality standards need to be maintained over long periods. Hand held battery operated professional digital pH meters are now available, designed with 1½ digit CD of 13 mm. These devices measure from 0-14 pH to the nearest point of 0.01.

Imitative devices: These are instruments designed to simulate mastication and bite. Lee et al. (1987) correlated sensory evaluation of several parameters by using both subjective and objective methods comprising of 11 instrumental methods for frankfurters and found a high correlation between them. Other studies too have been reported by Sharma and Wani (1995) for meat products.

Instruments however, usually analyze only a single component at a time, whereas the overall impression and taste of a food product can be properly assessed only by human sensory perception

(Winter, 1990). Objective testing therefore is used mostly by the food technologist, food processing industry and manufacturers for R and D work.

Therefore, even though highly sensitive and automated measuring instruments are now available to the food scientist, the importance of sensory analysis has grown over the years. This is because food and people always go together and it is their opinions which are paramount in assessing food acceptability.

Practice Exercises

1. Name the equipment that you would use to determine the density of milk.
2. What pH ranges are acceptable for cooking vegetables. Explain why?
3. List the equipment required for conducting objective tests in a food science laboratory.

References

Akoh, C.C. Fat replacers. *Food Technology*. 1998.52(3) : 47–52

AFST(I), Industry News. *Indian Food Industry*. 1999. 18(2) : 85.

Anon, (1999), *Indian Food Industry,* 8 (3) : 146.

Anon, (1999), Industry News, *Indian Food Industry,* 18 (1) : 10.

Brennan, J.G. Texture perception and measurement. In : Piggot, R.A. (ed.), *Sensory analysis of food*. 1984 London : Elsevier Applied Science Publishers. p. 59.

Brooker, B.E., **Food Theory and Applications**. 2nd ed. 1985, New York : Macmillan Publishing Company.

Charley, Helen, **Food Science**. 2nd ed. 1982, New York : John Wiley and Sons.

Dias, Fausto F., Tekchandani, Harish K. and Mehta, Darshan. Modified Starches and their use by food industry. *Indian Food Industry*. 16, (4) 1997 : 33–39.

Eapen, K.C., Shankaranand, R. and Vijayaraghavan, R.K. Review paper. The present status on the use of nisin in processed foods. *J. Food Sci. and Tech.* ed. 2. 1976.

Food Snippets, *Indian Food Industry* (2005), 24 (5) : 43, Sept.–Oct.

Gaman, P.M. and Sherrington, K.B. **The Science of Food**. 4th ed. 1996. Oxford : Butterworth-Heinemann.

Glasstone, Samuel. **Textbook of Physical Chemistry**. 2nd Ed. 1976. Madras : Macmillan Co. of India Limited.

Glicksmann, M. (1991). Hydrocolloids and the search for the oily grail. *Food Technology*. 40 : 94–103.

S, Hermansson, In Helen Charley. **Food Science**. 2nd ed. 1982. New York : John Wiley and Sons.

Glett, G.E. and Grisamore, S.B. Maltodextrin fat substitute lowers cholesterol. *Food Technology*. 40, 1991. :104–105.

Jacob, T. **Food Adulteration**. 1976. Delhi : Macmillan Co. of India Ltd.

Jellinek, G. In : **Sensory evaluation of food : Theory and Practice**. 1985. England : Ellis Howard Ltd.

Kalab, M. Microstructure of Dairy Foods : Milk products based on fat. *J. Dairy Sci.* 1985. 68 :3234.

Kalshian, R., Srikanth, B.R. and Shankar, M.S. Lethal condiments. *Outlook*. September 14, 1998, p. 67–74.

Kapadia, Payal, Smell a rat ? *Outlook*. April 17. 2000. p. 66–67.

Kent-Jones, D.W. and Amos, A.J. 6th Ed. **Modern Cereal Chemistry** 1996 London : Food Trade Press Ltd.

Khare, S.K., Nabetani. H. and Nakajima. M. Lipase catalyzed interesterification reactions and their industrial applications. *Indian Food Industry,* 2000. 19(1) : 29–35.

Kilgour, O.F.G. **Complete Catering Science**. 1986. London : Heinemann Professional Publishing Ltd.

Kinsalella, J.E. Functional properties of proteins: possible relationships between structure and function in foams. *Food Chem.* 1981. 7:273.

Kirk, Ronald R. and Sawyer, Ronald, 9th International Ed. **Pearsons Composition and Analysis of Foods.** 1991. England : Addison Wesley Longman Ltd.

Kon, S.K. **Milk and Milk Products in Human Nutrition**. 1959 Italy : FAO Nutritional Studies No. 17.

Kurien, V. India's Milk Production. *NF1 Bulletin.* 21, No. January 2000.

Lee, C.M. Whiting R.C. and Jenkins, R.K. Texture and sensory evaluation of frankfurters made with different formulations and processes. *J. Food Sci. 52 (4).* 1987. 896–900.

Lawless, Harry T. and Haymann, H. **Sensory Evaluation of Food : Principles and Practices**, 1998. Food Science texts Series. New York.

Lawson, H. **Food Oils and Fats**. 1997. New Delhi : CBS Pulishers and Distributors.

Lowe, Belle. 4th ed. **Experimental Cookery**. 1955. New York : John Wiley and Sons, Inc.

MacDonald, A. Diagnosis and Management of Food, Intolerance by Diet. *Nutritional Dis. mgt.* Update Series 8, Oct.–2000, CRNSS, N. Delhi.

Malik, RK and Dingra, K.C. **Handbook of Food Industries**. 1976. Delhi : Small Industry Research Institute.

Manay, N. Shakuntala and Shadaksharaswamy, N. **Foods : Facts and Principles**. 1987. New Delhi: Wiley Eastern Limited.

McWilliams, Margaret, **Foods : Experimental Perspectives** 3rd ed. 1996. London : Prentice-Hall International (U.K. Limited).

Meyer, Lilian H. Ed. (1987). **Food Chemistry** Indian ed. Delhi : CBS Publishers and Distributors.

Narasinga Rao, B.S. (2000): Nutritive Value of Rice Bran, *NFI Bulletin*. Vol. 21, Number 4, October 2000, p. 5–8.

Penichter, A.K. and McGinley, E.J. Cellulose gel for fat-free food applications. *Food Technology.* 1991. 45 : 105.

Phillips, M.C. Protein conformation at liquid interfaces and its role in stabilizing emulsions and foams. *Food Technol.* 1981. 35 (1) : (50).

Pomeranz, Yeshajhu and Meloan, Clifton E. **Food Analysis : Theory and practice**. 3rd ed. 1996. New Delhi : CBS Publishers and Distributors.

Potter, N.N. **Food Science.** 1987 Indian Ed. Delhi : CBS Publishers & Distributors. p. 699.

Potter, Norman N. and Hotchkiss, Joseph H. **Food Science**. 5th ed. 1996. Delhi : CBS Publishers. p. 33.

Pszczola, D.E. Fat replacers: Where do we go from here? *Food Technology*. 1997. 51(1) : 26.

Ranganna, S. **Handbook of Analysis and Quality Control for Fruits and Vegetable Products**. Ed. 2. 1986. New Delhi : Tata McGraw Hill publishing Co. Ltd.

Rana, L.; Sangwan, V.; and Rana, N., Nature and Extent of Adulteration in Pulses, *Proceedings of 86th Session of the Indian Science Congress Committee on Home Science*; 1999. Chennai p. 143.

Rees. D.A. Structure, conformation and mechanism in the formation of polysaccharide gels and networks. Advances in *Chem. and Biochem.* 1969. 24 : 324–326.

__ Polysaccharide gels : A molecular view. *Chem. and Ind.* 1972. 630–636.

Richert, S.H. Physical-chemical properties of whey protein foams. *Agric. Food Chem.* 1979. 27 : 665.

Roy, Susanta K. *Proceedings of National Symposium on Processing, Finance and Marketing in Food Industry.* 1996. Octorber 14. Abstracts p.xxx.

Sahoo, J and Verma, S.P. Quality Aspects of goat meat and meat products with special reference to refrigerated storage. *Indian Food Industry,* 1999. Vol. 15. (15).

Sathe, A. Y. **Food Analysis** 1999. New Delhi : New Age International (P) Ltd. Publishers.

Sauter, E.A. and Montocore, J.E., The relation of lysozyme content of egg white to volume and stability of foam. *J. Food Sci.,* 1972; 37 : 918–920.

Sen Gupta. Some simple and quick tests for adulteration in foods. *Indian Food Packer,* July-Aug. 1989. p. 24.

Shaefer, E. Etherton, P.P., Rools, B and Gordon, D. Fat Replacers : balancing the health benefits. *Food Technology.* 1996. 50 : 76–78.

Sharma, V. Arora, S. and Rai, T. Fat Replacers. *Indian Food Industry.* 1998. 17(2) : 89–97.

Sharma, V., Arora, S. and Sindhu, J.S. Flavour encapsulation application. *Indian Food Industry.* 1999. Vol. 18(1) : 39–48.

Sharma, B.D. and Wani, S.A. Sensory attributes of meat and meat products. *Indian Food Industry.* 1995. 14(3) : 22–26.

Shekar, S. and Bhat, G.S. Dissolved oxygen content of cow's and buffalo milk. *J. Fd Sc. Tech.,* 1984. Vol. 21, No. 5.p. 328.

Simopoulos, Artemis P. and Robinson, Jo. (1998), **The Omega Plan**, London: Harper Collins Publ.

Singh, L., Mohan, M.S. and Sankaran, R. Nisin as an aid for thermal preservation of Indian dishes. *J. Food Sc. & Tech.* 1987. Vol. 24, No. 6, p 277.

Singh, R.P., Heldman. D.R. and Kirk, J.R. Kinetic Analysis of light-induced riboflavin loss in whole milk. *J. Fd. Sci.* 1975.40: 164–167.

Sultan. W.J. **Practical Baking**. Ed. 2. 1972. Connecticut : AVI Publishing Co. Inc.

VanGarde, Shirky J. and Woodburn, Margy. (1999) **Food Preservation and Safety: Principles and Practice**. First Indian ex. Surabhi Publications, Jaipur, India.

Venugopal, V. By-products from Industrial Fishery Processing. *Indian Food Industry.* 1995. July–August, 14(4) : 22.

Winter, Q. Sensory perception. *Food Market and Technol.* 1990. 4(1) : 18–21.

Winton, Andrew L. and Winton, Kate Barber. **Techniques in Food Analysis.** 1999. New Delhi Allied Scientific Publishers.

Glossary

Bajra : is pearl millet considered as a coarse grain usually eaten in rural areas or by poor communities. Used extensively as fodder for animals.

Besan : This is the flour of split horse grim and or *chana dal.* extensively used as a batter, or for preparation of sweets in India.

Biolakton : Yoghurt like product developed for infant feeding. It protects infants from nosocomal infection and reduces incidence of lactose malabsorption and intolerance. It is also known to cure subnormal acidity.

Burfee : Indian sweet prepared from thickened milk and sugar and set in a tray 3-5 cm in height. When set it is cut into diamonds or squares and served as snack, candy or dessert. Depending on what other ingredient is added the sweet gets its name such as peanut burfee, spinach burfee, chocolate burfee and so on.

Chapati : Indian bread made from wheat flour dough, in which gluten is developed by kneading. It is rolled out into thin rounds V_4-V_8 cm thick and cooked on a hot iron griddle.

Chenna murki : A sweet snack prepared from cubes of cottage cheese, cooked in a syrup of 2-thread consistency. On air cooling recrystallization of sugar takes place on the surface.

Chikki : The local name for a noncrystalline brittle candy made by caramelizing sugar or jaggery. Some variations are marketed in which peanuts, roasted gingelly seeds or other nuts may be added.

Curd : A fermented milk product using a culture of lactic acid bacteria eaten with meals as such or sweetened for dessert.

Dal : A pulse preparation the consistency of curry, made by boiling pulse with 4-6 times the volume of water. After the desired consistency is reached it is topped with spices cooked in heated oil and or tomatoes as required.

Dalda : A brand of hydrogenated fat.

Desi : Traditional.

Dhokla : A savoury snack prepared from a fermented batter of two pulses and steamed in a **tray,** then cooled and garnished with green coriander. It is cut and served as sandwich or as plain squares or diamonds accompanied with a tangy sauce.

Dosa : A pancake like preparation made from a fermented batter of rice and split black gram both soaked and ground finely in the ratio of 3 : 1. A typically South Indian preparation now popular as snack or meal all over the country.

Garam masala : A mixtue of ground spices prepared for garnishing hot curries for flavour just before service.

Ghee : Clarified butter.

Gulabjamun : A sweet prepared from a mixture of thickened milk and cottage cheese made into balls, fried and soaked in syrup of 1-thread consistency. The sugar enters the sweet by osmosis and diffusion.

Idli : A steamed savoury snack food prepared from a fermented batter of ground rice and split balck gram mixed in the proportion of 2 : 1 and diluted to the right consistency for steaming in special moulds prepared to standardize the size.

Jal jeers : A spicy beverage made with roasted cumin seeds and other spices dissolved in water.

Jowar : A millet used as coarse grain, classed as a minor cereal.

Kadai : A utensil shaped like a chinese *wok,* commonly used in India for sauteeing foods or deep frying.

Kadhi : This is a North Indian curried preparation made from soured curd and bengal gram flour, garnished with whole coriander seeds, asafoetida, tomato and curry leaves.

Karachi halwa : A non crystalline sweet made from sugar and cornflour or other starch, having an elastic texture.

Keema : Minced meat. Can be used for preparation of curries, kababs etc.

Kefir : A cultured milk product manufactured in Russia for infant feeding. Exhibits anti-bacterial activity against *Staphyllococcus sepsis* in infants aged below 1 year.

Kheer : A desert prepared by boiling rice, other cereals or vegetables in milk till it thickens to the desired consistency. Sugar to taste is then added and cooked till it dissolves. It is then garnished with chopped nuts and served hot in winter and cold in summer. Depending on the ingredient added the preparation is known as rice kheer, pasta kheer, gourd kheer if gourd is used and so on.

Khoa : Milk is heated and thickened till it becomes a solid. This can then be refrigerated and used for making different kinds of sweets.

Kulcha : Baked Indian bread, prepared from fermented dough.

Ladoo : A sweet snack prepared with gram flour, fat and sugar syrup, usually associated with festivity. Different types of ladoos are prepared using cereal flours, seeds and nuts.

Lassi : Buttermilk taken as a sweet or spiced beverage.

Lobia : *Cow* pea botanical name *vigna catjang.*

Malas : Milk cream.

Mathri : A savoury snack made from refined flour dough which is shortened with fat to prevent gluten development and provide crispness.

Mithai : The general term for Indian sweets.

Mother Dairy : The name of the first national milk dairy established at Anand in Gujarat, under the umbrella of the National Dairy Development Board, by its chairman Dr. V. Kurien.

Murraba : Preserve made with sugar syrup or recrystallised sugar.

Naan : Indian bread made from fermented dough of refined wheat flour and baked in a traditional oven the *tandoor.*

Nimbu pani : A cold beverage prepared from fresh lemon juice, sugar and water.

Paneer : A term for fresh cottage cheese prepared from milk acidified for coagulation of proteins and then strained and cut into cubes.

Paraat : A steel plate with slanted edges of height 2-4 cm for kneading dough or making sweets.

Phirni : A dessert made from milk, Ticeflour and sugar thickened and set, usually in single serving portions.

Phulka : A bloated chapati made from wheat flour dough in which gluten is developed by kneading with the knuckles.

Pinni : *This is* a mixture of roasted wheat flour in clarified butter, followed by addition of sugar, nuts and some spices, and when still hot made into balls like ladoo.

Rabri : A sweet prepared from milk heated to evaporate most of its water, till it is the consistency that can be spooned. It is grainy in texture because of the partial coagulation of milk proteins.

Rasagulla : A sweet prepared from cottage cheese, made into balls and boiled in thin sugar syrup for 10-12 minutes. Served as a cold dessert or snack.

Rye : This is an important food crop in Europe usually used in bread making. The crop commonly cultivated is *Secale cereale*. It is also used for distilling liquors and animal feed.

Shakarpara : A fried snack prepared from wheat flour or refined flour, drained and dipped in syrup of one and a half or 2-thread consistency and then air dried. The sugar on the surface recrystallizes to give a fine snowy appearance.

Soya paneer : Tofu.

Tawa : This is a slightly concave iron griddle used for making chapati and phulka.

Thali : Round metal plate generally 1/2-1 inch in depth, used for serving meals in traditional Indian style.

Tikki : A round flattened kebab made of boiled mashed potato and stuffed with sauteed pulse and spices. It is generally shallow fried.

Vanaspati : Hydrogenated fat

Yoghurt : Similar to curd but fermented by a culture of *Lactobacillus bulgaricus* and *Streptococcus thermophilus* and held at 40-42°C for a few hours till set.

Abbreviations

AFSTI	Association of Food Scientists and Technologists (India)
Agmark	Agriculture marketing alpha
2-AFC	2-Alternative forced choice
ATA	Alimentary Toxic Abukia
B-	beta
BHA	Butylated hydroxyanisole
BHT	Butylated hydroxytoluene
BSI	British Standard Institute
BV	Biological value
°C	degree Celcius
CH	carbohydrate
CIFT	Central Institute of Fisheries Technology
CO_2	carbon dioxide
COOH	carboxylic
CMC	carboxy-methyl cellulose
A	Dextrose equivalent
A	decosahexanoic acid
DPCT	Difference paired comparison test
DW	distilled water
EFA	essential fatty acid
EPA	eicosapentaenoic acid
EPG	Esterified propoxylated glycerol
expt	experiment
FA	fatty acid
FAO	Food and Agriculture Organization
Fig.	Figure
FOP	Fruit Products Order
g	gram
H	Hydrogen
HCL	Hydrochloric acid
HDL	High density lipid
HTST	High temperature short time
H_2O	water
ICMR	Indian Council of Medical Research
ISI	Indian Standards Institution
K	Potassium
kJ	kilojoule
kcal	kilocalorie
KOH	potassium hydroxide
$KMnO_4$	Potassium permanganate
LCD	Liquid Crystal Display
LDL	Low density lipid
liq	liquid
MCT	Medium chain triglyceride
mg	milligram
mm	millimeter
MRL	maximum residue levels
MSG	Mono sodium glutamate

MUFA	mono unsaturated fatty acid	PUFA	Poly Unsaturated Fatty Acid
NaCl	Sodium Chloride	%	percent
NaHCO$_3$	Sodium bi-carbonate	RD	Relative density
NGO	Non-governmental organisation	R&D	Research and Development
NIN	National Insitute of Nutrition	t	table spoon
OTAI	Oil Technologists' Association of India	t	tea spoon
		tt	test tube
P	Phosphorus	temp.	temperature
pd	powder	TW	tap water
PFA	Prevention of Food Adulteration	UHT	Ultra High Temperature vegetable
pH	hydrogen ion concentration	VMA	Vanaspati Manufacturing Association
PIL	Public Interest Litigation	veg	vegetable

PRESERVATIVES

Preservatives are substances used and processes developed by which the keeping quality or shelf-life of food products is improved. These may be used in their natural form as food ingredients or chemicals which inhibit the growth of microorganisms in foods, maintaining their acceptability characteristics and wholesomeness. There are about 100 'anti-spoilants' which are in common use. Some are briefly mentioned here.

Antioxidants – These substances prevent the production of off-flavours and colours used for high fat containing products. For example – Benzoic acid in margarine, butylated hydroxy anisole (BHA) in fats, crackers, soups and potato chips.

Fungicides – These prevent mold and fungal growth on citrus fruits and their products.

Mold Inhibitors – These prevent mold growth in breads, cereals and their products. For example sodium and calcium propionate, sodium diacetate, acetic and lactic acids used in breads. Sorbic acid and sodium and potassium salts are preservatives for cheeses, syrups, pie fillings, etc. SOPRDAC is a brand developed for the specific purpose of preventing mold and rope-forming bacteria in bread and is cheaper and more effective than calcium propionate.

Index

Reader's Notes